OXFORD MEDICAL PUBLICATIONS

Commission of the European Communities
Health Services Research Series
No. 7

CEC Health Services Research Series

Series Editors

This book is one of a series concerned with health services research. It is an outcome of coordinated work by COMAC-HSR (Comité d'Action concertée) which reports to the CGC Medical and Health Research (Comité de Gestion et de Coordination) of the Commission of the European Communities, Directorate-General Science, Research and Development (DG XII).

The research is carried out by the 'concerted action' method. The Commission of the European Communities pays the costs of coordination and of bringing together researchers from various countries, while the actual research is paid for and executed by each country. The aim is to accelerate joint research activities by Member States in selected fields, such as health services research.

1. *Perinatal Care Delivery Systems: description and evaluation in European Community countries* Edited by Monique Kaminski, Gérard Bréart, Pierre Buekens, Henk J. Huisjes, Gillian McIlwaine, and Hans-Konrad Selbmann.
2. *Economic Appraisal of Health Technology in the European Community* Edited by M. F. Drummond.
4. *Technology Assessment and New Kidney Stone Treatment Methods* Edited by F. Kamper-Jørgensen, S. Challah, and T. Folmer Andersen.
5. *Expensive Health Technologies: regulatory and administrative mechanisms in Europe* Edited by Barbara Stocking.
6. *European Community Atlas of Avoidable Death* Second edition Edited by W. W. Holland.
7. *Home Care for Older People in Europe: a comparison of policies and practices* Edited by Anne Jamieson.

HOME CARE FOR OLDER PEOPLE IN EUROPE

A Comparison of Policies and Practices

Edited by

ANNE JAMIESON

Senior Research Fellow
School of Social Sciences
University of Bath

OXFORD NEW YORK TOKYO
OXFORD UNIVERSITY PRESS

This book has been printed digitally and produced in a standard specification in order to ensure its continuing availability

OXFORD
UNIVERSITY PRESS

Great Clarendon Street, Oxford OX2 6DP

Oxford University Press is a department of the University of Oxford.
It furthers the University's objective of excellence in research, scholarship,
and education by publishing worldwide in

Oxford New York

Auckland Cape Town Dar es Salaam Hong Kong Karachi
Kuala Lumpur Madrid Melbourne Mexico City Nairobi
New Delhi Shanghai Taipei Toronto
With offices in
Argentina Austria Brazil Chile Czech Republic France Greece
Guatemala Hungary Italy Japan South Korea Poland Portugal
Singapore Switzerland Thailand Turkey Ukraine Vietnam

Published in the United States
by Oxford University Press Inc., New York

Publication No. EUR 12997 of the
Commission of the European Communities,
Scientific and Technical Communication Unit,
Directorate-General Telecommunications,
Information Industries and Innovation,
Luxembourg

Reprinted 2011

ISBN 978-0-19-262050-7

Printed and bound in Great Britain by CPI Antony Rowe,
Chippenham and Eastbourne

Foreword

Raymond Illsley, Project Leader, Age Care Research Europe, School of Social Sciences, University of Bath

The research described in this book emerged from discussions held between policy makers and research workers across the European Community (EC) in the late 1970s. Cross-national research within the Community on health and social issues was then young and the machinery weak and slow moving. Yet the issues and the findings of this study, published 10 years after the first tentative proposal, are as live and relevant as they were then. This says very little about the foresight of the proposers, but a great deal about the power status of elderly persons and the long processes through which policy is formulated and implemented. Participants in our discussions and in COMAC-HSR recognized both the size and urgency of the problem—the need to mobilize resources and services more effectively to meet the growing demand for support and care of elderly persons. The debate has moved on—the complaint by physicians about the blockage of hospital beds, which they wished to use for other, more rewarding, patients, is now seen as the symptom of a larger problem, not an issue in its own right. The key role of home care in the maintenance of personal independence is well established and the volume of services has increased in most countries. But the two main hypotheses underlying the study continue to be as relevant as ever.

It was suggested that existing services were ineffectively deployed because of over-concentration of resources upon medical and institutional care rather than social and community care, and because of the fragmentation of planning, decision making and delivery between multiple organizations and professions. Adaptation to a large-scale demographic shift, and a change of priority from acute medicine towards care and support, entail a radical restructuring of arrangements for the funding, control, and administration of health and social service resources. These, and the very principles on which allocation is based, are seen to be deeply embedded in culture, ideology, legislation, organizational forms, and professional and service boundaries. In these respects, Community countries differ sharply from each other, and the value of this book is that it takes one limited set of services and explores these differences—not just differences in the volume and the quality of home care, but their place in the patterns of policy and services for elderly persons, and their relationship to health care and to welfare more generally.

In setting up the study we were surprised at how little experts about services in their own country (including ourselves) knew about practices, or even principles, pursued in other countries. Services had emerged nationally out of local culture, ideology, and historical events, not through cross-country observation and learning. Because systems, with all their local virtues or their organizational clumsiness, have developed in response to local circumstances, it is impossible to pick and choose and put together a mosaic of the best bits. It is, however, instructive to learn what is universal, what is nationally specific, to find that systems can operate efficiently with or without some features deemed indispensable in one's own country, or to perceive that other countries, through similar historical processes, have achieved what seemed uniquely bothersome in one's own system. Anne Jamieson adopts this cross-country learning perspective in the last part of the book as she identifies and discusses what, in all our countries, we have learnt about each other and ourselves in comparing home-care services. In later publications we shall extend those comparisons to other services for the elderly and to the policy process itself.

Contents

List of contributors xi

PART ONE: INTRODUCTION

1. **HOME CARE IN EUROPE: BACKGROUND AND AIMS** 3

Anne Jamieson

1. Age Care Research Europe (ACRE) 3
2. Home care in the context of the ACRE framework 6
3. 'Community care' or 'home care'? 6
4. The focus of the book 9

References 12

PART TWO: THE INDIVIDUAL COUNTRIES

2. **HOME-CARE SERVICES IN THE FLANDERS, BELGIUM** 15

F. Baro, L. Moorthamer, G. De Bruyne, H. Van den Bergh, and K. Magits

1. Introduction: home care in Belgium 15
2. Trends in policies for older people 16
3. The service system in the Flemish region: funding and organization 17
4. Present provision in the Flemish region 18
5. Home-care services in the study area of Groot-Antwerpen 27
6. Allocation of home help/cleaning help 29

Note 36
References 36

3. **THE HOME-HELP SERVICE IN DENMARK** 38

Bjorn E. Holstein, Pernille Due, Gert Almind, and Erik Holst

1. Home help for elderly people 38
2. The clients of home help 45
3. Decision-making for home help 49
4. Policy implications 59

References 60

4. THE HOME-HELP SERVICE IN ENGLAND AND WALES 63

Robin Lawson and Bleddyn Davies, with Andrew Bebbington

1. Introduction 63
2. The historical development of the service 64
3. The provision of domiciliary help today 69
4. The service in practice 78
5. Ways forward 91
6. Conclusion 96

References 96

5. HOME-CARE SERVICES IN FRANCE 99

Jean-Claude Henrard, Joël Ankri, and Marie-Claude Isnard

1. Historical development of *maintien à domicile* 99
2. Existing home-care services for elderly people 103
3. Informal support 112
4. Co-ordination 113
5. Conclusion 115

Notes 115

References 115

6. HOME-CARE SERVICES IN THE FEDERAL REPUBLIC OF GERMANY 118

6.1. Development of home-care services and policies for older people 119

Margret Dieck

1. The hierarchy of services and service systems 119
2. The history of the home-care services 119
3. The role of health insurance 122
4. The role of social welfare provision 123
5. Bridging the health and social-services systems: provisions for home care for frail people 124
6. The rationale behind service priorities, service hierarchies, and the inclusion or exclusion of elderly people 125
7. Organization and finance of formal home-care services 127
8. The extent of service provision 129

6.2. Allocation of home care in one federal state: a case study from Berlin (West) 131

Vjenka Garms-Homolová

1. The structure of the study 131

2. The functional capacity and structure of informal support as criteria of need for home help 133
3. Service provision in Berlin 136
4. Allocation and claim mechanisms 143
Notes 152
References 154

7. HOME-CARE SERVICES IN ISRAEL 157

Haim Factor, Brenda Morgenstin, and Denise Naon

1. Introduction 157
2. The development of home-help services 161
3. Provision of services today 164
4. Issues in the delivery of adequate services 169
5. Assessment and discussion of key issues 175
6. Summary 185
Notes 186
Acknowledgements 186
References 186

8. HOME-CARE SERVICES IN ITALY (WITH SPECIAL REFERENCE TO GENOA) 188

Carla Costanzi

1. Italy 188
2. Genoa 190
Notes 209
References 211

9. HOME-CARE SERVICES IN THE NETHERLANDS 213

Wim van den Heuvel and Hans Gerritsen

1. Introduction 213
2. The development of home-help services 214
3. Present provisions of home-help services 217
4. The home-help service and the care of the elderly 220
5. The home-help service in practice 224
6. The effects of policy 230
7. Concluding remarks 233
References 234

PART THREE: HOME CARE FROM A CROSS-NATIONAL PERSPECTIVE

Introduction to Part Three 239

10. HOME-CARE PROVISION AND ALLOCATION 240

Anne Jamieson

1. The aims of provision—the range of possibilities 240
2. The formal policy aims of home care 242
3. Home care in practice: patterns of provision and use of services 248
4. The process of service allocation 261

References 272

11. TRENDS IN HOME-CARE POLICIES 273

Anne Jamieson

1. An assessment of home-care measures 273
2. Past and recent trends 277
3. Factors affecting policies and their implementation 285
4. Conclusions 292

References 295

APPENDICES 297

Appendix 1: Demographic and economic background of the study in Belgium 299

Appendix 2: Background data from Denmark 302

Appendix 3: The pathways study—population and method (Denmark) 310

Appendix 4: Home-help referrals—typical trajectories (Denmark) 312

Appendix 5: Background data from the UK 315

Appendix 6: Background data from France 321

Appendix 7: Background data to the Berlin study 325

Appendix 8: Background data from Israel 328

Appendix 9: Examination of the need for help from others in care of the elderly (Questionnaire) (Israel) 337

Appendix 10: Background data from Italy 340

Appendix 11: A translation of an LIER assessment form (Netherlands) 342

INDEX 345

Contributors

G. Almind
General Practitioner, Institute of Social Medicine, University of Copenhagen, Denmark

J. Ankri
Laboratoire Santé et Viellissement, Université René Descartes, Paris, France

F. Baro
Universitair Psychiatrisch Centrum St. Camillus, Katholieke Universiteit, Leuven, Belgium

C. Costanzi
Scuola per Assistenti Sociali, Università di Genoa, Italy

B. Davies
Personal Social Services Research Unit, University of Kent, Canterbury, England

G. De Bruyne
Public Centre for Social Welfare, Antwerp, Belgium

M. Dieck
Deutsches Zentrum für Altersfragen, Berlin, Germany

P. Due
Institute of Social Medicine, University of Copenhagen, Denmark

H. Factor
Brookdale Institute for Gerontology, Jerusalem, Israel

V. Garms-Homolová
University of Osnabrück, Germany

H. Gerritsen
Department of Health Services, University of Groningen, The Netherlands

J-C. Henrard
Laboratoire Santé et Viellissement, Université René Descartes, Paris, France

E. Holst
Institute of Social Medicine, University of Copenhagen, Denmark

B. E. Holstein
Institute of Social Medicine, University of Copenhagen, Denmark

M-C. Isnard
Consultation de Gérontologie, Hôpital Sainte Périne, Paris, France

A. Jamieson
School of Social Sciences, University of Bath, Bath, England

R. Lawson
Personal Social Services Research Unit, University of Kent, Canterbury, England

K. Magits
Public Centre for Social Welfare, Antwerp, Belgium

L. Moorthamer
Universitair Psychiatrisch Centrum St Camillus, Katholieke Universiteit, Leuven, Belgium

B. Morgenstin
National Insurance Institute, Research and Planning Bureau, Jerusalem, Israel

D. Naon
Brookdale Institute for Gerontology, Jerusalem, Israel

H. Van den Bergh
Public Centre for Social Welfare, Antwerp, Belgium

W. van den Heuvel
Department of Health Services, University of Groningen, The Netherlands

Part One

Introduction

1
Home care in Europe: background and aims

Anne Jamieson

1. Age Care Research Europe (ACRE)
   1.1. Rationale and framework
   1.2. The ACRE project in practice
2. Home care in the context of the ACRE framework
3. 'Community care' or 'home care'?
4. The focus of the book
   4.1. What is home care?
   4.2. The aims and questions addressed in the home-care study
   4.3 The country chapters

References

1. AGE CARE RESEARCH EUROPE (ACRE)

1.1. Rationale and framework

This book forms part of a major study into care delivery systems in Europe, known as 'Age Care Research Europe'. The study has been funded by the European Community as a concerted action programme, in which research teams from nine countries have participated: Belgium, Denmark, France, Greece, Germany, Ireland, Italy, the Netherlands, and the UK. The study resulted from a research proposal and a research design formulated by Professor Illsley of the UK (who subsequently became Project Leader) and Dr Robert van Zonneveld of the Netherlands. The design is described in some detail elsewhere (Illsley 1987) and will only be briefly summarized here. From earlier discussions with policy makers and research workers, Illsley and van Zonneveld were aware that all countries were encountering difficulties in adapting the pattern of services and the distribution of resources to meet the increased demand on health and social services in a period of limited growth, and in the face of resistance from other service sectors. One major problem of common concern at the time was the blockage of the pathways into and through the services. Part of the blockage was undoubtedly due to the inadequacy of the total volume of services. They suggested, however, that a further and substantial part of the problem arose from the inappropriate use of those services that are available. This was caused, first, by a relative over-concentration of resources upon medical and residential institutions as opposed to the preventive use of support for people living in their own homes; and secondly, by widespread organizational and professional fragmentation in existing services.

European countries were known to differ in the size, composition and health status of their elderly population; in the structure of their health and social services; and in their policies towards the needs of and support for elderly persons. Any inter-country comparison concerned with the appropriateness of services and policies clearly required data on each of these three elements. Three related strategies of research were therefore proposed and have been pursued. The *first* aims to document the health status and social conditions of elderly people living at home, and to describe the availability and use of formal and informal support. This has been done through surveys of representative samples of the elderly population. The *second*, organizational, approach attempts to identify features of the structure and pattern of services within each country through the observation of the experience of clients and their carers in their interaction with the services. This has been done through case studies, documenting the decision-making processes at key points in the service systems. The *third* approach involves a review of policies, their formulation, and implementation, and of the structure of services relevant to the care of the elderly.

All three approaches (or 'sub-projects' as they were referred to in the research protocol (Illsley and Zonneveld 1984)) are, of course, interconnected. They can each contribute a particular perspective on a number of issues. Questions of service use or informal care can be illuminated by data from the survey, the pathways study, and the policy study. The study of policies (sub-project 3) forms the integrating core of our study, especially from a cross-national perspective. This is so because the overriding aim of the cross-national study is to compare policies and to understand similarities and differences between countries as regards the factors affecting policies, the motors of innovation, and the constraints upon change.

1.2. The ACRE project in practice

Cross-national comparison is a long-established method, as old as social science itself. It is the social scientist's substitute for controlled experiments. *Collaborative* research is a more recent phenomenon and has become increasingly common, following the improvement in means of communication and the generally increased international interdependence and integration. Collaborative research has the potential of providing us with inside knowledge and 'local' interpretations, which one scientist could not possibly develop. However, there are numerous practical problems in engaging in joint multinational research enterprise. Others (Berting 1986; Øyen 1990) have discussed many of these problems in some detail, and most people who have been involved in cross-national collaboration will recognize many of these. Berting points out the linguistic barriers, which often put a limit to the degree of participation in cross-national research. There are also cultural differences related to the style of organizing research and research meetings. The particular institutional and political circumstances of different countries lead to differences in research priorities and aims. There are differences of intellectual styles, some countries emphasizing paradigmatic exploration, others empirical description.

The research design anticipated difficulty in interpreting comparative data concerning services and social institutions, which, however similar their names, were structured differently and within distinctive administrative and cultural contexts that might crucially affect their operation. The design therefore refrained from specifying detailed data requirements from each of the three sub-projects. It did, however, specify in detail the objectives of each sub-project and the research questions it was expected to address (Illsley and van Zonneveld 1984). Comparability was therefore to be obtained by using whatever material was nationally relevant to examine shared and specific questions.

The funding for the participating national teams had to be obtained from their own national research councils or governmental bodies. This inevitably resulted in a great deal of divergence in the extent of funding obtained, and therefore in the amount of research that could be undertaken and in its timing. It also marked the beginning of divergence in design and foci. All these developments were unavoidable, given the particular organization and funding of this programme.

Without here entering into details, the extent of participation by the different countries can be summarized as follows. Four countries, Denmark, Germany, Ireland and Scotland, conducted a survey within the framework of the ACRE sub-project 1, although for Ireland funds did not stretch to a follow-up survey as planned. Italy and Greece participated by analysing survey material already collected as part of a World Health Organization (WHO) 11-country study. Belgium and the Netherlands were not successful in obtaining funds for this sub-project. Sub-project 2, the study of allocation of services, was conducted in all participating countries, except France, but with considerable variation in scope and some differences in emphasis and design. As regards sub-project 3, only one country, Germany, obtained funding to conduct a systematic study of policy formulation and implementation. However, all participants in the study of services undertook to analyse their findings in the wider context of their systems of health and social services and policies.

2. HOME CARE IN THE CONTEXT OF THE ACRE FRAMEWORK

The topic of this book cuts across all three sub-projects; its rationale derives from key questions specified in the protocol for each (for details see Illsley 1987). The survey (sub-project 1) focuses on the living conditions of older people living *at home*. Clearly, the different forms of care they receive in their homes constitute a central theme of our inquiry. From the point of view of policies for older people (sub-project 3), the question of home care seems to us to be one of the major themes in the debates in all countries, and we shall return to this below. But above all, the rationale for our choice of home care derives from the pathways study (sub-project 2), which is a study of the decision-making processes at key points in the service system.

Key points were defined as services at which decisions are made about admission, transference, or discharge, and at which the decisions made are likely to have a substantial effect upon the case load of other referring or receiving organizations. They should cover the major interfaces between health and social services, and between home and residential services. Because systems differ, key points as defined above are also likely to differ from country to country. Choice of key points was therefore deliberately left to each national team, using knowledge of their own system. It was acknowledged at the design stage that this might later create problems of comparison, but these were accepted as preferable to uniform choice of particular services. The project was concerned primarily with service systems rather than individual services.

However, when choosing their key points a majority of our colleagues in the different countries chose, as one of these, referrals to 'home help'. It was considered as a key service, both because it constituted an important link between institutions—especially hospitals—and the home, and because it was seen as a key service in relation to the stated policy aims of these countries, according to which older people should have the opportunity to remain at home for as long as possible.

3. 'COMMUNITY CARE' OR 'HOME CARE'?

Stated policy aims in most countries suggest that home care is absolutely central. However, most policy debates are couched in terms of *community care* rather than home care. Looking at the international literature, such as, for example, WHO documents, or any other discourse conducted in the *English* language, the concept of community care stands out. Most of us are familiar with this term, in the sense that it conjures up in each of us some image, but equally, most of us are aware of the problematic and contradictory connotations of the term. To quote Martin Bulmer from his book *The Social Basis of Community Care* (Bulmer 1987, p. 214), an excellent attempt to unravel the meaning of the concept:

> 'Community care' policy is a shambles, in part because 'community' has become a vacuous term, meaning all things to all people. It is very difficult to give the term consistent and useful meaning, yet it goes on being used because of its powerful and evocative reference.

When Bulmer says that 'it goes on being used', one needs to add 'at least in the English-speaking world'. What seems striking is that the precise equivalent of this term does not actually exist in all other languages. Although it is possible to translate the word 'community' into other languages, not only does it appear to have different connotations, but also, when put together with the word 'care' (which in itself is difficult to translate precisely), it often becomes impossible to find the exact equivalent. It seems to us that the debates which have been going on in the British context about the meanings of 'community care', about whether or not it is at all useful and so on, do not take place in, for example, Danish, French, and German. Instead, the common theme for all countries, which recur in policy debates, is the following aim: to enable people to stay in their own homes for as long as possible. Joan Higgens argues that the concept of 'community' 'is an unnecessary and complicating element in social policy analysis and can be abandoned without any real loss to meaning or understanding' (Higgens 1989, p. 15). Not everyone would agree with this in the British debate, but in *cross-national* analysis the concept may not be terribly helpful because of its ambiguities. Joan Higgens also argues that the real distinction is between the *institution* and *home*, and services are normally available either in the institution or from home (e.g. day care) or at home (in the case of domiciliary care). In our study this distinction certainly makes more sense than the distinction between 'community' and 'institution'.

This is not to say that the 'home/institution' dichotomy is simple and straightforward. Indeed, as will be argued in the final chapter, deliberate attempts to break down the difference between home and institution, in conceptual and practical terms, may well be an important aspect of future developments of services for older people. Thus, so-called sheltered housing, which already exists in most countries, constitutes an intermediate form of accommodation, which does not fit neatly into either category. For the purpose of our initial comparison between countries, we have decided to exclude sheltered housing, unless otherwise stated, and our main focus is on people living in their own private dwellings, as opposed to service-based accommodation, whether sheltered housing, 'homes for the aged', nursing homes or hospitals.

4. THE FOCUS OF THE BOOK

4.1. What is home care?

In Britain, the concept of home help is well known to most people, and the 'home-help service' is clearly identifiable and well defined in organizational terms. This is also the case in serveral other countries, in the sense that it is possible to identify a type of service that, in direct translation, means 'home help'—for example *aide domicile* in French; *hjemmehjælp* in Danish. However, the services delivered as 'home help' are not always the same in all countries. The tasks of home helpers overlap with those of other care providers in a variety of ways, and for this reason alone it does not make sense in a cross-national context to focus on home help only. Furthermore, in other countries, services exist that are not necessarily called 'home help', although they may perform similar functions. Finally, because of the centrality of the policy aim of supporting people in their own homes, it would not make sense to consider one particular service in isolation from other services delivered in the home. The starting point for this book, therefore, is upon the *kind* of help provided, irrespective of the legal/administrative manifestations of such help. These are divided into three core areas of help:

Nursing help, i.e., tasks that everywhere are seen as the domain of professionally qualified nurses. They include tasks like taking blood pressure, giving injections, insertion of catheters.

Personal care, i.e., help with tasks that everybody has to perform, like getting in and out of bed, bathing, washing, dressing.

Home-making, i.e., help with tasks in the house that, like personal care, we all have to do in our daily lives (shopping, cooking, cleaning, and administrative tasks to do with 'paperwork', filling in forms, paying bills, etc.). Tasks like snow clearing and gardening, though not relevant to all, should be mentioned here, although, as is argued here by several authors, they are often neglected by service providers. Finally, other activities, generally considered to be part of 'normal life', such as socializing or going for walks, should also be included here, although they are not instrumental tasks like the others. They are, however, important, and by some, though not all, service providers seen as part of their portfolio.

On looking at the *services* available to help with these various activities, the following picture emerges.

Professional nurses are found in all the countries studied and perform the 'technical' nursing tasks listed to people at home. In all our countries, nursing forms a separate entity in the range of services, although the extent of its separation from other services varies. Similarly, the extent to which nurses perform 'non-technical' tasks, such as personal care duties, varies between countries. For example, in the UK, nurses—or auxiliary nurses from the same organization—help bathe and wash people, whereas in most other countries this is done by others. In other words, the boundary between nursing and other services varies between countries.

Personal care and home-making services are delivered and organized in different ways. The most significant difference between countries is whether the two are integrated or divided up between different care providers. The concept of 'home help' as it is known in Britain is very similar in Denmark, France, and Genoa (because of the vast regional differences between regions within Italy it is not possible to generalize about the country as a whole). The home-help service provides help with personal care as well as home-making tasks. This is not the case in Belgium, the Netherlands, Germany and Israel. In these countries there is some kind of *separation*, broadly speaking, between personal care services and home-making. The degree and nature of the separation is not the same everywhere. In Belgium and the Netherlands the most significant feature is the existence of separate cleaning services. In Germany there is a very clear hierarchy of services, from technical nursing (*Behandlungspflege*), to personal care (*Grundpflege*), and at the 'bottom' of the hierarchy, home-making (*Haushaltshilfe*). In Israel, personal care and home-making services are separate, the former being the main focus of policy making and service development.

In a cross-national analysis of services, whatever concept one uses, it would not mean the same thing in all countries. In our discussion we will use the folowing terms: *home care* will refer to technical nursing, personal care and home-making services; *home help* will refer to personal care and home-making, even though for some countries this means that we are referring to more than one service. As the key focus of this book is upon help with activities of daily living, and in parallel with the chapters which follow on provision in individual countries, nursing will be discussed mainly in so far as it affects the provision and delivery of home-help services.

4.2. The aims and questions addressed in the home-care study

The overall *aims* of this study are to understand the role of home-care provision in supporting older people at home, and to assess and explain its success or lack of success in relation to stated policies for older people. The potential benefits from *comparing* a number of countries are several. At the purely descriptive level, many are interested simply in learning whether the situation in their own country is reflected elsewhere, and whether there are lessons that can be learnt 'from abroad' or models which can be transferred. Each national contribution serves an important function in its own right in relation to such aims. However, the purpose of bringing them all together and considering them from a cross-national perspective goes beyond that of description. We need to explain and understand the factors that bring about particular developments in policies and services, and we need to understand the constraints on change as well as the possibilities of change. Cross-national comparison offers opportunities, and this book represents an attempt to use these to improve our understanding of the plight of older people in need of care and to enable us to draw some conclusions regarding future developments, their desirability as well as their likelihood. Apart from a purely scientific interest in improving our insight, our practical need to understand each other better is obvious in the light of the increasing integration of the members of the European Community.

In writing about home care in each country, all our contributors were asked to address the same set of questions, which, briefly summarized are the following:

1. What, if any, are the formally stated policies of home care for older people?
2. What is the range of home-care services, the extent and nature of service provision, the kind of help available, the kind of personnel employed to deliver services?
3. How are the services organized and funded?
4. What are the formal policy aims for specific services, especially home-help type services? What is the target population? (What are the criteria of eligibility?)
5. What is the historical development of the home-help service?
6. How does the service operate in practice. How do people get home help? Who actually gets home help?
7. What is the relationship between formal care provision and informal care?
8. Assessment of the services: Do services meet the needs of older people? What are the shortfalls in provision and operation of the services? What is the relation between home-care provision and levels of institutionalization? What are the main achievements of the services?
9. What are the current policy issues and debates about the future of home-care services?

4.3. The country chapters

The chapters that follow on each of the countries included in this volume all address these questions. They do not, however, follow the same structure, and the emphasis given to each of the questions varies considerably. This, in our view, is inevitable; indeed any attempt to 'harmonize' the content of each chapter would be based on the mistaken assumptions that not only the nature of the service systems and policy issues have enough similarities for this to be meaningful, but also that the state of knowledge and analysis is similar in all countries. This clearly is not the case. To this must be added what we have already mentioned: in our particular study, the teams involved have diverging interests and experience, and the nature of their studies as well as the funding provided for these varied immensely.

4.3a. Some brief notes on each of the country chapters

Belgium. Although some general information about Belgium as a whole is included, the main discussion centres on the Flemish region, and in particular on the findings from the study of allocation of home help in Antwerp (sub-project 2). No survey was conducted for the ACRE study.

Denmark. The Danish contribution builds upon findings from the survey as well as the pathways study; the latter included case studies of referrals to home help in three areas of varying population density inside and outside Copenhagen.

France. No study was undertaken specifically on home help, nor was a survey conducted as part of the ACRE study. The chapter builds upon secondary material and focuses on policy developments and issues. It gives a broad overview of developments in France.

Germany (West). This chapter consists of two parts. The first addresses policy issues and gives an account of developments in the Federal Republic as a whole (before unification with East Germany). The second builds upon detailed research carried out in West Berlin, where our colleagues conducted a survey as well as case studies of home-care service allocation at community centres (*sozialstationen*).

Italy. The Italian contribution is based on research conducted in and around Genoa in the region of Liguria. It brings in some general material from Italy as a whole, but as for Belgium, the regional differences within the country makes it difficult to generalize about the country as a whole. Most of the chapter is concentrated on Genoa. The design of the research here differed from that of our teams. The information about services derives partly from general interviews with key managers and professionals in the system and partly from a survey specifically focused on service use. Thus no case studies of the decision-making process were conducted.

The Netherlands. This chapter is based primarily upon existing research in this country and thus gives an overview of policy and service issues nationally. It reports the findings from a number of studies of home-help clients.

The UK. This contribution comes from the team at the Personal Social Services Research Unit in Canterbury, where a great deal of research has been conducted into service allocation. It draws upon many of these findings, as well as the wealth of information already available for the UK.

Israel. Finally, a chapter on Israel has been included. This country, although not a member of the EC, has been affiliated to our programme. We have included Israel in this volume because some interesting developments have taken place in the area of home care, and because a great deal of research has been conducted, which adds to our understanding of trends across Europe.

REFERENCES

Berting, J. (1986). Language and culture in cross-national research. Unpublished paper delivered to the Cross-National Research group, Aston University, Birmingham.

Bulmer, M. (1987). *The social basis of community care.* Unwin Hyman, London.

Higgens, J. (1989). Defining community care: realities and myths. *Social Policy and Administration*, **23,** 3–16.

Illsley, R. (1987). Pathways into and through services for the elderly in Europe: a research design, *Revue Epidemiologie et Santé Publique*, **35,** 339–48.

Illsley, R. and van Zonneveld, R. (1984). Care delivery systems for the elderly. Research design and proposal. Unpublished document.

Øyen, E. (1990). *Comparative methodology*. Sage, London.

Part Two

The individual countries

2
Home-care services in the Flanders, Belgium

F. Baro, L. Moorthamer, G. De Bruyne, H. Van den Bergh, and K. Magits

1. Introduction: home care in Belgium
2. Trends in policies for older people
3. The service system in the Flemish region: funding and organization
   3.1. The administrative structure of the Flemish health and social services
   3.2. Organization of home-care services
4. Present provision in the Flemish region
   4.1. Home-help services
   4.2. Cleaning services
   4.3. Home nursing
   4.4. Service centres
   4.5. Other services
5. Home-care services in the study area of Groot-Antwerpen
   5.1. The spectrum of home-care services
   5.2. Home-help and cleaning services
   5.3. Allocation of home-help and cleaning services in the study area
6. Allocation of home help/cleaning help
   6.1. The cases selected
   6.2. The decision-making process for cleaning- and home-help

Note
References

1. INTRODUCTION: HOME CARE IN BELGIUM

This chapter focuses on the home-help services in Flanders;[1] the findings discussed relate to these only as far as they have participated in the study. Belgium is divided into three regions, each with their own language and cultural characteristics: (i) the Flemish region, (ii) the Walloon region, and (iii) the Brussels region. The German community is part of the Walloon region. Appendix 1 describes the population in the three regions. In the fields of 'home care' and 'community care', different concepts exist within Belgium. These are not always exactly defined, neither was there complete similarity between those definitions we could find. In a policy note from the

Ministry of Social Affairs (1987), one of the main objectives of the health policy for the coming years was to put greater emphasis on financial support for home care (*thuiszorg*). This support is expected to reduce the number of admissions to general hospitals or to homes for the elderly, and to shorten the length of stay in general hospitals. The same note also declares: 'health care at home (*thuisgezondheidszorg*) can help sick people and those in need of care to stay in their own environment with all the care they need'.

In the literature in this field, we find the same concepts of home care and health care at home, both including services provided to people in their own homes or as out-patients (Spinnewyn and Pacolet 1985; Dooghe 1987; Dooghe and Van Den Boer 1987). Sometimes 'home care' is limited to health care (like home nursing) and does not include different kinds of service, but this is not a general trend. All help provided by family, neighbours, and friends—so-called informal care—is referred to as *mantel-zorg*. In the policy note mentioned to above, it is not clear whether home care also includes informal care. A distinction is made between professional care and non-professional care (including informal care and self-help). The note says: 'Measures undertaken to support home care should not replace informal care.'

In the scientific literature the concept of home care is defined very broadly to include professional as well as non-professional care. In our review of home care in Belgium, the following services will be described: home-help services, cleaning services, hot meals services, services centres, and home nursing. Excluded here are the general medical practitioner, social workers, private nurses, and other private carers.

2. TRENDS IN POLICIES FOR OLDER PEOPLE

A number of different stages can be distinguished in the post-war development of the welfare services (Dooghe 1987; Dooghe and Van Den Boer 1987). The *first stage* was characterized by an emphasis on *institutional care*. A major part of the overall health-service budget was spent on the hospital sector, and community services came to be regarded very much as a poor relation. Even in 1983, as much as 56 per cent of the aggregate expenditure under the general scheme for sickness and disablement insurance was on institutional care, whilst the community services received a meagre 16 per cent.

During the *second stage* of development in the 1960s and early 1970s, at a time when the welfare state was expanding, there was a massive growth in the number of professional services and facilities, in both the institutional and community-services sector.

The welfare services are now well into a *third stage* of development. There is a tendency to move away from institutional care provided outside the patient's normal environment towards the provision of care within and by that environment. There is now a broad consensus that large numbers of elderly people are capable of continuing to live at home, thanks to spontaneous, non-professional help provided by relatives, neighbours, and friends. Self-help and community help are now being stimulated.

Many arguments have been raised in recent years in support of a more rapid expansion of home care: 'Both psychological reasons, such as the advantages of being nurses at home by relatives, and financial considerations have helped to step up the importance of this type of service, which offers elderly people the possibility of retaining their independence and freedom, to which they attach a great deal of importance, for as long as possible' (Dooghe 1987a; Dooghe and Van Den Boer 1987). However, there is still a discrepancy between budgets provided for the acute hospital sector on the one hand and for the chronically ill and handicapped on the other. Hospital care remains the main cost in the total expenditure on health. Elderly patients stay in acute hospitals longer than necessary: first, because there are not enough alternatives for adequate care; secondly, because hospital treatment is free for patients (reimbursed by sickness insurance), unlike home help or residential care (Dooghe 1987).

3. THE SERVICE SYSTEM IN THE FLEMISH REGION: FUNDING AND ORGANIZATION

3.1. **The administrative structure of the Flemish health and social services** (Baro *et al.* 1990)

During the last two decades, Belgian administration has become increasingly decentralized. Step by step the unitary state has been transformed into a federal state in which only few matters are still the responsibility of the central government. From 1980 the Flemish and the French communities have had their own constitutions. Their governments (called Executives) are autonomous in certain matters. In law, these matters are defined as the 'matters concerning the person' (Dutch, *persoonsgebonden materies*). These areas are: health policy, social services, policies related to the elderly and the disabled, and applied scientific research. But the communities do not have full authority in these matters: they operate within a framework of national legislation and regulation.

Within the Ministry of the Flemish Community, two Administrations have been created: the Administration for Health Care and the Administration for Social Welfare and the Family, each headed by a Community

Minister. The Administration of Health Care has, among others, responsibility for hospitals, combined rest- and nursing homes, and home nursing. The Administration for Social Welfare and the Family has responsibility for all social services for the elderly (home-help services, services centres, housing, and residential homes).

3.2. Organization of home-care services

Within the legal framework set up by the Flemish government, different private and public organizations can provide the various kinds of home-help services.

The main *public body* providing home help and other services is the Public Centre for Social Welfare (PCSW; Dutch=OCMW), regulated by a national law of July, 1976. According to this law, each municipality should have its own PCSW. The social policy of the PCSWs is related to the following tasks—the organization of:

social services in general;
residential homes for the elderly, nursing homes for the elderly and housing for the elderly;
hospitals;
services for home help in the family and for the elderly;
meals services;
community centres for mental health care.

The municipalities themselves have their own social policy, also concerned with matters related to elderly people. To ensure the best possible co-ordination, the municipalities, by law, have the authority to control the budget of the Public Centres and every decision by the Public Centres to develop services, as far as this has financial implications.

In the *private sector* there are various organizations. First of all, the sickness insurance funds can organize home help. Five funds exist: the Catholic, the Socialist, the Liberal, the Neutral, and the Fund for Occupational Diseases. Other important private organizations are: the Catholic Pensioners Union, the Catholic Women's Organization, the White and Yellow Cross, and other religious groups.

4. PRESENT PROVISION IN THE FLEMISH REGION

4.1. Home-help services

4.1a. Formal policy aims

The main professional bodies active in the field of services provided in the home are the home-help services. They started to develop some 40 years ago, after being based on private initiative, charity, and voluntary work. The need for family help grew before and during the Second World War and soon the need to professionalize these initiatives emerged. As a result, in 1949, the services for family help gained official recognition and received subsidies: the home-help services were started as services for domestic help.

In 1954, a Royal Decree brought about the first important alteration. The aims of home help were extended to aged couples or elderly people living alone. This extension even resulted in separate regulations for the home-help services for elderly people in 1965. From 1973 the same regulations have applied to family- as to home-help services for the elderly. People caring for a sick, older person living with them, and thereby overburdened, could appeal for family or home help. The cases in which help could be given were thereby extended to informal carers.

In 1976 the existing regulations were regionalized and since then the Flemish community has had its own regulations (Steyaert 1986). The home-help services are now regulated by the Decree of 22 June 1988 of the Flemish Executive Committee (the Flemish government): regulation of the recognition and subsidy of the services for family- and home-help assistants. According to the Decree the function of family and home help for the elderly is 'to provide temporary home help to families and people living on their own—in the first place to those who need it most and to those who are less well off financially—who request this help, because they are unable or have difficulties in performing their tasks in the family, especially their domestic tasks, because of the absence of one of the parents, because of mental or physical disability or other special social circumstances, one of the aims being to stimulate families and people living on their own to help themselves' (Flemish Executive decree 1988).

The home-help service presents itself as a front-line service. Its primary task is to support older persons so that they are able to continue living in their own environment. The home help is well placed to help people with specific problems of a medical, psychological, and/or social kind by referring them to the relevant services, and to help them to restore their social and domestic contacts.

4.1b. Trends in home-help provision

Table 2.1 gives an overview of the development of the home-help services in the Flemish community in the last 10 years (Steyaert 1986). Detailed information on the frequency and intensity of care on the one hand, and on user profiles on the other, is not available for the Flemish community as a whole. The increased cost to the state in the period 1980–85 is especially due to the labour cost (mainly social security) and not to an increase in the care provided. There is an increase in the number of hours of help

Table 2.1. Evolution of some characteristics of the home-help services in the Flemish community between 1975 and 1985; absolute numbers

	1975	1980	1985
Hours of help (× 1000)	6 105	8 862	8 666
Clients	37 543	37 979	33 121
Hours/year/family*	163	233	262
Services	70	133	125
Home helps	5273	7009	7441
Cost for the state (million BF)	748	1880	2875
Subsidy/hour	172	197	312
Cost in BF/family	37 855	49 496	86 794

* Hours/year/family = number of hours provided in each family on a yearly base.

provided but a decrease in the number of clients, which reflects the fact that an increasing number of hours of help is provided to each family. The rise in the budget is to a large extent due to inflation. The mean cost per family has more than doubled: in 1985 the real cost of one hour of help is estimated to be 457 BF.

4.1c. The tasks of home helpers

The tasks that may be performed by the home helps are mainly oriented towards household activities. Four groups of tasks are defined:

(1) home-making activities: preparing meals, washing dishes, washing and ironing, cleaning;
(2) some personal care activities like bathing, chiropody, manicure, first aid, etc.;
(3) moral support; counselling and advice;
(4) general and family support: contacts with other care-givers, administrative support, shopping.

The social worker (or social nurse) is responsible for:

(1) the first contact with the clients;
(2) the intake, including the social inquiry;
(3) the work schedule of the home helps;
(4) the follow-up of each client.

The service manager is in charge of the general organization of the service, all financial activities (for the clients as well as for the personnel), staffing, and external contacts.

4.1d. The clients

Every aged person can apply to get home help. But it is the decision of those responsible for the different services that determines whether the applicant gets this help or not. The needs of the applicants are evaluated through a social investigation. It is clear that the way in which the social investigation is conducted and how it is reported will have a very important impact on the decision. In its Decree, the Flemish Executive Committee (1988) says that 'the help is given on request and according to the real needs of the applicant'. Obviously such a vague definition leaves room for interpretation. The Decree also says that this help should in the first instance be given to the most needy and those of low financial means.

Our interviews with service managers showed that in practice the financial situation of the applicant is of no great importance, at least not in deciding on the extent of help required. The income of the applicant is assessed in the report of the social worker because it serves as a basis upon which to calculate the client contribution.

As far as the clientele is concerned, local studies have revealed that 78 per cent of those using the home-help services are women, whilst two-thirds of them have reached the age of 75 years or above. Two out of three are widowed and almost seven out of ten live on their own. No less than 35 per cent of users are without children. The profile of the clientele of home-help services is that of the most vulnerable categories of elderly people: those living on their own, the oldest elderly people, elderly people in a multi-pathological state of health, elderly people without children, and elderly people who are financially weak (Dooghe and Van Den Boer 1987).

4.1e. The amount and frequency of help provided

The Decree defines the distribution of home help as follows. Two periods of care are distinguished. During the first 13 weeks, there is no limitation on the help that can be provided. From the fourteenth week onwards, home help is limited to 32 hours a week for each person. If more than 32 hours of help are given during this period, this must be limited to a maximum of 2 per cent of the hour quota (see below) and each service has a minimum of 400 hours to fill in this need.

Home help is given during the day between 7.00 and 20.00 hours. Depending on the needs of the aged person the care can be given in packages of two to eight hours a day. In practice, from interviews with the home-help services in the research region (Antwerp), it became clear that the services themselves make their own agreement about minima and maxima of help provided. As far as home help is concerned, all the services provide a maximum of between 8 and 16 hours per week. Some services spread this help over two half-days a week. Other services only provide one full day to reduce travel costs (which are not subsidized and thus reduced to a minimum).

4.1f. The qualifications and training of the family- and home-help assistants
The Decree defines the conditions which a home helper must fulfil. To work in a recognized service for family and home help, the home helper must have one of the following: training as a family social-worker, a family and health worker, or a children's nurse; a certificate as a family- and home-help worker from an acknowledged training centre; a certificate from outside the Flemish community of equal merit.

The training required must include moral, psychological, hygienic, social, and domestic knowledge. It must include 500 hours of theoretical training and 150 hours of practical training in various health and social institutions. In addition to this, home helpers must also undergo some in-service training every two years.

4.1g. The funding of home help
A basic principle for the financing of the home-help services is that of 'divided responsibility'. The Flemish government is responsible for 70 per cent of the cost of these services. The remaining 30 per cent is met by local government and the clients themselves. The amount of client payment depends on the net family income. There is no repayment from sickness insurance. Client contributions were 13.5 per cent of the total income of the services in 1984. The average contribution for clients in 1987 was 60 BF per hour.

Seventy-six per cent of the home-help services are provided by public-sector bodies, whilst 24 per cent are private organizations (Provinciale Welzijnscommissie Antwerpen 1986; Dooghe and Van Den Boer 1987). The majority of the public services are organized by the Public Centre for Social Welfare; there are still a few services run by local governments (municipalities). The private services are organized by the different sickness insurance funds (Catholic, Socialist, Liberal), by the Catholic Pensioners Union and by the Catholic Women's Organization. An organization can be officially recognized as a home-help service if there are at least three full-time home helpers:

for every 150 families who receive help, one full-time social nurse can be appointed;

for every additional 75 families, there can be one extra half-time social nurse;

for every 150 home helps one manager can be appointed: a social worker or a social nurse, or someone with a university degree.

In practice, large differences can appear as far as the organization of each service is concerned, depending on its size and on whether it is a public or a private service.

Services authorized by the Ministry receive government funding in the form of an allowance towards wages and operating costs for work at a certain rate per hour. Therefore they have to meet certain conditions:

all the hours used must be within the quota that can be subsidized (see below);
a social inquiry must be carried out in which the needs of the applicant are examined, before the help is actually granted;
home help must be provided in the residence of the applicant.

Since 1980 the number of performance hours that can be provided by a service for family and home help has been fixed by the Flemish government at a total of nine million. Each service has a certain quota of hours that can be subsidized. The reasons for fixing a maximum number of hours of family- and home-help service that can be subsidized were twofold. First, financial reasons: the government did not manage to free the necessary funds for the continuous growth of the home-help services. Secondly, policy reasons: because of the fast growth of the home-help services, the original aims became less and less clear. The government no longer had a clear picture of which clients were being reached. By limiting the number of hours, the government hoped to have more impact on the services. 'Blocking the performance hours to be subsidized was and is an instrument to create selectivity and put forward priorities' (Steyaert 1986).

The services for family and home help therefore came under great pressure because of the increasing number of applicants. A solution was seen in the use of programmes to stimulate employment. The aim of these programmes was to let long-term unemployed people do community work (minimum two years of unemployment and fully entitled to unemployment benefit work in non-commercial organizations; wages and social insurance contributions were paid by the state [Ministry of Employment]). By employing these people, services have been able to increase their hours by as much as 40 per cent. Because of their lack of qualifications these people have been employed in the cleaning service (see below).

The Flemish government wishes to have a clear profile of the clients (and potential clients) of the home-help services before they will consider a change. The pressure on providers forces them to be more selective in the granting of help. This selectivity is carried so far that several categories of people who qualify for help (e.g., elderly living with their children, overburdened informal carers) do not get any (Spinnewyn and Pacoler 1987).

4.2. Cleaning services

4.2a. Development

Before the development of the cleaning services, it had become clear that the home-help services were frequently limiting their activities to cleaning help. The potential of the home-help services was only partly used. In this context, the creation of cleaning services was seen as an important development.

As mentioned already, a scheme was launched at the end of the 1970s whereby the long-term unemployed could be asked to do community work. Special home-cleaning services were set up as temporary experiments. About 3800 cleaners were appointed at the beginning of the 1980s, all people who had been unemployed for at least two years. They are attached to the existing home-help services, their wages and the social security are paid by the government (Provinciale Welzijnscommissie Antwerpen 1986).

4.2b. The clients

As for the home-help services, every older person—living alone or in a family—can request cleaning help. For each request, a social inquiry will be made by the social worker. Although not formally defined, there is a consensus that priority should be given to the most needy and those with least financial means.

As for home help, there is a graded scale of co-payment. Most of the cleaning services use the same income scales as the home-help services. There is no repayment from sickness insurance. Again, no formal regulation determines the amount or frequency that can be provided. As a consensus, all the cleaning services provide care for four hours per week, concentrated on one day. In the research area, one cleaning service even provides one day (eight hours) every two weeks in order to reduce the travel costs, which are not subsidized (Hedebouw *et al.* 1988).

4.2c. The relation between the home-help and cleaning services

The cleaning and home-help services are closely related in two ways. First, cleaning help is *organized* within existing home-help services. Those responsible for the home help are usually also responsible for cleaning help. Secondly, cleaning services have grown out of the home-help services and are defined as an *alternative* to home help for those who only need home-making help.

Cleaning help has in part replaced home help. In practice, services will never provide cleaning *and* home help to one person. Elderly people may try to ask for cleaning help from one organization and home help from another, but only in exceptional cases will they succeed in obtaining both services.

4.3. Home nursing

The basic objective of home nursing is to provide patients with the care they need in their own environment, in order to prevent the need for hospitalization, or to enable early discharge from hospital.

The Flemish government is responsible for home services and provides subsidies for the personnel, co-ordination, and management. These subsidies are only a very small part of the total expenditure. Most of the funding for home nursing services is provided by the State Institute for Sickness and Invalidity Insurance (Dutch=RIZIV). By law only well-defined nursing tasks can be reimbursed by the RIZIV: these are especially of a medico-physical kind. All other activities—done by home nurses—are not paid for, as these are all psycho-social. One of the largest organizations in Belgium active in the field of home nursing is the White and Yellow Cross (about 80 per cent of all home nursing activities). It consists of 132 different services distributed over the whole country. It employes 2686 nurses; almost half of the staff work part-time. In addition to this the sickness insurance funds (Socialist, Liberal), the PCSW, and private nurses organize home nursing.

In general, home nursing services were used on no less than 15.4 million occasions in 1984, 11.5 million of which related to users in the Flanders region. Although home nursing services are provided to all sections of the population, three-quarters of the patients are aged between 55 and 85 years (Dooghe and Van Den Boer 1987).

A survey conducted by the White and Yellow Cross in 1982 found the following. Two-thirds of those calling in home nursing were aged 65 years or above. Over one in four was even older than 80 years. Almost two out of three patients were women. Four per cent of patients were bed-ridden and 9 per cent confined to a wheelchair or chair. In other words, 13 per cent of the patients were more or less unable to move without assistance. A further 29 per cent were unable to move around or go out without help. The survey also revealed that a large number of the clientele (44 per cent) only received home nursing after having spent some time receiving treatment in hospital. This finding emphasizes the importance of the service in providing post-treatment care.

Most of those elderly people being nursed at home (58 per cent) were visited at least once a day by a nurse. The average duration of nursing is 12 months. The main nursing activities are injections (58 per cent), personal care (42 per cent), and attending to sores (21 per cent). Some patients receive a combination of two or three nursing activities. Generally speaking, infirm elderly people being nursed at home can rely on receiving assistance from relatives or neighbours. Only 5 per cent of all patients live on their own and cannot count on receiving any help from relatives or neighbours (Dooghe and Van Den Boer 1987).

4.4. Service centres

In order to allow a broad range of services to be provided to elderly people, either in their homes or from a central location in the area in which they live, special service centres were set up to act as co-ordinating points. According to a Decree of 1985 the main task of a service centre is to increase the accessibility of the following kinds of help: family and household care, physical care, information and social care, and material help (Ministry of Flemish Community 1985).

The service centres can function in two ways: either to refer people to existing services (like home help, nursing, etc.), or to set up these services themselves if they do not yet exist (Provinciale Welzijnscommissie Antwerpen 1986).

Funding for the building of service centres is provided by a Flemish fund for the construction of hospitals and medico-social institutions. The Flemish government provides subsidies for the daily functioning of the service centres. Public and non-profit organizations can set up service centres. In order to get official recognition, the following conditions must be fulfilled: the centre must be centrally located; it must be open 32 hours a week, and it must provide services for the elderly in their immediate environment through close co-operation with other services.

4.5. Other services

Among other services for older people should be mentioned 'meals-on-wheels'. Table 2.2 describes the evolution of the number of services in the

Table 2.2. Evolution of services for meals-on-wheels in the Flemish community from 1977 to 1985; absolute numbers

	1977	1980	1985
Services	64	118	98
Hot meals/week	9833	30172	25490
Deep freezing/week	8215	16265	11365
Total number/week	18048	46437	36855

period 1977 to 1985. The decline in the 1980s is a result of funding restrictions (Provinciale Welzijnscommissie Antwerpen 1986; Dooghe and Van Den Boer 1987). With only one exception, all the services are public-sector entities.

5. HOME-CARE SERVICES IN THE STUDY AREA OF GROOT-ANTWERPEN (GREATER ANTWERP)

5.1. The spectrum of home-care services

Table 2.3 gives an overview of the number of ambulatory services available in the study area, with an indication of the public or private character of these services.

Table 2.3. Number of ambulatory services in Groot-Antwerpen according to the organizing body; 1988

	Public sector	Private sector	
		Sickness insurance	Private
Hot-meals services	1*	0	?
Service centres **	17	0	2
Services for home nursing	1	2	6
Services for cleaning help	1*	4	0
Services for home help	2***	4	3

* Only PCSW.
** All service centres are provided by the PCSW.
*** One service by the PCSW and one service by the city of Antwerp.

The largest service for home nursing is the one organized by the White and Yellow Cross, a private service which works in close co-operation with Catholic Sickness Insurance. Also the Socialist and the Liberal sickness insurance organizations provide home nursing, as do private nurses.

5.2. Home-help and cleaning services

The PCSW organizes home and cleaning help. It is a rather exceptional situation that in one and the same city two public services exist: aside from the PCSW the city of Antwerp also organizes home help but no cleaning help. The Socialist and the Liberal sickness insurance organizations have their own services for home and for cleaning help. The Catholic Sickness Insurance does not organize home or cleaning help: they refer people to the service for home help and for cleaning help provided by the Catholic Pensioners Union. There are several other private services, but these reach a much smaller number of elderly people.

Table 2.4 gives an overview of the number of elderly (60 +) currently receiving help from the services for home help and for cleaning help.

Table 2.4. Number of elderly people (60+) receiving home help and cleaning services in Groot-Antwerpen; December 1987

	Cleaning help	Home help
PCSW	2448	1193
Municipal service	0	316
Total (public sector)	2448	1509
Catholic Pensioners Union	500	308
Liberal sickness insurance	504	359
Socialist sickness insurance	600	412
Total (private sector)	1604	1091
TOTAL	4052	2600

Except for the municipal service for home help, all the services for home help or cleaning help mentioned in this table participated in the study.

5.3. Allocation of home-help and cleaning services in the study area

The following is a brief description of the steps in the procedure for dealing with service requests in the study area. In general this process looked the same in all four organizations:

(1) the request: by the elderly person, by relatives, by professional services;
(2) first selection by the person who receives the request, based on the reasons for the request;
(3) social inquiry by the social worker (at home);
(4) report of the inquiry, written by the social worker, used as a base for the final decision about kind and frequency of help that will be provided;
(5) final decision about whether the person will receive help, whether it will be cleaning help or home help, whether the help will start immediately or not, and about the frequency of help.

A more detailed account of these five steps is as follows.

1. The request for cleaning or home help can be made by the elderly people themselves or by their relatives. Other professional services (social services, general hospital, general practitioner) may also contact the services.

2. Immediately after this request, the person who receives it makes a primary selection. During this first contact, the reasons for the request will be looked at carefully to decide whether cleaning or home help will be useful. At this stage, requests can be refused for several reasons:

if it is obvious that the person is too frail and that neither cleaning nor home help is enough, he/she may be referred to other services (home nursing, residential care, etc.);

if there is thought to be a great deal of informal support or private care, a request for cleaning or home help can be refused;

financial reasons are also important, especially for a request for cleaning help: if the clients are well-off, they are advised to find a private cleaner because the cost of the cleaning service will be higher for them. This is not the case for a request for home help, because it is almost impossible to find a private one.

Variations in the size of the services cause differences in the composition of the personnel. In practice this means that in smaller services, the person in charge also does much of the social work (social inquiries at home), whereas this is not the case in larger services. In most of the services participating in the study, the request for cleaning or home help was, at the first stage, dealt with by the social workers. Only one service (Socialist Sickness Insurance) had a separate employee who answered personal or telephone requests. In other words, the social worker has a crucial role in deciding whether a social inquiry will be made or not.

3. If a request has not been rejected, the social worker of the service will visit the elderly person for an assessment.

4. On the basis of this inquiry the social worker will write a report, describing the life circumstances, the health status, the availability of informal care, and the financial situation of the elderly person.

5. The final decision about the kind and the frequency of help to be provided is based on the report written by the social worker. This means that again the social worker has a great deal of influence. How this decision is taken differs between the services. In the Catholic Pensioners Union and the Socialist and Liberal sickness insurance organizations the social worker takes the final decision about the kind and the frequency of the help to be provided. The person in charge of the service always gives his/her final agreement, which mostly tends to support the decision of the social worker. In the PCSW the decision is taken by a separate committee but based on the report of the social worker. Mostly the recommendations of the social worker are accepted.

6. ALLOCATION OF HOME HELP/CLEANING HELP

6.1. The cases selected

In this section we will describe the main results from our study of the decisions regarding allocation of home-help and cleaning services. The following services co-operated in our study:

the PCSW services for cleaning and home help;
the services of the:
Christian Association for Pensioners,
Socialist Sick Fund,
Solidarity for the Family (Liberal Sick Fund).

Altogether 38 cases were studied (15 home help and 23 cleaning help). Two types of older people (over 75 years) living in Greater Antwerp were selected:

(1) people requesting help, but put on a waiting list after a social inquiry;
(2) people for whom cleaning/home help had already started, either immediately after the request or after having been on the waiting list.

In all cases, the elderly person and a key professional were interviewed. Interviews were also sought with informal carers, where relevant. However, only in 14 of the 38 cases did we interview an informal carer. In 9 cases there was no informal carer, and in 15 cases no interview was possible because the older person (12 cases) or the carer (3 cases) refused permission. The most frequent reason for refusal given by the elderly people themselves was that they did not want their relatives 'to be bothered'.

Figures 2.1 and 2.2 show the pathways of the cases. They were constructed on the basis of the following questions:

1. Was the decision to allocate a cleaning or a home-help service?
2. Was the person on the waiting list or had the service already begun?
3. Was the help temporary or permanent?
4. Was it an acute request or not?

The decision as to whether a request was acute or not was left to the judgement of the social worker who has made the official inquiry; the services do not have a clear definition of 'acute or urgent' requests. In practice it was clear that those who were defined as 'non-urgent' were put on the waiting list.

Our interviews with service managers showed that waiting lists are a reality. This was confirmed by our case studies. As Figs. 2.1 and 2.2 show, only a minority were allocated help immediately without having been on a waiting list. This was more so in the case of cleaning services.

Most requests were for permanent help; only in three cases were they for temporary help. In these cases there was an acute request and help was given immediately. All these cases were people discharged from acute hospital care (e.g., with a broken arm), and without home care they could

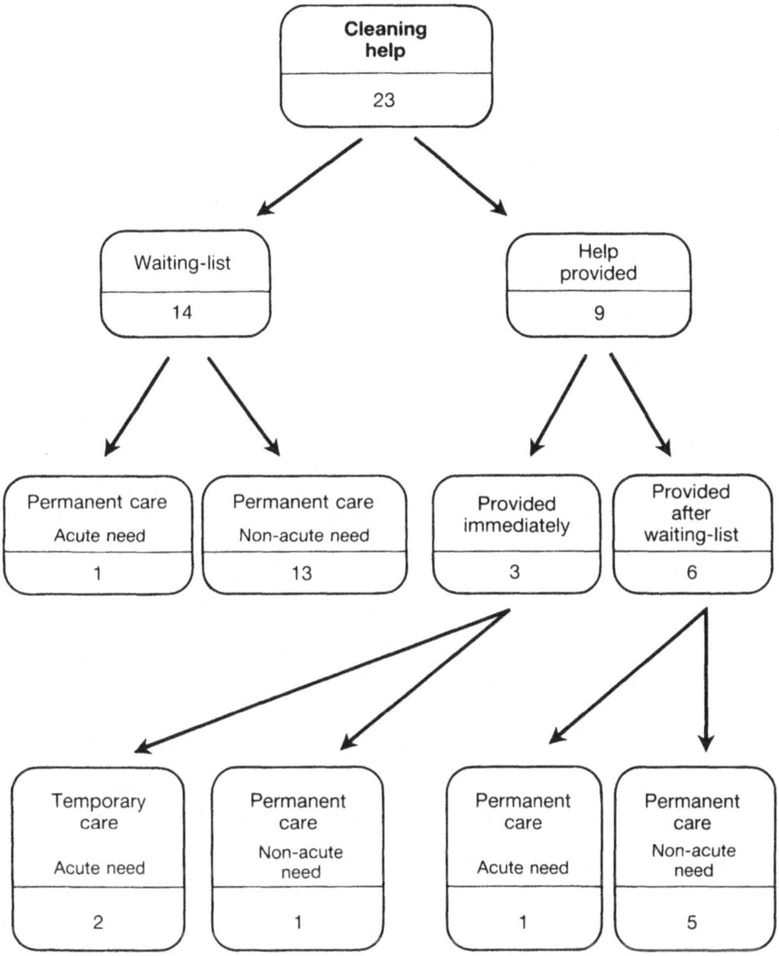

Fig. 2.1. Cleaning help.

not have been discharged. On the other hand, as Figs. 2.1 and 2.2 show, some elderly people with an acute request for help were still on the waiting list.

6.2. The decision-making process for cleaning- and home-help

The process underlying a decision to provide help (and determining the kind and the amount of help) can be divided into three phases: (i) *the starting situation*: why did an elderly person decide to ask for help from

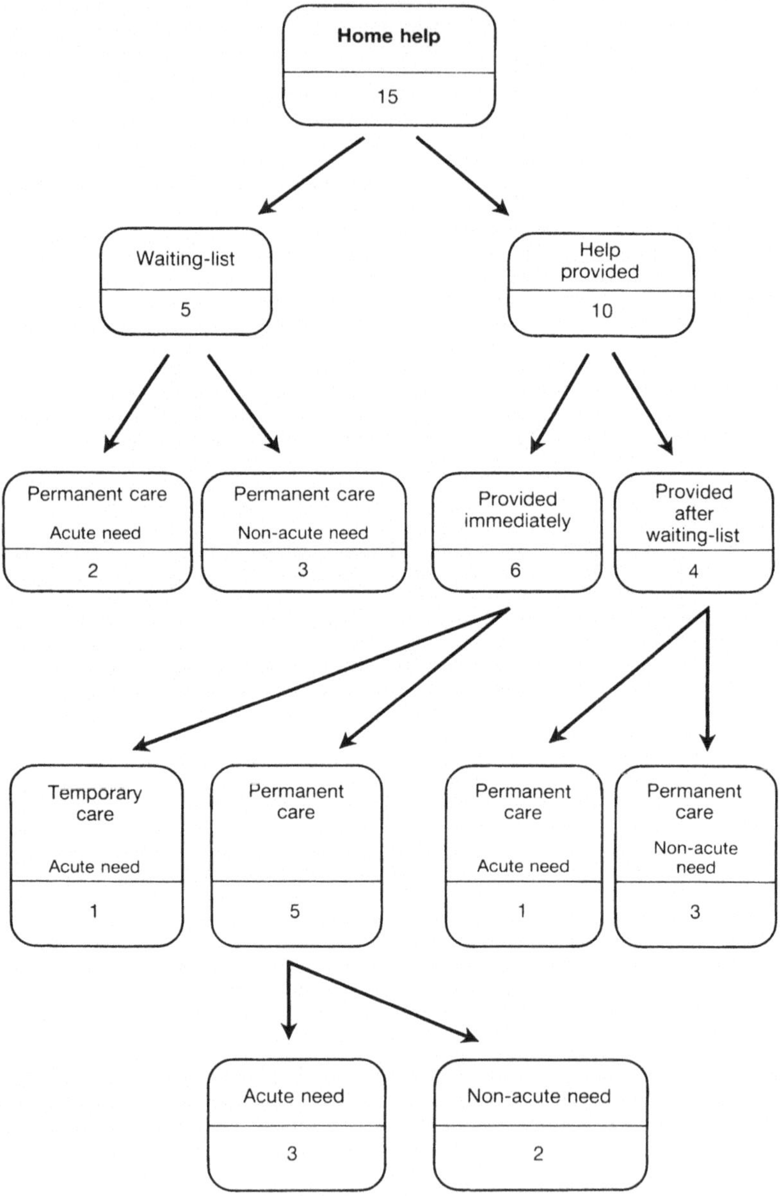

Fig. 2.2. Home help.

professional service? What was the background for seeking help?; (ii) *the request for help*: what kind of help was requested? What alternatives were considered?; (iii) *the decision*: what decision was taken in the end? Who had the decisive influence? How was the new situation evaluated by the different parties involved?

The starting situation

The group applying for cleaning help comprised 12 men and 11 women. The majority of those applying for home help were women (10 women and 5 men). The average age of the cleaning-help cases was 79.5 years; the average age of the home-help cases was 82 years.

The reasons/motives/circumstances behind the request for help, can be classified into four groups: (i) the physical condition of the elderly person; (ii) their mental condition; (iii) social factors; and (iv) practical reasons. More than two-thirds of the elderly people mentioned physical reasons; two-thirds also mentioned practical reasons, mainly problems in performing domestic tasks. The most important social reason was the health condition of the spouse. The loss or decrease of informal care was mostly mentioned by the professional carer. In most of the cases all the participants pointed to a combination of different reasons.

The request for help

We asked each of the three types of 'actors' involved—the older person, their carer, and the professionals—which solution they preferred. Table 2.5 compares their preferences with the care actually provided (whether immediately or in the form of acceptance for the waiting list). In most cases there was agreement between the three parties. It is particularly important to note that many professionals interpreted a *request* for help as meaning a *need* for help. To them, it was not a matter of choosing *whether* a person should have help, but merely *what* kind of service to allocate.

In 41 per cent of the cases the referral was made by the elderly people themselves or their carers. In the other 59 per cent, other professionals were involved. In all cases of acute need the family or others were always involved.

When asking about possible alternatives and whether any had been considered, we found that many elderly people and their carers did not know or could not think of any. Thus almost half of the elderly respondents saw no alternative solutions (n = 15), 14 mentioned one alternative and 4 mentioned two alternatives. Admission into a residential home was the most important alternative mentioned. Because of the negative attitude of the elderly people to residential care, this possibility was not considered any further. In some cases the alternative was another service for cleaning or home help, but it could not be realized because of waiting lists. In a few

Table 2.5. Relation between the preference for care and the actual care that is or will be provided; absolute numbers

Preference for care	Actual care provided	
	Cleaning help	Home help
Elderly		
Cleaning help	20	3
Home help	1	9
Cleaning help or home help	1	0
Care in general/no opinion/opinion of children is best	1	3
Informal carer		
Cleaning help	6	0
Home help	1	3
Residential care	0	2
No opinion	1	0
Professional carer		
Cleaning help	21	1
Home help	0	10
Cleaning help or home help	0	2
Residential care	0	1
Care in general/only informal care	1	1

cases, (more) support from the informal carers would be the alternative to professional care. In these cases the overburdening of the informal carer was a reason to call in professional help.

The professional carers in the cleaning and home-help services mentioned more alternatives than the elderly people. Only one-fifth of the professionals did not mention any alternatives ($n = 6$); 14 professionals mentioned one alternative and 14 others mentioned two or three alternatives. Help from the informal carer or a private cleaner were the most important alternatives mentioned by the professionals, a different pattern from what we found with the elderly—informal care was not available or could not continue because of overburdening.

The decision

In most cases there was general agreement about the decisions taken. As already mentioned, the professionals accepted a request for help as a need for help. Disagreements only arose as to whether it should be cleaning or home help. In cases of disagreement the views of the professionals tended to prevail over those of the older person, unless informal carers were also involved in the process. When they were the preferences of the older people and/or their carers tended to prevail.

The outcome of the decision-making process was the following:

For cleaning help, most cases were referred to the waiting list; some cases received help immediately as they were already on the waiting list; only very few cases received acute help.

For home help, one-third received acute help; one-third were put on the waiting list; and one-third received help immediately as they were already on the waiting list.

Our case studies showed that health and functional ability were the most important criteria in determining whether a person was allocated help, and whether the help was cleaning or home help. Thus the home-help cases were elderly women; elderly poor who could not count on informal care; and those whose informal care mostly came from partners (who in most cases needed help themselves) or from the neighbours. Generally those allocated home help had more health-related problems than the cleaning-help cases. However, there was some overlap, which can be explained by the availability of informal care. Thus the cleaning-help cases, especially those with a higher ADL (activities of daily living) score could rely more on informal care. This means that the availability of informal care can be an important factor in the decision about the kind of help that will be granted.

All those over 81 years were granted home help immediately. The only exception made was a 78-year-old woman who had broken her arm and who could only stay at home with ambulatory care. In our general interviews with managers they had emphasized that the cleaning services were hardly ever able to respond to acute requests because of a shortage of personnel. Yet we found four elderly people for whom the cleaning service was started immediately after their request. Two of these had broken arms and two other cases were lucky that at the moment of their request one cleaner was free.

About half the applicants were satisfied with the decision taken. These were mainly people who were allocated help immediately, some of whom might have been on a waiting list for some time. Not surprisingly, those unhappy with the decision were those who were put on the waiting list. This meant that they would have to wait for one to six months before any help could be given. A considerable number of these either did not have any informal support at all, or their health problems presented an enormous burden upon the informal carers.

Although a larger proportion of those receiving immediate help had problems in performing the tasks of daily life than those put on the waiting list, many of the 'waiting-list clients' had problems of equal severity. It would seem that 'need' defined in terms of health problems and availability of informal care was taken into account mainly in choosing between home-help and cleaning services. Once this choice had been made, and unless there were special, acute circumstances, providers were perhaps guided as much by the principle of 'first come, first served' as by any clear measures of need. This is certainly a possibility which we will consider in our further analysis of the case study material. Until this has been done it is not possible to draw any firm conclusions or to discuss policy implications.

NOTE

[1] The Belgian study was conducted by the Catholic University of Leuven (Prof. Dr. F. Baro). The research region was Groot-Antwerpen. The project was undertaken in co-operation with the Public Centre for Social Welfare of Groot-Antwerpen (Mr G. De Bruyne, secretary, Elderly Public Policy Centre).

REFERENCES

Baro, F., De Bruyne, G., Magits, K., Moorthamer, L., and Van den Bergh, H. (1989). *Het funktioneren van bejaardenvoorzieningen. Een studie over het besluitvormingsproces bij het toekennen van hulpverlening aan bejaarden.* (The functioning of the home-care for the elderly; the decision-making process.) Onderzoeksrapport 5, De General Interviews: overzicht van de voornaamste bevindingen. Leuven–Antwerpen (internal document, OCMW Antwerpen).

Baro, F., De Bruyne, G., Magits, K., Moorthamer, L., and Van den Bergh, H. (1990). *Het bejaardenbeleid in Vlaanderen.* (The policies for older people in Flanders.) Leuven–Antwerpen (internal document, OCMW, Antwerpen).

Dooghe, G. (1987). *Raming van de behoeften naar non-profit voorzieningen voor bejaarden in Vlaanderen: 1985–2000.* (The estimation of the needs for no-profit services for the elderly in the Flanders.) Onderzoek in opdracht van de Gemeenschapsminister van Gezin en Welzijnszorg. Brussels, CBGS.

Dooghe, G. and Van Den Boer, L. (1987). *Care for the elderly in Belgium.* Brussels, CBGS werkdocument, No. 37.

Flemish Executive decree (1988). *Het besluit van 22 juni 1988 van de Vlaamse Executieve tot regeling van de erkenning en subsidiering van de diensten voor gezins—en bejaardenhulp en van de opleidingscentra voor gezins—en bejaardenhulp en van de opleidingscentra voor gezins—en bejaardenhelp(st)ers.* (Decree of 1988 concerning the services for cleaning help and home help.) Bijlage A: Statuut (B.S. 1 July).

Hedebouw, G., Winters, S., and Pacolet, J. (1988). *Ondersteuning van de draagkracht van de mantelzorg bij bejaarden.* (Support measures for informal care of the elderly.) Onderzoek in opdracht van de Gemeenschapsminister van Volksgezondheid en Leefmilieu. Leuven, Hoger Instituut voor de Arbeid.

Ministry of Flemish Community (1985). *Naar een nieuw Vlaams beleid inzake bejaardenzorg. Normen voor erkenning en subsidiering van voorzieningen voor bejaarden*. (Towards a new Flemish policy for the home care of the elderly; criteria.) Brussels.

Ministry of Social Affairs (1987). *Beleidsnota van de Minister van Sociale Zaken in verband met de ziekenhuizen, de rust—en verzorgingstehuizen en de thuisgezondheidszorg*. Brussels. (The health-care policies for older people in Belgium.)

National Instituut voor de Statistiek (1981). *Algemene Volks—en Woningtelling van 1 maart 1981*. (National Statistics on Population and Housing, 1981.) Brussels.

Provinciale Welzijnscommissie Antwerpen (1986). *Naar een geintegreerd beleid voor thuisverblijvende bejaarden*. (Towards an integrated home-care policy for the elderly.)

Spinnewyn, H. and Pacolet, J. (1985). *Kostprijs van de thuisgezondheidszorg*. (The cost of home care in Belgium.) Onderzoek in opdracht van de Landsbond der Christelijke Mutualiteiten en van de Nationale Federatie van de Wit-Gele Kruis Verenigingen. Leuven, Hoger Instituut voor de Arbeid.

Spinnewyn, H. and Pacolet, J. (1987). *Een financiele tegemoetkoming in de thuisgezondheidszorg. Modaliteiten en budgettaire implicaties*. (Subsidized home health care.) Onderzoek in opdracht van de Minister van Sociale Zaken. Leuven, Hoger Instituut voor de Arbeid.

Steyaert, R. (1986). *Home huishoudhulp op mensenmaat. Aanzet tot een nieuw beleid inzake gezins—en bejaardenhulp*. (Humanizing home care; a new policy.) Kabinet van de Gemeenschapsminister van Gezin en Welzijnszorg, Brussels.

3

The home-help service in Denmark

Bjorn E. Holstein, Pernille Due, Gert Almind, and Erik Holst

1. Home help for elderly people
   1.1. The historical development of the home-help service
   1.2. The current legislative basis: target population
   1.3. The range of services offered by local authorities (communes)
   1.4. Home-help provision
   1.5. The tasks of home helpers
2. The clients of home help
   2.1. Previous studies
   2.2. The ACRE study
3. Decision-making for home help
   3.1. Formal pathways
   3.2. Framework and method of the pathways study
   3.3. The decision-makers' perspective
   3.4. Results from the case studies
4. Policy implications
   4.1. Our proposals for changes to improve service allocation

References

1. HOME HELP FOR ELDERLY PEOPLE

1.1. The historical development of the home-help service

This chapter focuses mainly upon the home-help service in Denmark. The service has been and is the backbone of home-care policies over the years. The context within which it operates is as follows. Counties are responsible for the funding of hospitals, general practitioners, and a number of specialized institutions such as psychiatric nursing homes. Most other health and social services are organized and financed by the local municipalities ('communes'). Access to general practitioners is free and unrestricted, and the practitioner refers patients to hospitals, practising specialists, physiotherapy, and home nursing. Access to social services is decided by the local social services department. Tables 1 and 2 in Appendix 2 provide data on expenditure for health and social services in Denmark.

The first legislation on home help in Denmark appeared in 1949. The aim was to give financial support to local municipalities, which established 'substitute housewife' arrangements, primarily to support families with children during a mothers' illness by providing short-term help, usually of no more than two weeks. This service was free for families of limited means and there was a co-payment for families with average or high incomes. Elderly people were not regarded, at this stage, as a target group for this service.

This legislation was slightly modified in 1963, introducing 1968 as the time limit for the local government to organize 'substitute housewives' *and home help*. Home help was intended to assist disabled and elderly people in need of more permanent support at home. There was state reimbursement of 80 per cent of the local governments' expenses until 1970. Since 1970 the state reimbursement has been half.

The guiding principle for elderly people, often described by the term 'as long as possible in your own home', became manifest in the early 1970s, and was part of the wider move to de-institutionalize disabled, mentally ill, mentally handicapped, and elderly people. As far as elderly people are concerned, the following changes took place. First, the Social Security Act (1972) underlined the obligation of the communes to organize permanent home-help services for the elderly. Secondly, that Act changed the legislative basis of institutions for elderly people in order to restrict institutional care to those with the most pronounced need. Until 1973 there were two kinds of institutions, (a) the so-called old age homes, which were meant to be residential institutions for elderly people who were not in acute need of nursing care, and (b) 'homes for the old and the sick'. The new legislation removed the state reimbursement for 'old age homes' but provided state reimbursement for 'nursing homes', residential institutions for impaired elderly people in need of nursing care. Thirdly, the first experiments with 24-hour domiciliary care appeared in the mid-1970s and gained enormous publicity and public interest. Finally, the need of comprehensive policies for elderly people that could meet the challenges of the apparent demographic and social changes became still more evident throughout the late 1970s and resulted in the government setting up, in 1979, a commission to review these policies. This commission completed its work in 1982.

A number of factors facilitated the development of public domiciliary care. The reorganization of local government in 1970, whereby the 1379 Danish communes were merged into 275 larger communes, meant that each was big enough to organize and run a comprehensive set of social services. The general ideological climate facilitated the broad growth of public-welfare expenditure during the 1950s, 1960s, and 1970s. Demographic changes, especially the rapid growth of the population of oldest old, became apparent, and general knowledge about elderly people were growing. In particular, the results of a general survey of the elderly, conducted by the National Danish Institute of Social Research and published in the early 1970s, showed that the vast majority of them were able to live independently (Stehouwer 1968, 1970).

Another factor was the supply of housing, which grew faster than the population in the post-war period. As a consequence, a growing proportion of the population obtained their own dwellings, which they did not have to share with others. Therefore, still more older people now live alone, and the proportion living together with children or other relatives is declining. The proportion of those living with a child was 21 per cent in 1962, 11 per cent in 1977, and 4 per cent in 1986 (Stehouwer 1970; Platz 1981; Holstein *et al.* 1988). This development has reduced the role of the family as carers. An inter-Nordic study focused on the numbers of women, 45 to 59 years old, as these seem to be the most important source of informal care (apart from spouses) (Daatland and Sundström 1985). This group has decreased from 1100 per 1000 elderly in 1940 to less than 600 per 1000 elderly in 1980. Moreover, a growing proportion of this population group has become involved in the labour force. During the latest decades the support and help for dependent elderly relatives from their social networks has been changing from a regular, almost daily help (shopping, cooking, cleaning, etc.) to a more episodic kind of help (gardening, repairs, economic advice, etc. (Holstein *et al.* 1988).

1.2. The current legislative basis: target population

The legislative basis for today's home-help service is the Social Security Act, which was introduced in 1973. By law, communes must organize a number of social services including home help, home nursing, equipment for the handicapped, nursing homes, and day-care facilities (The Social Security Act 1972; Appendix to the report from the Parliament's Committee on Social Welfare regarding the proposed Act). The distinction between 'substitute housewives' (for short-term support) and home help (for long-term support) was maintained but the terminology was changed to *provisional home help* and *permanent home help*. Permanent home help was meant to meet the needs of those chronically ill and elderly, and was considered to be a major preventive service (preventing the need for nursing-home and other institutionalized care). Until July 1989, home help was free for those with low income (regular old-age pension plus minor supplements) and there was co-payment for those with higher income. Home help exceeding six hours a week was free regardless of income. Since 1 July 1989, home help has become a free service for everybody in need, although local authorities are allowed to charge those receiving the service as a temporary measure. As mentioned above, the state reimburses half of the local government's expenses for home help.

By law, home help is to be provided to everyone who is unable to perform regular daily activities because of a permanent disease, disability, or impairment. Before Parliament's agreement to this law, two important points were made clear by the Minister of Social Affairs:

Home help should be provided on the basis of need for assistance with daily activities, regardless of economic situation.

Home help should be provided on the basis of an evaluation of the family's total situation. In reality this means that the presence of a healthy spouse will be taken into consideration in the evaluation of need.

1.3. The range of services offered by local authorities (communes)

1.3a. Residential care

Apart from hospital care, the communes are responsible for the provision of residential care. All communes have a number of nursing homes for persons in need of extensive care. Nursing homes are free for elderly people on low income (old-age pension), and until recently their pension was replaced by pocket money as board and lodging are free. For elderly people with additional income there is a co-payment arrangement. The local communes control access to institutional care.

Many communes have further supply of service flats and other residential premises for disabled and impaired elderly people. Most communes have decided to replace (some or all) nursing-home facilities with extensive, 24-hour, domiciliary care. The tendency now is to redefine a nursing home from being a building with a certain amount of nursing care and other services available to being a range of services which can be provided where it best suits the clients and/or their relatives.

Six per cent of elderly people in Denmark (65+ years) now live in nursing homes. The proportion increases with increasing age: 65–69 years, 1 per cent; 70–74 years, 2 per cent; 75–79 years, 4 per cent; 80–84 years, 11 per cent; 85–89 years, 24 per cent; 90–94 years, 43 per cent; and 95+ years 62 per cent. (Elderly Commission 1981). The proportion so living has decreased slightly since 1975 for each age group. The number of nursing-home beds has been almost stable (49 500) during the 1980s, but is now declining slightly. It is believed that nursing-home residents have had increasing disability over the last two or three decades, but there is no statistical information available to document this trend. The most likely explanations for this possible increase in disability are (i) that the composition of the elderly population has changed (relatively more old elderly and fewer young elderly); and (ii) that the supply of domiciliary care has increased significantly, making home help and home nursing available for those who would need institutional care if they had not received them.

1.3b. Home-care services

Home nursing is usually for short-term assistance after discharge from hospital or during episodes of acute illness. The home nurses' typical functions are to give drugs and injections, care for wounds, and give advice on health. Entry into home nursing is decided by the general practitioner, the hospital which discharges the patient, or by the commune. Seventy per cent of all visits by home nurses were made to individuals of 65 years or older, and 12 per cent of the elderly population receives home nursing one or more times during a year. Most of these elderly, home-nursing patients receive this service for a few weeks or a few months. Home nursing is free of charge (Statistik om hjemmesygeplejevirksomheden 1981).

Equipment which facilitates the daily activities of disabled persons (such as hospital beds, wheelchairs, walking sticks, handles, special kitchenware, toilet facilities, etc.) can usually be borrowed from the local social services department.

Most communes, but not all, have a number of *additional services* available: meals-on-wheels, day-care centres, clubs, laundry service, chiropody, gardening service, snow-clearing service, free or subsidized transport, occupational therapy, physiotherapy, and education.

Most communes, but not all, have *24-hour domiciliary care* (or at least domiciliary-care services from 7.00 to 23.00 hours). This service provision is organized in a number of different ways. Often it includes the provision of home nursing and home help, day and night (Andersen 1980; Hansen and Werborg 1983–1984, 1985).

Most communes but not all offer 'respite care', which is a temporary admission to a nursing home. Relief beds are used for three main purposes: (i) recovery or rehabilitation after an illness or discharge from hospital; (ii) care during an illness that does not require hospital treatment; (iii) temporary care of chronically impaired patients in order to give relief to a spouse or prevent their exhaustion.

Day centres are provided in many communes but the extent of this service is insignificant compared to other kinds of care. The staffing (full-time equivalents) in nursing homes is 50 800; home help, 25 500; and day centres, 1900.

Home help is the most important home-care service and will be described in detail next.

1.4. Home-help provision

There is no public statistical information on home-help provision before 1977. In 1972 there were 13 800 home helpers (full-time equivalents) (Elderly Commission 1981), and the population aged 65+ years was 600 000, which gives a ratio of 23.0 home helpers per 1000 inhabitants of 65+ years. In 1984, the corresponding figures were 25 500 home helpers, 749 000 65+ year-olds, which gives a ratio of 34.0 per 1000 (Samordning i sundhedsvaesenet 1985). The number of home helpers grew by 85 per cent during these 12 years, whereas the population above 65 years old grew by a quarter. The growth in home-help provision has been modest since 1980 (Kähler and Madsen 1985).

How many elderly households (at least one member over 65 years) were receiving home help before 1977 is unknown. A national survey in 1962 indicated that less than 5 per cent of elderly people received provisional assistance from a 'substitute housewife' during an illness. Nobody was reported as having permanent home help (Stehouwer 1968, 1970).

The number of elderly households receiving home help was 79 000 in 1977, and approximately 125 000 in 1984. This means that approximately 17 per cent of the population above 65 years receives home help. The proportion receiving home help in various age groups in 1984 were (Kähler and Madsen 1985): 67–69 years, 6.0 per cent; 70–74 years, 11.3 per cent; 75–79 years, 21.6 per cent; 80–84 years, 34.0 per cent; 85+ years, 38.2 per cent.

As indicated above, home help is provided as a provisional or as a permanent service. Of those elderly people who receive home help, approximately 95 per cent receive permanent help. Most elderly people (86 per cent) only receive the home-help service during the day on weekdays; the remaining 14 per cent are considered so dependent on help that they receive help at weekends and/or during the evening or night (Appendix to the report from the Parliament's Committee on Social Welfare regarding the proposed Social Security Act 1972).

For the period in which statistical information is available the majority of the households receiving home help had relatively few hours of help a week. Table 3.1 indicates the distribution of weekly home-help hours by age; in all age groups the majority receive less than 7 hours a week.

The distribution of home-help services has changed in recent years in several ways. First, still more older people receive home help (as indicated above). Secondly, equality among geographical areas has increased. By law, every local government 'commune' must organize home help, but the amount is left open. As a consequence of the autonomy of local governments, the provision of home-help services varies considerably from one to another. In 1971, the ratio between regions was 2:1, based on home-help

Table 3.1. Number of hours of permanent home help by age, Denmark 1983. (Source: Samordning i sundhedsvaesenet 1985.)

Hours per week	67–79 years (%)	80–84 years (%)	85+ years (%)
1–6	84	79	67
7–12	11	14	20
13+	5	7	13

hours per 1000 individuals of 65+ years (Kjerkegaard 1976). More recent nationwide data on inequality in provision are not available but a recent study of home-help provision in 12 communes shows a ratio of 2:1 (Olsen and Gregersen 1988). A document from the National Board of Social Affairs reports that there was a change from 1981 to 1984: staffing was stable or increasing in 175 communes, and decreasing in 100 communes. The communes with a decreasing number of home helpers were, generally speaking, communes with a higher than average number of home helpers in 1981 (Kähler and Madsen 1985). Thirdly, there has been a slight shift in provision of home help from the young old to the old old. In 1981, 36.1 per cent of the population of 85+ years received home help; in 1984, the proportion was 38.2 per cent (Kähler and Madsen 1985). Fourthly, there has been a reduction in average number of hours of help per week. In 1981, 76.2 per cent of households receiving home help received 1 to 6 hours; the corresponding figure for 1984 was 79.4 per cent (Kähler and Madsen 1985). Finally, there are signs of increasing professionalization of home helpers. An increasing proportion of home helpers work full-time. The typical 'housewife substitute' during the 1960s was a housewife with a few hours of employment a week. The typical home helper of today is a woman employed full-time (Elderly Commission 1981). Another trend is the increasing educational effort. The typical 'housewife substitute' during the 1960s had no formal training or education; the majority of today's home helpers are still women with no more than basic school education, and no occupational or theoretical education. The requirement of today, however, is that home helpers must undertake a basic training lasting 7 weeks and often one or two additional 1-week courses.

1.5. The tasks of home helpers

According to the social security legislation, the home helpers' work is *home-making* and *personal* care, i.e., shopping, cleaning, cooking, bed making, assisting with toileting, dressing, washing, bathing, hair combing, and other aspects of personal hygiene, and outdoor walks. The local government may introduce restrictions on some of these activities, but generally speaking this is what the home helpers do (The Social Security Act 1972; Kähler and Madsen 1985). The local government may also introduce additional home-help services such as snow-clearing and gardening. Many communes accept that *socialization* (conversation, walks) is an integral part of the home helper's job. Some of the personal care is sometimes provided in day centres, but home help is by far the most important provision. Home helpers do not undertake *nursing* activities such as injections, bandaging, administration of medicine, and surveillance. These are done by home nurses.

Two recent empirical investigations confirm this picture. Hendriksen *et al.* (1984) describe the home helpers' work-load in terms of working hours used for a variety of tasks. Figure 1 in Appendix 2 presents the findings, which show that cleaning is the main task. Approximately 37 per cent of the home-help hours are used for cleaning, about 43 per cent for other domestic activities, 13 per cent for conversation, and 6 per cent for personal care (dressing, washing, etc.). The study also reports that most elderly people are satisfied with their regular home helper but unhappy about changing helpers.

Olsen and Gregersen (1988) draw a detailed profile of the elderly people receiving home help in 12 communes. There are major differences between communes in the amount of help provided (ratio between 'best' and 'worst' commune, 2:1). Ninety per cent of the home-help consumers have received help for more than one year. Their study also confirms that the majority are satisfied with their home helper, but that changing helper causes dissatisfaction. The reasons for satisfaction are mainly the practical help received, but the personal contact is also mentioned by many people as a positive factor. In most cases there are good relationships between the elderly people and their home helpers. The most satisfied home helpers serve the most satisfied clients.

From recent studies of 24-hour domiciliary care, we know what functions the home helpers undertake during the evening and night hours (Andersen 1980; Hansen and Werborg 1983–1984). Data from Hansen and Werborg's study in regard of 113 000 visits during these are shown in Appendix 2, Table 3. The most frequent activities were giving medication, observation, changing clothes, helping into or out of bed, serving dinner, personal hygiene, helping with toileting, and preventing bed sores.

Recent studies have evaluated the impact of 24-hour domiciliary care. For elderly people receiving this service, it increases the feeling of comfort, security, and life satisfaction. Moreover, these people have significantly fewer hospital and nursing-home admissions than others of similar age and functional ability. Cost–benefit analyses show that savings in hospital- and nursing-home-bed days exceed the costs significantly (Hansen and Werborg 1983–1984).

2. THE CLIENTS OF HOME HELP

2.1. Previous studies

Some Danish studies have described which categories of elderly receive home help. Hansen (1982) and Platz (1981) describe met and unmet needs for home help in a random sample of the Danish, community-based, elderly population in 1977. The proportion receiving home help was largest among the oldest, women, those living alone, and those with reduced functional ability and in poor health. Among those living alone, more men than women received home help. Approximately 10 per cent of the study population over the age of 70 thought they needed (more) home help and the proportion in need of help was larger among incapacitated or ill elderly people. The majority of those who thought they needed home help already received some help. Among those who do not get help, only 1 to 3 per cent thought they needed this kind of service.

Avlund and Schultz-Larsen (1990) describe a population of 70-year-old people in Glostrup. Seven per cent of men and 10 per cent of women received home help. Individuals had a high probability of receiving home help if they had poor functional ability, were living alone or with a disabled spouse, were social class IV to V (low), had few personal resources, and were receiving help from their informal social network.

Olsen and Gregersen (1988) made a comprehensive study of the elderly home-help clientele in 12 communes. Approximately 90 per cent had received home help for more than one year, the majority (86 per cent) during the day on weekdays only. Two-thirds of the clientele were women, three-quarters were single. The group had numerous health problems and contacts with a general medical practitioner, a high intake of medication, and a high frequency of loneliness and weak social relations.

A study of 470 ill elderly people aged 75 years or more (Almind *et al.* 1987) showed that more than two-thirds of this group had received home help. The health and social profile of recipients differed in many ways from that of elderly people receiving other services, such as frequent contact with a general practitioner or home nursing. Those who received home help had, generally speaking, fewer resources: weak social networks, weak psychological resources, poor health, and poor functional ability.

2.2. The ACRE study

Late in 1986, a random sample of non-institutionalized elderly people, 70 to 95 years old, was investigated by means of a postal questionnaire. The sample was drawn from four communes: Hvidovre, an urban area in the capital; Slagelse, an urban area in a small town; Dianalund and Stenlille, two rural communes. The sample is representative of the distribution of the total population of Denmark in that approximately one-third live in the metropolitan area of Copenhagen, one-third in urban areas (towns of more than 10 000), and one-third in villages and rural areas. The sample was of 1835 individuals, of whom 1261 (69 per cent) returned the questionnaire. The response rate, which was not associated with gender, was highest in the rural area, and among the younger elderly people.

In one commune the non-respondents were approached for personal interviewing and 60 per cent of this group were interviewed, increasing the total response rate in that commune from 68 to 78 per cent. Respondents to the postal questionnaire and the personal interviews were compared in respect of 228 variables and shown to be alike in most respects. Among those personally interviewed there was an over-representation of single persons and individuals with reduced social, psychological, and health resources.

The questionnaire included 228 questions (variables) on demographic and social characteristics, living conditions, health and functional capacity, social network and social support, psychological resources, life-style, use of health and social services, perceived unmet needs, and perceived future needs and solutions.

The main findings are presented in Tables 4 to 12 in Appendix 2. The data confirm that the health services are used extensively by elderly people in Denmark: during one year, 84 per cent were in touch with their general practitioner one or more times, and three-quarters used one or more of the other health and social services (Table 4). Women, the oldest, those living alone, and elderly people with health problems used more services than other groups (Table 7). Table 8 shows the relationship between the functional ability and home help. Instead of looking at the aggregate ADL (activities of daily living) index we focused on three specific tasks: the ability to leave the house without help, the ability to clean the house, and the ability to wash and bathe oneself. The table shows four important results: first, that irrespective of the indicator of functional ability, relatively more of those living alone receive home help. Second, there is a steep increase in home help with decreasing functional ability. Third, even among those without functional impairment we find a few who receive home help. Fourth, even among those who are unable to leave their house, do their cleaning, or wash and bathe, a small proportion do not receive home help. This is true for people who are living alone and those who are not. Self-assessed health is an excellent predictor of the utilization of services. When health is defined in this way, there are only small groups with a poor fit between need and use.

The investigation shows that home help generally is provided in accordance with two formal criteria: impaired functional ability and lack of relatives who can provide help and care.

We want to comment on five issues regarding home help. First, the study confirms other Danish (Platz 1981; Hansen 1982; Almind and Holstein 1987; Olsen and Gregersen 1988; Avlund and Schultz-Larsen 1990) and Scandinavian studies on home help (Daatland 1982; Tornstam 1982; Waerness 1983; Daatland and Sundström 1985). For instance, it confirms gender differences: among those living alone more men than women receive home help; among those living with a spouse more women than men do so (Table 7). The immediate interpretation is that men cope less well with daily activities than do women. Therefore, they need more home help than do women living alone. The married men manage with the help of their spouse. On the other hand, married women need home help more often than men because they cannot manage with only their husband's help. However, variance analysis showed that gender and household composition are less important predictors for use of home help, and that most of the variations can be explained by age and functional ability.

Second, the relationship between social network and home help is remarkable (Table 11). Formal home help and home help from the social network seem to complement each other. In the international literature on domiciliary care for elderly there is a tendency to interpret home help as an indicator of poor informal support (Amann 1980). Formal home help is seen as a substitute or compensation for lack of informal support. Our data do not confirm this interpretation.

Third, the strong association between formal home help and poor quality of life is remarkable (Table 12). Home help, then, is provided to elderly people who feel lonely, old, forgotten, superfluous, in poor spirits, without future perspective, and with poor self-assessed health and life satisfaction. We assume, therefore, that home help is an important resource for those who have the poorest personal/psychological resources.

Formal home help is not necessarily the best kind of help for this category of elderly people, nor are the formal criteria for provision of home help beneficial for those with poor psychological resources. One possible solution is to differentiate between home-making (help with domestic tasks like cleaning, shopping, etc.), and the provision of human/social contacts and personal support. This distinction could be included in the process of referral in order to find a home helper who meets the needs of the individual elderly person. We do *not* suggest two separate organizations, one for home-making and one for socialization. We think this provision should be combined in one organizational structure which orders a larger number of individually designed solutions.

Fourth, we find it interesting that perceived unmet needs for home help are almost exclusively present in the groups of elderly people already using home help (Table 6). Our interpretation of this finding is that the communes provide home help to practically all elderly people in need of this service but that often the provision is too scarce.

Fifth, the association between usage of home help and household income indicates that elderly people who have to pay a certain proportion of the cost are more cautious in their demand for help (Table 9). This constitutes a potential risk of insufficient support for those elderly people with modest additional income. The new legislation in Denmark, which made home help totally free for the elderly by July 1989, might reduce this problem.

3. DECISION-MAKING FOR HOME HELP

3.1. Formal pathways

Decisions about home help are made by the local government (the commune). The local social services department assesses the applicant's need for home help and decides on the amount of help to be provided.

There are no formal regulations for this assessment, except the very general statements in the Social Security Act mentioned earlier. Usually the local government decides some general policy for provision of services, and the need for home help is assessed by the home-help manager or supervisor by a visit to the applicant's home. The educational background of these managers or supervisors is either in nursing or administration.

Application for home help can happen in several ways. The most common is direct application by the elderly persons themselves or by their relatives. In many instances, help is applied for by the general practitioner or by the hospital on discharge. Some communes may have health visitors for the elderly who identify unmet needs for home help and apply for help.

3.2. Framework and method of the pathways study

The study we present in this section aims at understanding (i) the decision-making process regarding services for the older people, in this case the home-help service; and (ii) the co-ordination between agencies involved in the provision of services for the elderly. It focuses on the pathways from one kind of service utilization to another (the 'pathway study').

One of the basic ideas is to analyse the decision making within an organizational framework: how do the numerous and separate units and professional groups collaborate in serving elderly people, and what are the consequences for the clients of the mixed and fragmented.

Another basic idea behind the study is to describe health and social policies for the elderly not only in formal terms but also as they work in practice. What manifest and latent principles are displayed in policies when studied in this way, and how do these principles fit the formal policy statements and intentions?

Third, the study is organized within a framework of decision-making processes. Ideally, the process includes three parties: (a) the elderly client; (b) one or more informal care-givers; and (c) one or more professional care-givers and managers. Ideally, these three parties engage in six stages of decision: (i) identification of problems; (ii) review of alternative solutions; (iii) involvement of relevant parties in the choice of solution; (iv) choice of solution; (v) implementation; and (vi) evaluation and, if needed, modification of chosen solution.

In order to understand the decision-making processes, and the factors affecting them, two sets of data were collected. First, key decision makers in the system were interviewed about general policies and problems. Secondly, 53 case studies were made of referrals to home help. In these cases, clients, professionals and, where possible, a relative were interviewed (see Appendix 3 for details of the method).

3.3. The decision-makers' perspective

During the interviews with the key persons in the four communes we focused on the strengths and weaknesses of the care delivery system for older people. The group of respondents were remarkably unanimous in their evaluation of the system.

3.3a. Structural strengths and weaknesses

The home-help service for the elderly had very few problems in its administrative and practical structure. The most serious problem was the lack of education of the home helpers. Of the four communes studied, three are introducing team-based home help, which means that helpers and home nurses work closely together within the same local area and make decisions collectively. This new structure entails more responsibility for the home helpers, as they are expected to make ongoing assessments of the clients' need for help. However, so far the home helpers have no training in how to do this.

The interviews with key decision-makers confirm what we found to be the strength of the home-help service.

First: All people who apply for home help, receive it, that is, everybody receives some kind of help from the beginning, and the assessment of need is made once the home help has started. This policy implies that nobody is refused or has to wait, which we consider very important for people in difficult, acute, or stressful situations.

Second: In three of the four communes the leaders consider it important to have an assessment of need for home help. In the fourth commune they have instructions concerning cleaning, laundry, cooking, and shopping. The leaders stressed this principle of flexible assessment in order to meet the individual wishes and needs of each elderly person.

Third: The people working in the area of home help and home nursing take a lot of new initiatives. The idea of collective home help is one; others are mental training for demented elderly people, training/education for everybody working with old people; giving payment/salary to family members looking after dying elderly relatives, etc.

3.3b. Entry to and exit from home-help service

One of the main strengths of home help is its flexibility—the possibility of meeting individual needs in each situation. Therefore, the existence of other services is important. There were relief beds in three of the four communes, and among the professional decision-makers this service is considered very important. It makes it possible for people to have more intensive and continuous help for a short period of time during illness or while a spouse is in hospital. If this service did not function the home-help service would have to take over a task for which it was not created and which would hardly be fulfilled.

Twenty-four hour domiciliary care is another example of a neighbouring service which creates a great deal of flexibility in the system. It fills the difficult gap between hospital/nursing home on the one hand and home help on the other. The service providers regard it as very important. There is, however, a financial problem: the domiciliary care department has the right to initiate 24-hour care but does not get any extra money to run this service. This type of service enables very impaired people to stay in their own homes, but it also puts a strain on the resources available, and leaves the rest of the elderly with a worse service.

Many professionals state that lack of options for rehabilitation in their communes puts undue strain on the home help. Either the home helpers try to provide some training, or they have to do work which the elderly people themselves could easily do if they had a few weeks of rehabilitation therapy. This gap in service provision leads to inappropriate use of the home-help resources.

Other deficiencies in provision are of gardening and well-functioning day centres.

Waiting lists for hospital treatment and nursing homes are other unnecessary barriers which lead to impairment of the elderly person's health and everyday life (at least for a period) and use a great deal of home-help resources.

The weaknesses mentioned so far are mainly due to economic and political decisions made by the communes or by the regional government (county). These problems could be reduced by decisions made in the local area, although the scarcity of resources provided by the state makes the task very difficult. However, there are problems that are almost impossible to solve, because of the existing structure of the health system (Fig. 3.1).

First, the political and economic separation of the county and the commune and their different responsibilities in the health-service system create

County (regional)	Communes (local)
• Hospitals	• Home help
• Psycho-geriatric nursing homes	• 24-hour domiciliary care
• General practitioners	• Ordinary nursing homes
	• Home nursing
	• Meals-on-wheels
	• Equipment

Fig. 3.1. Examples of services for the elderly administered by the regional and local government.

serious obstacles in attempts to reach satisfactory holistic solutions for older people. The two often have incompatible interests. The following three difficulties in particular were often mentioned by the service providers:

1. *Discharge from hospital.* The elderly person might or might not want to come home, yet for cost reasons the hospital (i.e., the county) wants to discharge them as soon as possible when medical treatment is no longer necessary. The domiciliary service department (i.e., the commune) wants to have some days' notice before receiving them, as they have to plan their work and also because of scarce resources.
2. *Care of the chronically ill or dying.* This could be improved: the service providers agree that these people should be able to die in their own homes, but in some communes this is still not possible because no resources (i.e., 24-hour domiciliary care) follow the patient from the county hospital to the commune.
3. *Assessment for psychogeriatric or general nursing home.* From the interviews with the service providers it appears there are discrepancies between professional judgements of the mental state of the elderly person when it comes to the question of where they should stay. The service providers find these differences of opinion mainly arise because of the economic separation of the nursing-home service, whereby psychogeriatric homes are funded by counties, and the general homes are funded by the communes.

Second, the service providers point out the lack of formalized cooperation among the professionals. It seems that all groups of professionals consider this a serious problem. In most of the communes they have made their own experiments in order to try to solve this problem; in some cases these have been successful, for example in relation to procedures for discharge from hospital. Among general practitioners in particular the lack of co-operation is a major problem as they are not paid for these activities via their regular fee-for-service payment; they are only paid for patient contacts.

3.4. Results from the case studies

Fifty-three cases of referrals to home help were selected for study. Only referrals for four hours or more of home help were selected, and all of them were successful. We are not aware of any cases referred but not admitted. Entry into domiciliary care in Denmark is completely unrestricted, but those who enter the system without a need are discharged quickly. Most of the cases were referred from the hospital (37 of the 53 cases) but the local social services department was always involved in the decision. The remaining 16 cases were initiated by the elderly people themselves, sometimes assisted by the general practitioner, or a relative, or a friend. Appendix 4 shows typical trajectories regarding referral to home help.

3.4a. The respondents

Two-thirds of the elderly people were women. The median age was 79 years (range 68 to 102 years). Of the men, approximately half were married and the other half lived alone. Of the women, three-quarters lived alone. The group was generally characterized by a high level of functional disability. Practically all needed help for daily activities and one-third needed help for every one of the five activities that we asked about: moving outdoors, shopping, light housework, heavy housework, and personal hygiene. In addition, half the respondents had impaired hearing, one-third impaired vision, at least one-fifth had severe problems in remembering their daily programme. They thus constituted a group of old people with very poor functional ability. The psychological resources of the respondents were classified according to their answers to seven questions. We defined these resources as poor when they had at least four of these seven characteristics: loneliness, feeling old, unhappy about social contacts, unhappy with life as such, no future plans, anxious, and depressed. Those with at least six of the opposite characteristics were classified as having strong psychological resources. By this classification, approximately one-third of the respondents had poor psychological resources, one-third strong resources, and the remaining third formed a middle group.

3.4b. The cases

The cases varied considerably in their background, trajectory, and outcome. In applying for home help, they had two dominant categories of problem:

(1) those that arose in relation to discharge from hospital, the most frequent reasons for hospitalization being fractures, pain resulting from falls, stroke-induced hemiparesis, or social causes (unmet need for care);

(2) those that arose without prior hospitalization because of acute breakdown of the elderly person's social network and/or progression of existing chronic disease such as rheumatoid arthritis, asthma, or bronchitis.

Most cases could be regarded as serious, *acute problems* of care, which in combination with poor functional ability constituted a very serious threat or problem for the elderly client. There is no doubt that home help, in a number of these cases, probably most, prevented serious events such as social breakdown, hospitalization, or admission to a nursing home. Domiciliary care seems to function effectively as a *secondary preventive* effort. Domiciliary care was not, in any of the cases begun as an *early preventive measure*. We selected only cases who had at least 4 hours of home help. Those having less help, for example, two hours of home help per week, may include some whose home-help provision was an early preventive effort. In a number of our cases we saw in retrospect an earlier, unmet need for domiciliary care. We therefore believe that the primary preventive aim of the home help is not always fulfilled. We also found a number of cases where there was an obvious need for help, but where the clients or their household decided to leave the provision of domiciliary care because it could not give what was needed, e.g., transportation, rehabilitation. This, of course, reduces the preventive impact of the care.

We analysed the decision-making process by referring to the model in Fig 3.2. Ideally, the elderly clients:

(1) should know what alternative solutions are available to solve the actual problem (arrow 2);
(2) should engage in thorough and balanced discussions with the relevant professional decision-makers (arrow 3) and informal care-givers (arrow 4);
(3) should make the decision themselves (arrow 7).

None of the cases complied fully with all these criteria, which means that the elderly clients were not fully involved in the decision about domiciliary care. Approximately half the cases complied more or less with one or two of the criteria, which means that the elderly person had some influence on the decision. The material allowed us to analyse reasons for the lack of influence; we have identified five kinds of non-influence:

- The client voluntarily leaves the decision to somebody else (usually some relative).
- The client is pushed aside by the professional decision maker (the decision maker decides what is best regardless of the client's different perception of needs).
- The informal social network removes initiative and decision-making from the client.

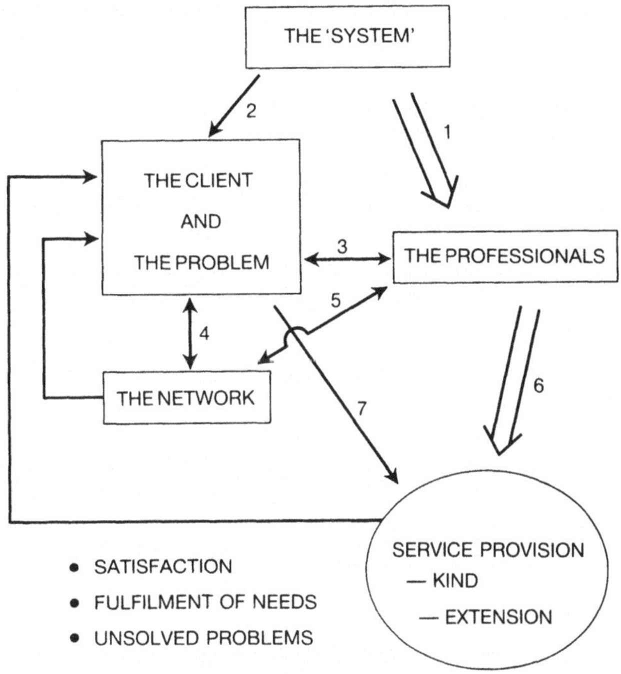

Fig. 3.2. The decision-making process.

- The client is pushed aside by an alliance between the professional decision-maker and the informal social network
- The client is under pressure to make a decision which he or she does not really want.

3.4c. Which solutions are considered?

Most of the elderly respondents claimed that no solution other than home help had been considered. Some mentioned a nursing home or service flat as an alternative which had been considered, and some mentioned some kind of rehabilitation facility. When we compared the answers to this question by the clients and the professionals there were often considerable differences. There was no clear tendency for either party to mention further consideration of alternative solutions. Neither party appears to have really discussed alternative solutions to the acute problem with one another.

3.4e. Who is involved?

We asked both the elderly people and the professionals two questions: one about the parties who had been involved and the other about the contribution they had made. Again, we found major discrepancies in their answers. These show that neither party was aware of whom the other had involved.

The home-help manager was always involved in these cases. This category of person, however, was only mentioned by two-thirds of the clients. The hospital (or some staff members at the hospital) are mentioned in most of the cases which began on discharge from hospital. The general practitioner was mentioned only in a few cases, family members in approximately half the cases, and friends/neighbours in very few of the cases. The roles of these parties differ considerably. The role of the hospital is to refer the elderly person to the social services department, which then assesses the situation and decides on the amount of help to be allocated and on the practical details of the provision. The general practitioner often functions as the client's advocate, trying to convince the social services department of the need for help. Family members, friends, and neighbours also function as mediators between the elderly client and the professional decision maker. In a few of the cases a family member has been successful in an active attempt to avoid outside help.

3.4f. The problems solved

Practically all cases were examples of domiciliary care that seemed to be absolutely necessary to avoid institutionalization. The elderly clients were so impaired and/or their informal social network so frail or so worn out that they could not manage on their own at home. The study really showed the potential of domiciliary care. Some of the clients were so impaired that they needed help with practically everything, and in many instances there were no resources that could be mobilized from the informal social network.

We saw a number of exemplary cases, those with a thorough assessment of needs and of the capacity of the elderly person and their social networks, worked out in co-operation between hospital staff, the communes' social services department, the client, and their social networks. Contrary to what is usually said about the Danish health and social services sector, we saw a number of excellent examples of co-operation between the hospital and the commune in fact, it is our view that these cases generally speaking function better than those where the commune's home-help service acts alone. This observation might not be generally valid. We included cases of transfer from hospital care to domiciliary care after more than two weeks of hospitalization. A number of these patients were from departments that specialized in the discharge of elderly patients (so-called long-term medicine departments). We believe these discharges represent the most excellent examples of co-ordination between hospital and primary health care. Moreover, we believe that many discharges after a short stay in hospital are considerably less well co-ordinated. The interviews with the key persons/decision makers confirmed this. The realistic alternative to domiciliary care for most of these clients was to stay in the hospital until their functional ability had improved considerably or to go to a nursing home, temporarily or permanently.

Basically, the two formal criteria for the delivery of home help—impaired functional ability and lack of a caring social network—seemed to be the main guidelines for the professional decision makers. There were, however, important differences in the way the four communes administered this policy. The most pronounced differences related to three factors: (i) the level of service provision; (ii) the flexibility of provision; and (iii) local restrictions on the home-help functions.

The level of service provision. The four communes have different levels of services for their elderly population, which of course affects the amount of help provided. During the year of data collection all four communes went through serious cuts in their budgets and, therefore, we observed a change in help provided from the start of the study to the end.

Flexibility. The four communes had different degrees of flexibility in their provision of help. One of the communes provided help on the basis of a rigid assessment of needs, defined as inability to perform daily activities. This leaves no room for further, individually adapted solutions, but has the advantage of securing the individual a minimum provision of help when needed. Another commune provided help in a more flexible way, which may be beneficial but which may give too little help, for example to an impaired elderly person with a healthy spouse.

Local restrictions. The most obvious example of these in our study material is that one of the communes resisted providing home help for rehabilitation such as mobility training. The reason for this attitude was that this provision is formally the responsibility of the hospital and therefore of the county not the commune. Another example was the resistance of one of the communes to the provision of terminal nursing care. Again, the reason was that terminal care is seen as a hospital function, i.e., the responsibility of the county and not the commune.

3.4g. Unsolved problems

Most of the clients expressed gratitude and satisfaction with the solution. However, in most cases there were unsolved problems (not including unresolved health problems). These unsolved problems were diverse:

too little help for regular domestic activities;
lack of rehabilitation/mobility training;
lack of recreation facilities;

too many/changing home helpers;
alienated contact with the professional decision-maker;
inability to move out of doors and nobody to help;
unfinished solution;
change of residence needed;
total dependence on help from spouse who him/herself needs help;
lack of relief for spouse;
lack of transportation;
lack of 'medicine card' (no access to free medication);
inability to do the gardening;
lack of equipment (e.g., emergency call apparatus);
uncertainty about the future;
uncertainty about medication dose.

We analysed the reasons for these unsolved problems and found five kinds of barrier to efficient problem solving:

- structural problems, such as lack of opportunity for rehabilitation, lack of opportunity for having one and the same home helper all the time, lack of services such as window cleaning, gardening, etc;
- co-ordination problems between hospital and agencies responsible for primary health care and social services;
- insufficient professional competence (e.g., the professional has not taken the time to see through the real problems; the professional lacks knowledge about elderly people with poor psychological resources);
- insufficient help in the initial stages causing irreversible damage to the rehabilitation process;
- the social network is in itself a source of strain for the elderly person or lacks the resources needed to provide support on a daily basis;
- poor psychological resources of the elderly people themselves.

The presence of one of these problems constitutes a potential barrier to a satisfactory solution. Frequently, two or more of these barriers occur together which, of course, makes it more likely that unsolved problems will occur.

The unsolved problems indicate something about how policies for elderly people work in practice. Some of the barriers derive from structural characteristics of the system, which result in lack of co-ordination. Other barriers relate to the extremely complex nature of many older people's problems; for example, the problems induced by strained social relations or by elderly people with poor psychological resources (dementia, depression, passivity, lack of ability to express desired solutions, lack of ability to predict which solutions are needed).

Still other barriers may reflect lack of resources or lack of professionalization among the management staff. Generally speaking, we found that the managers and supervisors who made the assessments were competent and dedicated to their job. They do, however, operate under conditions which are not ideal: pressure on time, insufficient resources, and political pressure to further savings. These conditions may well result in solutions that are not ideal for the elderly clients.

4. POLICY IMPLICATIONS

Three main conclusions can be drawn from the studies presented here: first, that home help seems to be provided to those most in need; secondly, that home help (together with other domiciliary care services) has the potential to care for severely impaired people at home; and thirdly, that the elderly clients' influence in decision-making about home help is limited, and the provision of home help often leaves them with unsolved problems.

The first point is shown by our survey of older people living at home. The proportion of those who need help with daily activities and do not receive home help is very small. The proportion who receive home help but do not need help with daily activities is also very small. Those who get help are generally speaking those who need it because they are unable to perform daily activities. It is more difficult to conclude anything about the kind and amount of help provided. The case studies show several examples of insufficient help where the commune does not provide the correct kind of help. This applies to rehabilitation, to certain kinds of domestic assistance (e.g., snow clearing, gardening), and to care of demented or psychologically frail elderly clients. The survey study shows that 24 per cent of those receiving home help think they are in need of more help. This indicates that the provision of help is scarce compared to the need.

The second point is demonstrated by the massive problems of the applicants for home help; most of them are unable to look after themselves at home—yet it is possible to care for them at home by means of efficient domiciliary care.

Finally, the pathway study shows that the decision-making process for domiciliary care is the domain of the professional decision maker, in this case the home-help manager. Very often neither the clients themselves nor their social networks are really involved in shaping the domiciliary care solutions. The frequent presence of unsolved problems a few weeks after admission into domiciliary care may reflect insufficient follow-up by the decision-makers in the social services department. It may, however, also reflect the relatively poor involvement of the elderly clients in the decision. We assume that meaningful involvement of elderly clients in decision-making should include their own evaluation of the service provided and a joint effort to adjust the service provision to their needs.

4.1. Our proposals for changes improve service allocation

Our main findings lead us to four suggestions for adjustment of the present service provision, two concerning the daily allocation of services and two referring to the structure.

1. We consider it of great value to involve the clients themselves much more in the decision-making process. The large number of unsolved problems might be avoided by discussing all possible solutions with the elderly person before the decision is made, and/or by reassessing the situation at a later stage.
2. Lack of flexibility in service allocation is, in our view, the most important reason for not reaching the optimal solution in most cases. We therefore propose that the communes think in terms of more flexible solutions and perhaps try to avoid the tendency to prescribe home help, whatever the problem. The need for flexibility might be more apparent to the decision makers if there was a more rigorous, systematic, and comprehensive follow-up assessment of the original solutions.
3. The service providers indicated the need for a formalized structure to enhance collaboration between the agencies and professional groups involved (social services departments, hospital, general practitioners). This was not indicated by our case studies—indeed we think that the co-operation in most of our cases was acceptable or even excellent. But this may be due more to individual attitudes than to formal structures, which could be better integrated.
4. There is a need to stimulate economic collaboration between the agencies involved. The best and most economical solution is often not chosen because of separated budgets. The separation of the community care budget (the communes) from the hospital budget (the county) hardly provides any financial incentive for the communes to take over patients ready for discharge from hospital as early as possible. In many cases, therefore, patients remain in hospital longer than they need because of the cost implications for one part of the system, the commune, although from the point of view of the costs to the system as a whole, discharge would be the cheapest solution.

REFERENCES

Almind, G., Holstein, B. E., and Larsen, B. S. (1987). *Syge ældre mennesker i eget hjem* (Ill non-institutionalized elderly). FADLs Forlag, Copenhagen.

Amann, A. (1980). *Open care for the elderly in seven European countries*. Pergamon, Oxford.
Andersen, A. S. (1980). *Døgnplejeforsoget i Viborg—en analyse og vurdering* (24-hour domiciliary care in Viborg—analysis and evaluation). AKF, Copenhagen.
Avlund, K. and Schultz-Larsen, K. (1990). What do 70-year-old men and women actually do? And what are they able to do? *Comprehensive Gerontology* (in press).
Daatland, S. O. (1982). *Den offentlige ældreomsorgen i en norsk bykommune* (The public services for the elderly in a Norwegian urban commune). Norsk Gerontologisk Institut, Oslo.
Daatland, S. O. and Sundström, G. (1985). *Gammal i Norden* (Old in the Nordic countries). Nord, Stockholm.
Elderly Commission (1981). *De ældres vilkar* (The living conditions of the elderly). Ministry of Social Affairs, Copenhagen.
Hansen, E. B. and Werborg, R. (1983–1984). *Døgnhjemmeplejen i Naestved I–II* (24-hour domiciliary care in Naestved I–II). AKF, Copenhagen.
Hansen, E. B. and Werborg, R. (1985). *Hjemmesygepleje hele døgnet—Et forsog på Amager* (24-hour domiciliary care—an experiment in Amager). AKF, Copenhagen.
Hansen, G. (1982). *Sociale serviceydelser for ældre* (Provision of social services for the elderly). Socialforskningsinstituttet, Copenhagen.
Hendriksen, C., Lund, E., and Stromgaard, E. (1984). Hjemmehjaelpere og deres arbejdsomrade (Home helpers and their job activities). *Ugeskrift Laeger*, **146,** 138–41.
Holstein, B. E., Almind, G., Due, P., and Holst, E. (1988). *The elderly in Denmark. Health and Social Situation*. Institute of Social Medicine, University of Copenhagen.
Kähler, M. and Madsen, A. (1985). *Personaleforbruget på ældreomradet 1981–1984* (Staffing in the elderly service sector 1981–84). Socialstyrelsen, Copenhagen.
Kjerkegaard, E. M. (1976). *Levevilkar i Danmark 1976* (Living conditions in Denmark 1976). Danmarks Statistik & Socialforskningsinstuttet, Copenhagen.
Olsen, H. and Gregersen, O. (1988). *De ældre og hjemmehjælpen* (The elderly and the home help). Socialforskningsinstituttet, Copenhagen.
Platz, M. (1981). *De ældres levevilkar 1977* (The living conditions of the aged, 1977). Socialforskningsinstituttet, Copenhagen.
Samordning i Sundhedsvæsenet (1985). Den sociale og sundhedsmaessige indsats over for aeldre (Co-ordination in the health system: social and health services for the elderly), Appendix A in the report No. 1044. Samordningsudvalget for Sundhedsvaesenet, Copenhagen.
Social Security Act (1972). Copenhagen.
Statistik om hjemmesygeplejevirksomheden 1981 (Statistical information on home nursing activity 1981) (1984). Sundhedsstyrelsen, Copenhagen.
Stehouwer, J. (1968). *Living conditions of the aged*, Vol. V, *Mobility and incapacity for self-care*. Socialforskningsinstituttet, Copenhagen.
Stehouwer, J. (1970). *Living conditions of the aged,* Vol. VI, *Family contacts*, Socialforskningsinstituttet, Copenhagen.
Tornstam, L. (1982). *Självständigt boende. En undersökning om äldres boende,*

flyttningsmönster och behov av social service (Independent living. An investigation on housing, mobility, and need for social services among the aged). Sociologiska Institutionen, Uppsala.

Waerness, K. (1983). *Kvinnor och omsorgsarbete* (Women and caring activities). Prisma, Stockholm.

4
The home-help service in England and Wales

Robin Lawson and Bleddyn Davies, with Andrew Bebbington

1. Introduction
2. The historical development of the service
   2.1. Post-war origins and development
   2.2. The Seebohm Report and local government reorganizations
   2.3. The 1980s
   2.4. Overview
3. The provision of domiciliary help today
   3.1. Summary of provision
   3.2. The home-help service
   3.3. Home/community nursing
   3.4. Interfaces between services
4. The service in practice
   4.1. Who receives home help?
   4.2. What do clients receive?
   4.3. The efficiency of targeting
   4.4. Assessment and allocation
   4.5. The outcomes of home help
   4.6. Inter-agency co-ordination
   4.7. Managing the service
5. Ways forward
   5.1. Summary of issues that require attention
   5.2. Some ways forward
6. Conclusion
References

1. INTRODUCTION

Services for elderly people have come under increasing scrutiny in the UK in the 1980s because of the increasing numbers of frail elderly people in the population, constraints on resources, and the national policy of caring for vulnerable people in their own homes for as long as possible. If the home-help/care service is to be the cornerstone of community care, as the

* With contributions from H. Charnley, A. Fitzpatrick, A. Netten, and A. Whitley.

Social Services Inspectorate (SSI) (1988) proposed, a number of changes will be required, including the provision of more personal care, more flexible provision, and co-ordination with other services both within and outside social services departments (SSI 1987, 1988).

Section 2 outlines the historical development of the home-help service to the present day. Section 3 describes the provision of home-help and related services today, including the nature of the provision, organization, and allocation. Section 4 covers the same issues in practice, although, because there are few formal, national instructions for the provision of home-help services in the UK, a clear distinction cannot be made between what should happen and what actually happens in practice. Section 5 summarizes the key issues for the home-help service today, and indicates some ways forward.

2. THE HISTORICAL DEVELOPMENT OF THE SERVICE

2.1. Post-war origins and development

The home-help service in England and Wales was first embodied in a statutory power in the Maternity and Child Welfare Act of 1918. The domestic focus of the service was established through its definition as one substituting for the mother's duties in a home (cleaning, cooking, washing, general child care) during her lying-in period. The service was funded by local health services and was limited legally, during the next quarter century, to maternal support work, despite mounting pressure to extend it. However, wartime economic needs demanded that younger supporters of frail elderly people should be freed for war work, and that demand for overstretched residential resources should be damped down. Maintaining high morale among civilians and service personnel was also considered a priority. Finally, after pressure from Ernest Bevin and senior officials from the Ministry of Labour and National Service, the need for a formal extension of domestic-help provision was recognized in December 1944 (Ministry of Health 1944), and the setting up of such a service was legitimized and encouraged, though initially the structure and funding of the old and new services diverged. The organizational tasks involved were (i) to maintain a register of approved home helps; (ii) to assess and rank applicants' need of service; and (iii) to assess applicants' ability to pay, and make policy decisions concerning the proportion of costs that charges were to cover. It was thought that the service was needed most in urban areas, and that similar rural schemes should only be set up after consultation with the Ministry of Health. The National Health Service Act (Ministry of Health 1946) granted to local authorities permissive power to provide domestic help:

for households where such help is required owing to the presence of any person who is ill, lying in, an expectant mother, mentally defective, aged, or a child not over compulsory school age.

The system thus became fully unified, under the aegis of the local health services, and grant-aided on the same basis as other local authority health services.

Expected primarily to serve young families, the sick, and the mentally disordered, the home-help service became largely one for elderly people within five years of the day when the National Health Service (NHS) was launched, and, by the mid-1960s, three cases out of four were elderly. Many had come to receive services for five years and more, resulting in the silting up of resources in the support of persons not currently in high need. But growth was rapid: more than 6 per cent per annum in the number of elderly cases, a rate exceeding the rate of growth of the very elderly population (Davies 1968). However, it was argued that provision fell short of the need for a service which could make admission to residential care unnecessary. Townsend and Wedderburn (1965) estimated that a trebling in scale would be necessary to meet needs. Most health authorities gave little attention to the service's potential as a nucleus about which could be created a service meeting needs for personal and household care, so reducing the probability of admission to residential homes. Typically, responsibility for it was seen as a purely administrative, almost clerical, task; and internal organization varied greatly. Contemporary critics also complained that bodies of techniques and criteria of need were not established, tested, and promulgated (Davies 1968). Much was left to the front-line managers—untrained home-help organizers.

2.2. The Seebohm Report and local government reorganizations

In the late 1960s, the search for greater efficiency and effectiveness in service delivery brought into question the diverse provision of services caused by lack of co-ordination among separate agencies. In 1965, the Seebohm Committee was set up. Its brief was to review the organization and responsibilities of local authority personal social services. When it reported in 1968, it pointed to shortages in the amount of services, and the frequently inadequate and poor quality service caused by lack of available resources. This shortage was attributed to small-scale agencies, divided responsibilities, and lack of research into and evaluation of services. Research commissioned by the Seebohm Committee argued that services for elderly people had developed better where responsibility had been consolidated in a department other than the local health authority (Davies 1967).

The Seebohm Report (1968), therefore, proposed that a single department should be responsible for all social care services, and that it should be run directly by the local authority. These recommendations met considerable opposition initially from the home-help organizers, who feared that they would lose resources and status by the transfer of responsibility from the local health departments to the new social services departments. Also it was argued that most referrals were from the health services, and that co-ordination with community and primary health services was very important for many cases in great need. The Seebohm Committee paid scant attention to these issues. The Seebohm reorganization was closely followed by the consolidation of local authorities into the largest local government units in the Western world. Within five years, the managers had moved from small organizations with clear and often straightforward functions to run giant organizations with broad policy-making ambitions and a wide variety of functions and services for every group in the community; doing so without any training in management. The result was that for a decade the home-help service was largely left to its own devices by the social services departments as it had been by the old local health departments, although there was an increase in home-help numbers up to the mid-1970s, and some discussion about who should receive help (Davies 1981).

2.3. The 1980s

In the 1980s, however, as growth in demand and pressure on resources increased, community-based care, including home-help services, became a focus of attention and criticism, as it consumed substantial resources and could be used to make admission to institutions for long-term care unnecessary. Consequently, there has been a series of national government reports in the 1980s on community care in general, and on services for particular client groups such as elderly people.

The most influential critique was from the Audit Commission for England and Wales, which, as part of a series of 'value for money' projects, studied local authority services for the elderly over a number of years. The resulting report, *Managing services for the elderly more effectively* (Audit Commission 1985), was concerned about the increases in residential facilities in contrast to community care, and sought to establish a better balance between the two. It identified the need for better management to overcome the problems of inappropriate use of residential care, poor targeting of services, which failed to supply those who needed the service most, poor co-ordination of services by the variety of provider agencies (especially social and health services), and waste through inefficient organization of services.

This focus on better management is evident in much of government policy for the public sector in the 1980s, as well as in the private sector, and the term 'new managerialism' has been coined.

In 1986, another Audit Commission report, *Making a reality of commun-*

ity care, proposed that services should be local, integrated, and based on team-work and partnership with the non-statutory and informal sectors. It suggested that, for services for elderly people, there should be a single budget held by one manager in a district/authority to buy in services from any source, in order to overcome the fragmentation of services between the local authorities and health authorities.

This idea was rejected for a number of reasons. In 1986, the Secretary of State for Health and Social Services asked a leading figure in commerce, Sir Roy Griffiths, 'to review the way in which public funds are used to support community-care policy and to advise me on options for action that would improve the use of these funds as a contribution to more effective community care'. The resulting report *Community care: an agenda for action* was published in 1988. It recommends that local authorities should take over responsibility for all community-care services, leaving the NHS as a purely health-related service, and that the social services departments should be able to buy in services from a variety of sources, maximizing the potential of the non-statutory (including private) sectors to provide care in order to promote choice and competition. The idea is that social services departments would purchase and co-ordinate care, and manage cases, but not necessarily provide the care services. At the same time, potential clients are encouraged to try and get help from their own social network and other community resources before approaching the social services, and it is proposed that clients pay for services where they can afford to, although not for the 'case management' component. The report also proposed that central government should provide a direct grant to social services departments to cover 40 to 50 per cent of the estimated cost of community care.

While the report has received much support from various quarters, the key proposal of making local authorities responsible for community care is unpopular with the Tories, who have been reducing the powers of local government since they came into power in 1979. However, after looking at alternatives, on 11 July 1989, 15 months after the Griffiths report was published, the Government finally announced that it would be making local authorities responsible for community care, although it has yet to clarify funding arrangements and whether additional resources will be made available. Many commentators fear that without substantial injections of money, the transfer of responsibility for community care to local authorities will merely mean the transfer of blame for inadequate services from central to local government. Given the delay since the report was published, many local authorities have, however, been establishing systems which anticipate the mixed economy of supply envisaged by Griffiths.

Finally, the SSI has produced a series of reports since 1987, on the home help service (SSI 1987, 1988). These focus on making the service more efficient and effective as a cornerstone of community care, catering not only for elderly people, but increasingly, in future, for other people with special needs. The key recommendations are that the service should shift away from domestic care to personal care, and should be targeted more rigorously on frailer clients with greater and more complex needs. The reports suggest how this change can be managed, focusing on more rigorous policy development translated into clear and achievable objectives: better budget management, better case management, improved front-line management and improved working structures for home helps. The second report stresses the need for more resources if such improvements are to be achieved.

2.4. Overview

This section has described how a home-help service intended for one clientele was, within five years, serving another. It describes how initially it was an unimportant part of the domain of an organization with a wide range of responsibilities, headed by public-health physicians who generally failed to see the service's potential for development; and who were content to leave its management to senior clerks without policy training. It also shows how it was (unwillingly) transferred to the new departments in 1971 and a new authority in 1974, separating it from its primary focus of identification and the source of most of its referrals, the community and primary-health services. The newly responsible social services departments had managers who had, within five years, been catapulted without training from small, simple organizations for the administration of a few standard services into large, complex entities with ambitious and diffuse responsibilities for policy making and financing, and for the provision of many and varied services for the entire population. The home-help service was neglected by management and remained a 'Cinderella' service. Indeed, in some areas, the reforms of the mid-1970s actually set back developments by making health and social-care agencies look in on their own interests rather than on the development of services for users who often need their careful co-ordination. The consequences for effectiveness have been described well in review after review (Goldberg and Connelly 1981; Dexter and Harbert 1983; Davies and Challis 1986). However, community-based social and health-care services came to be recognized as being of key significance in new managerialist critiques of health and social care in the 1980s. It was thought that they might substitute for inefficient and ineffective, institution-based modes of long-term care, the demands on which already consumed vast public resources and the demands of which were likely to increase rapidly.

3. THE PROVISIONOF DOMICILIARY HELP TODAY

3.1. Summary of provision

Table 4.1 indicates the range of services providing domiciliary care to elderly people (see also Appendix 5). The main providers in terms of cost and number of clients are the home-help/care services, run by local authority social services departments and funded by central government through the block grant system and through local rates; and the home-nursing service, run by district health authorities (DHAs) and funded by central government from general taxation. These two services are the focus of this chapter and are described in greater detail below. While public services continue to dominate domiciliary care, there have always been private

Table 4.1. Types and sources of domiciliary care for elderly people (see also Table 1 in Appendix 5)

Activities	Who delivers
Personal care (feeding, dressing, mobility, bathing)	Home help (SSD[1] or private); auxiliary nurse (DHA[2]); OT[3]—provide aids to personal care
Home-making (cleaning, laundry, cooking, shopping, administration—including pension collection)	Home help (SSD); domestic help (private); volunteers unpaid (voluntary organization) including meals-on-wheels
Nursing (injection, bandaging, administration of medicines)	District nurse (DHA); private nursing (paid from private insurance or client's own pocket)
Surveillance	Health visitors in some authorities (DHA); street wardens (SSD); sheltered housing wardens (local authority, voluntary, private); social workers (SSD); alarm systems (SSD and/or local authority housing departments); home helps in some authorities (SSD); meals-on-wheels volunteers (voluntary, funded by SSD); GPs may screen elderly people on their registers, but not common (Family Practitioner Committees, part of NHS)
Socialization (conversation, walks)	Home help; volunteers (voluntary organizations); day-centre staff (SSD, voluntary organizations)

[1] Social services departments; [2] District Health Authority; [3] occupational therapist.

Day centres provide social activities, food, and sometimes shopping and access to care, e.g., chiropody, occupational therapy, bathing.

nursing agencies, and in recent years many small, and a few large, private home-help agencies have sprung up in wealthier areas throughout the country. The voluntary sector does not seem yet to be heavily involved in the provision of home-help/care services, but is active in the provision of meals-on-wheels, lunch clubs, day care, and in sitting/social-contact services.

The pattern of who provides which services is already changing and is likely to change further as the Government increases its emphasis on choice and competition between providers, and is shifting responsibility for payment back towards the user (Griffiths 1988).

3.2. The home-help service

3.2a. Structure

Local authorities have a statutory duty to provide a home-help service through their social service departments, but there is no obligation on an individual client basis (Hedley and Norman 1982). In other words, a client has no statutory right to receive a service from a social services department. The internal organization of home-help services varies between authorities with regard to line management and relationship to social-work teams. The service is also affected in its links to other services by whether the social services department within which it operates is organized on a functional (e.g., field-work or residential care) or client-group (e.g., elderly and physically disability) basis (Bebbington *et al.* 1986).

Home-help services usually comprise a number of senior home-help organizers, one to cover each geographical sub-area of the authority; each of these seniors would have one or more organizers assisting them; each organizer is responsible for a number of home helps. Again, the division of tasks between the senior organizer and the other organizers varies, as does the organization of home helps. Generally speaking, however, each organizer deals with individual case management (if these tasks arise), staff supervision, and balancing the budget. There are moves in some authorities to give organizers more control over and responsibility for budget management.

3.2b. Finance

Finance for the home-help service provided by local authority social services departments is via central government grant allocations and is also raised through local taxation. In addition, the National Health Service Act (Ministry of Health 1946) and the accompanying Ministry of Health (1947) circular 118/47 made allowance for charges to be imposed to contribute to the costs of the service, although this was to take into account the means of the individual. Historically, the proportion of the cost of the service raised in this way has never been large and has declined since the 1950s.

In the financial year 1986–7, for instance, a quarter of the 116 local authorities provided the service free of charge, just over a quarter charged a flat rate, and the remainder charged according to the means of the individual, 20 of these authorities imposing a minimum charge. Income raised in this way recovered averages of 10.4, 4.7 and 5.2 per cent of the cost providing the service in shire counties, metropolitan districts, and London boroughs, respectively. The highest recovery was 22.5 per cent in one of the shire counties (SSI 1988).

For a brief period in the 1980s, central government-funded social security payments in the form of 'domestic assistance allowance' for disabled elderly people were allowable to cover the cost of privately purchased domestic care.

With the changing political climate favouring an ethos of individual responsibility, charging for statutory home-help services is becoming more common, and is promoted by two recent Government reports:

- People should be charged for services where they can afford it, but not charged for the assessment and care planning (Griffiths 1988).
- Charging may be used to recoup costs, charge economic rates for those consumers who are assessed as able to pay (SSI 1988).

Charging arrangements vary between authorities, and there has been no national guidance on this, although recent Government reports are pushing for charging to be used more commonly for various public services (see 3.5). Five types of charging arrangement can be identified, and these are:

(1) free service—client pays nothing;
(2) flat-rate charge (usually per week) at any level of service—each client pays the same amount regardless of means;
(3) two-tier system whereby those on supplementary benefit (or equivalent income) receive a free or cheaper flat-rate service, while those above supplementary benefit level pay a higher flat rate;
(4) a means-tested sliding scale of charges whereby payment is according to means.

There is nearly always allowance for charges to be waived in exceptional circumstances where an organizer feels this to be appropriate, although this happens very rarely. (Types (1) and (2) are subject to the payment of maximum charges by those who refuse to declare their means.)

3.2c. Policy

There are no formal eligibility criteria for the home-help service. There is no third-party reimbursement: finance and allocation are consolidated at the level of the individual social services department, and responsibility for assessment and allocation lies with the street-level bureaucrat (home-help organizers), with few rules and guidelines to follow. Policy and practice varies from authority to authority, therefore. However, broad national guidelines are as follows.

Who is the service for? Successive central government statements have emphasized the role of the home-help service as a service to help disabled people to remain in the community, and it is targeted on people who have difficulty with the activities of daily living and who lack other sources of support in the community, and particularly, in their household (see Section 4.1, 'Who receives home help'?).

The most recent statement of this kind came from the Government's SSI, which is pushing for the home-help service to cover a greater range of client groups in order to support people with special needs living in or moving into community settings.

> The great majority of current domiciliary service clients are elderly. Development of a 'home care' service will require diversification of services with a view to meeting the needs of physically and mentally handicapped people, for whom institutional and residential care alternatives are increasingly regarded as inappropriate (SSI 1987, p. 26).

The Inspectorate is also pushing for the targeting of home-help resources 'on consumers who require more frequent and varied support, if they are to be an effective substitute for residential care services for more people than at present'. The Inspectorate found, in fact, that authorities are still favouring cover (extensiveness) to intensity of service, and that any increase in resources tends to go towards increasing cover, not intensity (SSI 1987) (see also Section 4).

What should home helps provide? In order to meet the needs of increasingly disabled clients, the home-help service is shifting its emphasis from domestic to personal care targeted on those considered most in need. The report *From home help to home care* (SSI 1987) was all about how to achieve this change. New national guidelines for the job description and pay structures for home helps have been developed in recognition of their changing role:

> The duties will include: domestic duties (including cleaning, cooking and washing), physical tasks approximating to home care (including dressing, washing and feeding clients), and social duties (including talking with clients, helping clients to maintain contact with family, friends and community, assisting with shopping and recreation), aimed at creating a supportive, homely atmosphere where clients can achieve maximum independence (National Joint Council for Local Authorities' Services [Manual Workers], September 1985).

It is up to individual authorities whether and when to implement these changes. While home helps are becoming known as home-care attendants and other titles in recognition of their changing role, the term 'home help' is used throughout this chapter to avoid confusion.

3.2d. Staff and training

Home helps are mainly middle-aged women, although there are now a few male home helps and organizers. Work has been on a part-time and mainly casual basis, with limited opportunities for a guaranteed number of hours per week, although this depends on the policy of the particular local authority. Training is minimal and may consist of a simple induction course, accompanying an existing home help, or the provision of a series of in-service courses on particular aspects of caring and safety (Dexter and Harbert 1983). There are no legislative requirements for qualifications or training to be given (Hedley and Norman 1982; Clarke 1984). Again, the amount of training offered varies between authorities, with growing emphasis on training accompanying the shift to a personal-care service.

3.2e. Extent of provision

As the formal home-help service is almost entirely the responsibility of social services departments (though there are some recent experiments in private provision), so it is possible to assess the extent of the service from local authority statistics. The following figures include designated home-care staff, but exclude marginal categories such as people in 'good neighbour' schemes, street wardens, etc.

At 30 September 1985 there were 55 537 whole-time equivalent home helps in England and Wales (nearly all home helps work part-time); and 2854 organizers. This is equivalent to 1.1 home helps per 1000 population, or more relevantly, 17.2 home helps per 1000 people aged 75+. Home helps work on an hourly basis, and an estimated 92 million hours were received nationally by clients during the same year. There were an estimated 690 000 active cases on 11 November 1985, approximately 12 per whole-time equivalent home help (Chartered Institute of Public Finance Accountancy 1987).

Gross expenditure nationally on the home-help service in the year ending 31 March 1986 was £347m, which represented 0.14 per cent of the gross domestic product of 1985 (Central Statistical Office 1987). About 10 per cent was recovered from charges.

Numbers of home helps in each of the 116 autonomous local authorities are shown in Table 4.2. These vary considerably, from 7 per 1000 people aged 75+ in the southern county of Surrey to 41 per 1000 people in the northern city of Sunderland. The general pattern is that provision is higher in the north than the south, and higher in urban areas, particularly inner

Table 4.2. Whole-time equivalent social services home-help staff for each local authority area in England and Wales at 30 September 1985: total and rate per 1000 people aged 75+

Authority	No	Rate	Authority	No	Rate
North			*West Midlands*		
Cleveland	616	23.4	Hereford & Worcs	617	16.0
Cumbria	623	18.8	Shropshire	260	11.3
Durham	824	23.0	Staffordshire	958	18.1
Northumberland	450	23.2	Warwickshire	499	18.8
Gateshead	334	26.3	Birmingham	1356	22.6
Newcastle upon Tyne	676	34.1	Coventry	449	25.9
North Tyneside	290	23.2	Dudley	305	18.8
South Tyneside	209	20.9	Sandwell	327	17.9
Sunderland	633	41.1	Solihull	159	16.6
			Walsall	226	17.8
Humberside and Yorkshire			Wolverhampton	313	21.1
Humberside	1104	20.9			
North Yorkshire	695	13.4			
Barnsley	357	28.3	*East Midlands*		
Doncaster	466	30.3	Derbyshire	1465	25.7
Rotherham	402	31.1	Leicestershire	730	14.3
Sheffield	1076	27.9	Lincolnshire	505	13.7
Bradford	726	25.1	Northamptonshire	309	9.7
Calderdale	330	24.4	Nottinghamshire	1245	21.2
Kirklees	534	23.0			
Leeds	1066	22.5	*Thames and East Anglia*		
Wakefield	359	21.5	Bedfordshire	412	16.6
			Berkshire	612	17.3
North West			Buckinghamshire	487	16.7
Cheshire	863	16.7	Cambridgeshire	504	14.3
Lancashire	1585	16.0	Essex	1280	13.5
Bolton	354	22.5	Hertfordshire	656	12.3
Bury	225	20.6	Norfolk	671	12.4
Manchester	779	26.8	Oxfordshire	468	14.9
Oldham	354	26.8	Suffolk	456	10.3
Rochdale	326	27.6			
Salford	343	21.6			
Stockport	308	17.1	*South*		
Tameside	399	30.7	Dorset	541	8.6
Trafford	258	18.6	Hampshire	977	10.5
Wigan	473	28.8	Isle of Wight	93	7.4
Knowsley	207	29.6	Kent	989	9.6
Liverpool	672	20.4	Surrey	465	6.9
Sefton	405	19.2	East Sussex	658	8.4
St Helens	337	34.0	West Sussex	560	8.4
Wirral	324	13.8	Wiltshire	377	11.4

Table 4.2. (*contd.*)

Authority	No	Rate	Authority	No	Rate
South West			*Outer London*		
Avon	1162	17.9	Barking	194	18.3
Cornwall	362	10.2	Barnet	218	10.1
Devon	804	9.2	Bexley	260	19.7
Gloucestershire	431	12.4	Brent	419	28.9
Somerset	433	12.7	Bromley	219	10.8
Wales			Croydon	234	12.3
Clwyd	387	13.6	Ealing	242	14.1
Dyfed	337	14.7	Enfield	303	16.1
Gwent	633	24.8	Haringey	415	34.3
Gwynedd	267	14.5	Harrow	213	14.5
Mid Glamorgan	863	28.8	Havering	215	16.8
Powys	114	14.9	Hillingdon	272	18.8
South Glamorgan	399	16.1	Hounslow	163	12.9
West Glamorgan	578	23.6	Kingston upon Thames	73	7.0
Inner London			Merton	208	16.0
Camden	410	32.5	Newham	294	24.7
Greenwich	417	31.6	Redbridge	187	11.4
Hackney	403	35.7	Richmond upon Thames	144	11.1
Hammersmith	252	23.8	Sutton	117	9.2
Islington	254	24.7	Waltham Forest	384	24.0
Kensington	113	13.0			
Lambeth	492	32.6			
Lewisham	493	31.0			
Southwark	466	32.4			
Tower Hamlets	218	23.7			
Wandsworth	411	23.2			
Westminster	287	21.3			
City of London	8	26.6			

Sources: DHSS *Personal social services local authority statistics: staff of local authority social services departments at 30 September 1985*, Table 1.

Y Swyddfa Gymreig *Staff adrannau gwasanaethau cymdeithasol: blwyddyn yn diweddu 30 Medi 1985*, C.1.3.

OPCS *Monitor PP1 86/2: Mid 1985 population estimates for local government and health authority areas of England and Wales*, Table 2.

cities, than in rural areas. An exception is the suburban areas around London, which are among the lowest.

There is, as we have explained, no statutory right to receive home help, and there is no national advice on entitlement in terms of type or amount of care. The amount of service allocated varies according not only to assessment of individual 'need' but also to criteria (if any) devised locally by individual authorities, which vary enormously. These are described in Section 4.

3.2f. Pathways into and through home-help services

People can gain access to home-help services via a referral from a variety of sources including general practitioners, community nurses, hospital staff, social workers, and relatives. A home-help organizer will, in theory, conduct an assessment of the person's needs and then allocate a service in numbers of hours. It is rarely that anyone requesting a service is turned away, resulting in low-intensity services, an issue addressed by the SSI (1987, 1988). Most social services departments have a local policy of reviewing each case, usually every six months, but the size of case loads and organizational inefficiency mean this is rarely possible so that care is poorly monitored and cases are rarely closed. The term 'case management' has been coined to cover the range of tasks from case finding (a rare phenomenon in social services departments), through assessment, care planning, provision, and monitoring/review, to case closure, and the improvement of performance in these core tasks of case management is a key theme in recent Government documents (SSI 1987; Griffiths 1988) in the quest for greater efficiency.

3.3. Home/community nursing

Community nursing is the responsibility of DHAs and is funded by central government from general taxation. It is always free at the point of use. Each DHA is organized differently, but most have a community unit within which community nursing is located. There will normally be a unit nursing officer, and a number of senior nursing officers in charge of community nursing, which covers district nurses, nursing auxiliaries, health visitors, and school nurses. District nurses provide treatment and monitoring in the client's home; auxiliary nurses are involved with more caring functions, particularly getting the patient up and dressed, and bathing, although district nurses may also provide such personal care. District nurses and auxiliaries provide this service for all client groups. Now that home helps are providing more personal care, there is a blurring of the boundaries of roles, particularly between them and the auxiliary nurses. The blurred area of overlap focuses on getting patients up, bathing, and helping them to bed (Davies *et al.* 1990). While the move into personal care by home helps could reduce the health service work-load and expenditure, it is a threat to auxiliaries, and tensions in this area have caused some social services departments to hold back from promoting personal care.

Health visitors are concerned mainly with the under-5 (pre-school) age group, but in some DHAs they are beginning to work with elderly clients, monitoring well elderly people and advising them on keeping healthy.

Community nurses may be based in local premises such as health centres and local hospitals, and are sometimes attached to doctors' practices. The concept of the primary care team, involving, for instance, district nurses, social workers, and general practitioners, is developing in some authorities.

Referral to community nursing is made by general practitioners, hospital staff, and social workers—a similar range as for home helps. District-nursing care tends to be allocated shorter term than home help, visits being curtailed once the clients are considered to be 'back on their feet' (a district nurse will commonly be allocated after discharge from hospital, for instance, and is withdrawn once the client seems to be able to cope on their own again). Auxiliary-nurse care might continue for longer.

District nurses and health visitors receive a 3-year, hospital-based training, and further training for community nursing. Auxiliary nurses receive training on the job. Changes are being introduced whereby more highly trained, specialist nurses receive additional salary increments. The trend in nursing is towards ever increasing specialization and professionalization, to the detriment, some feel, of the caring aspect of their work.

Two other significant groups of community nurses are the community psychiatric nurses, who are generally attached to priority-care units in health authorities, and health visitors. Occasionally health visitors may work with elderly people at home, monitoring and advising them on their health, but this group of nurses usually works with the under-5 age group; there is a group of them that works full-time with elderly clients and are called geriatric visitors.

3.4. Interfaces between services

Pressure on the home-help and community-nursing services are not only coming from the increases in client numbers and levels of disability caused by demographic change. Health authorities, with their own financial problems, lack of beds, and their belief in prevention of admission and early discharge to speed rehabilitation and prevent dependency, tend to discharge elderly clients into the community earlier than in the past, leading to ever greater need for co-ordination between hospital medical and nursing staff, hospital social workers, general practitioners, community nurses, and the home-help service.

At senior management, policy-making levels, co-ordination is achieved by means of a formal joint planning and consultative machinery between social services departments and DHAs at the local authority level. This may include voluntary-sector representation at the statutory sector's discretion. The joint groups have available to them funds called 'joint finance', which are controlled by DHAs, and are used to start up joint initiatives and those involving the transfer of responsibility for services from DHA to social services departments. The funding of such schemes must be picked up by the local authority or another agency, such as a voluntary organization, after the first few years.

However, at the field level, there is no nationally defined, formal, collaborative structure, so that ways of co-operating are developed locally and vary greatly. They include case conferences and improved communication between different professionals involved with the same client, but while excellent examples of local collaboration exist, overlaps and gaps in services persist, causing inefficiency and confusion. The blurring of roles between home helps and auxiliary nurses is just one example of where problems can arise.

Private-sector care (for instance, private nursing and private home help to supplement statutory provision), and voluntary input (such as meals-on-wheels and sitting services) also need to be co-ordinated with statutory provision.

This problem of co-ordinating services has been raised in a number of government documents in the 1980s (see 2.3); the recent Griffiths report (1988) proposes extending the use of non-statutory provision, which will make effective co-ordination yet more important. It puts forward the concept of a care manager to oversee assessment, allocation, and review functions, and to manage the care, from a variety of sources, for each individual. It also proposes a key worker for each client to monitor changes in a client's circumstances, and to ensure efficient use and co-ordination of care. Ideas close to this model have been tried in various authorities throughout the country.

4. THE SERVICE IN PRACTICE

This section focuses primarily on the home-help service; on how it looks and how it operates in practice.

4.1. Who receives home help?

From Table 4.3, it can be seen that 9 out of 10 home-help recipients are elderly. The *1985 General Household Survey* provides a picture of elderly recipients. Ninety-five per cent of people aged 65 and over live in private households, and of these 9 per cent reported that they were currently receiving the home-help service. The service goes particularly to the very elderly: it is received by one in four of those aged 75+. Tables 4.4 and 4.5

Table 4.3. Analysis of home-help service client types (from CIPFA, 1985/6)

Client type	Percentage
Persons aged 65–74	22
Persons aged 75+	68
Families with children	1
Physically/mentally handicapped	6
Mentally ill	1
Other, unknown	2

Table 4.4. Persons over 65 receiving the home help in 1985, by degree of disability, living alone, and social isolation

Disability[3]	Not living alone (%)	Living alone; not isolated (%)	Living alone; isolated (%)[2]	All (%)
None/low	1 (1690)[1]	7 (581)	9 (336)	3 (2607)
Moderate	12 (191)	46 (96)	58 (66)	30 (353)
High	16 (236)	58 (88)	78 (32)	32 (357)
All	4 (2117)	18 (765)	19 (435)	9 (3317)

[1] The figures show the proportion of people of given disability and social support who receive the home-help service: for example, of 1690 elderly people who were not living alone and had none/low disability, 1 per cent were receiving the home-help service. (Source: reanalysis of the *1985 General Household Survey*.)

[2] Social isolation: is visited by, or goes to visit, friends and relatives weekly or less often.

[3] Disability: unable to manage without help the following tasks—shopping, cleaning paintwork, cleaning windows, sweeping floors, jobs involving climbing, small amounts of laundry, going up/down stairs, getting around the house, taking a bath, walking outdoors. None/low = able to manage 8–10 tasks; moderate = able to manage 5–7 tasks; high = able to manage 4 or less tasks.

give details of people over 65 years of age receiving home help by degree of disability, social isolation, and household structure.

There is also an awareness of the increasing burden of work undertaken by relatives, neighbours, and friends (often called 'informal carers') in enabling elderly people to stay at home. This is due to rapidly increasing dependency ratios, combined with the reduction in family size in the twentieth century. Some authorities are trying to find ways of supporting them in their task, including allocating hours of home help to provide respite for informal carers. The Griffiths report (1988) encourages the support of informal carers and other providers (the private and voluntary sectors). The balance between public and private responsibility for care is likely to remain a major debate for some time.

Table 4.5. Distribution of home-help service among elderly people by household structure

Household structure	Receiving home help (%)	All elderly (%)
Living alone	73	46
Living with spouse only	20	38
Living with spouse and others	1	5
Living with children only	5	8
Living with others (not children)	1	2
Sample size	275	2962

Source: re-analysis of *1985 General Household Survey*, persons aged 65+ living in England and Wales.

Characteristics predicting the use of home help include age, disability, and lack of alternative sources of support. Although the service is provided for domestic duties, disability with personal tasks is a weak predictor of who will get services. Table 4.4 shows that elderly people living alone or with a partner only are the main recipients. There are now only small differences between sexes and social classes in receipt, though what there is seems to attract hot debate (see, for example, Townsend and Davidson, 1982; Arber *et al.* 1988). In Section 3.2 it was noted that more service is provided in cities and Inner London: Bebbington with Moennadin (1989) show that this is true, even after allowing for differences in disability and lack of support.

4.2. What do clients receive?

There is variation among authorities in the specificity of tasks done by home helps. In some areas, tasks are prescribed, while in others home helps are left to do whatever seems most necessary on the particular day.

Table 4.6 shows the distribution of tasks in a recent survey of elderly recipients of home help. It indicates that domestic tasks still dominate the use of home-help time, although there has been a widening of function in recent years to include personal care such as bathing and rehabilitation. The SSI is keen to encourage this trend (see 2.3). Some authorities are using special staff or projects to introduce these functions, while others are opting for mainstream changes (Lawson 1989).

In terms of amount of help received, minimum allocations in theory are 1 to 1.5 hours per week, although in practice shortage of staff, for instance through sickness, means that some clients receive a spasmodic service. Maximum allocations are more likely to be subject to stricter guidelines.

Table 4.6. Tasks undertaken by the home-help service

	Regularly (%)	Sometimes (%)	Never (%)	Would like (more) (%)
Housework (clean and tidy)	98	0	2	13
Lighting coal fire	5	1	94	0
Laundry	23	9	67	1
Cooking meals	7	5	88	1
Shopping	36	9	55	1
Collecting pension	14	4	82	0
Personal care	7	3	90	1
Writing letters, etc.	10	4	86	0
Giving medicine	4	1	95	0
Popping in to check	7	2	91	1
Take for walk	2	3	95	0
Rehabilitation[1]	9	2	89	0

Source: Bebbington *et al.* (1986). Tasks undertaken for 356 clients of the home-help service in England and Wales, and tasks for which help or more help would be liked.

[1] Assisting clients to undertake tasks for themselves.

Some authorities set clear limits of hours while others operate a principle of providing whatever service is required to keep an individual in their own home. The latter approach is often time limited and there is general concern not to exceed the cost of a residential place.

In 1986/7 the average number of hours provided weekly in the shire counties was 3.3 per client (average range, 2.1 to 5.0), for the metropolitan districts the average was 3.3 hours (average range, 1.8 to 4.7) and in the London boroughs, 3.2 hours (average range, 2.5 to 4.3) (SSI 1988).

4.3. The efficiency of targeting

There are no formal eligibility criteria for the home-help service allocated by home-help organizers within locally run social services departments. Needs' assessment by organizers is a major determinant of whether and how much service is provided. However, with local autonomy in allocation, there has been increasing public concern about variation in standards, and to ensure that the service should be targeted effectively. The two major recent revews by the Audit Commission (1985) and the SSI (1987, 1988) both conclude that improvement could be made, in particular by concentrating a greater proportion of available resources to the most needy and not spreading the service so thinly. Table 4.7 illustrates the reason for concern, by comparing actual receipt with a variety of definitions of who

Table 4.7. Target efficiency of the home-help service for the elderly, by three definitions of need

Definition 1.	Appreciably disabled. Persons over 65 who have difficulty getting up/down stairs; getting wound the house (except stairs); getting in/out of bed; cutting toe-nails; bath or shower; walking outdoors. Score 1 for each task causing difficulty and 2 if it can only be done with help. A score of 6+ counts as appreciably disabled.	
	Elderly who are appreciably disabled:	11%
	Elderly appreciably disabled who get home help:	32%
	Elderly home help clients who are appreciably disabled:	36%
Definition 2.	Domestic difficulties. Persons who could not manage at least one of the following: cleaning windows inside; sweep or clean floors; wash small amounts of clothing by hand.	
	Elderly who have domestic difficulties:	20%
	Elderly domestic difficulties who get home help:	31%
	Elderly home-help clients with domestic difficulties:	67%
Definition 3.	Disabled lacking support. Persons living alone who: are appreciably disabled as defined above; or cannot walk outdoors; or have difficulty getting round indoors; or have difficulties getting up/down stairs; or cannot open bottles; or cannot sweep/ clean floors; or cannot use a frying pan. Persons living with one other elderly person who: cannot sweep/clean floors, open bottles, use a frying pan, and the task is not done by the partner: or who are appreciably disabled or unable to get round the house. Persons in other households who: are aged 75+, appreciably disabled, and not helped by other household members; or bedfast; or unable to feed without help; cannot sweep/clean floors, open bottles, use a frying pan, and the task is not done by another household member.	
	Elderly who are disabled lacking support:	15%
	Elderly disabled lacking support who get home help:	34%
	Elderly home-help clients who are disabled lack support:	51%

Source: Re-analysis of *1985 General Household Survey*: 2962 people aged 65+ in England and Wales.

might be provided with the service. Though no such questionnaire-based definition can give the insight into individual cases of a professional assessment, and therefore we could not expect an exact match, nevertheless the lowness of the target accuracy, particularly for the third definition, is a surprise.

Table 4.7 suggests that there are twice as many elderly people not receiving the service whose needs seem to be just as great as those getting the service. Very few of these are getting equivalent help from elsewhere. But it would be difficult to conclude quite such a high level of unmet need. Recent consumer studies do not reveal large numbers of disabled elderly people who either do not know about the service or who have tried but failed to get it. Even in extreme cases, Levin *et al.* (1986) found that only one in four supporters of demented elderly people without the service would accept it if offered. The home-help service is popular, but acceptance can have psycho-social implications in terms of role definition and loss, and therefore many people prefer to manage for as long as possible without. Among recipients, comparatively few want extra help (see Table 4.6, extreme right-hand column).

An alternative interpretation of Table 4.7 is that as there are many people not getting the service who have greater needs than those who do, perhaps many of those who get the service do not really need it. It is impossible to discriminate between these disparate conclusions without a full understanding of the outputs (benefits) of the service; at present, studies of effectiveness are in their infancy. However, Davies *et al.* (1990) have found that 10 per cent of recipients do not appear to be benefiting at all by any of a number of criteria (e.g., indicators of life satisfaction and morale). Frequently this is because the service was provided at a time of crisis, but although the elderly person has since recovered the service has been retained. Home-help cases are often not reassessed for long periods, perhaps several years, and even when they are, home-help organizers are often reluctant to withdraw services against the client's wishes. However, apart from ensuring that reassessments take place, some authorities are introducing time-limited care for clients with rehabilitation or other short-term needs (Personal Social Services Research Unit [PSSRU] Domiciliary Care Project 1990).

There are signs that some authorities are now introducing more explicit criteria for service receipt as a way of tightening up on the targeting of services to those deemed locally to be 'most in need', and to help in the monitoring of allocations. For instance, an authority participating in a recent study of change had introduced three categories for targeting purposes, based on the need for long-term, short-term, and rehabilitative home care. Its assessment form incorporated explicit criteria for provision of help based on specific tasks and standard allocations of these, any variation from which had to be justified.

Another authority has introduced four categories of client in descending order of priority, based on level of vulnerability and need for different types of service. This is used alongside a document outlining criteria for service receipt; people meeting the criteria are eligible for service, subject to degree of need, alternatives available, and their category of priority as described above.

Yet another authority is developing a care-planning system whereby each home-help task has a standard time attached (e.g., assisting to get out of bed/dressing is allocated 10 minutes per day). After assessment, a care plan is drawn up. A discrepancy between the standard time allocation and the actual time taken to care for a client over a 3-week period should then, in theory, spark off a case review. The sum of the time allocations gives rise to the categorization of clients into four groups depending on the hours they need. This system is being developed for information/monitoring purposes at present and not for targeting (PSSRU Domiciliary Care Project 1990).

4.4. Assessment and allocation

As already stated, the number of hours allocated to clients is determined, in theory, through some kind of locally developed assessment of their 'need'. Home-help organizers allocate services after assessing potential clients for the extent of their 'need'. While the above developments in tightening criteria for allocation should become an integral part of the assessment, the effect of this will take some time to become established. In the meantime, it is clear that elderly people with fewer sources of informal help do receive more home-help hours. Other criteria for allocation demonstrated by the modelling of service inputs are reduced levels of self-care, an inability to do housework, the responsiveness of home-help organizers to expressions of depression and loneliness, and to poor housing conditions, which exacerbate the handicapping effect of impairment (Davies *et al.* 1990).

Interviews with home-help organizers in a 1985 study of domiciliary-care services demonstrated the catholic acceptance of referrals for the home-help service, with more than 95 per cent of referrals leading to service allocation (Bebbington *et al.* 1986). The concept of prevention rests heavily with many organizers, who feel that low-level intervention at the early stages of deteriorating ability may effect a form of monitoring and prevent breakdown leading to unnecessary institutional care. Home-help organizers in all areas responded to referrals quickly, with only clearly non-urgent cases waiting two weeks for an assessment visit (Davies *et al.* 1990).

Assessment is a vital task of case management in ensuring that services are allocated to those who need them, and yet in only 3 of the 10 study areas was explicit attention paid to needs- or problem-based assessments. Despite the use of checklists to guide assessments of need, allocation of service was often based on demand within the existing minimum and maximum allocation limits. An example of good practice was the use of a weekly task time-sheet displaying the key activities of daily living on a daily basis. The sheet is completed by entering the name of the person who ensures that this activity happens. This could either be the elderly person themselves, a spouse, neighbour or relative, a home help, community nurse, volunteer, etc. In this way, unmet needs are identified and can be addressed in the process of putting together a package of care (Davies *et al.* 1990).

The assessment process has been criticized for assessing clients for standard types of service, and allocating standard amounts and types of care (Challis and Davies 1986; Davies and Challis 1986). There are moves in many areas now, however, to make services more responsive to the needs, preferences, and circumstances of clients, by carrying out a 'problem-based' assessment, developing more flexible services, including evenings and weekends, and improving the co-ordination of care provided by different practitioners and agencies (Challis and Davies 1986; Davies and Challis 1986; SSI 1987). The SSI is pushing for improved management of the service to achieve this.

4.5. The outcomes of home help

There is little objective evidence that the service prevents institutionalization, partly because evaluation is so difficult. Many people who are institutionalized will have previously had the home-help service, so studies correlating the two often imply an association. Gorbach and Sinclair (1981) found that once differences of need had been taken into account, there was no correlation between the scale of the home-help service and the amount of residential care provided in individual local authorities.

Davies *et al.* (1990) examined the situations of 482 elderly people who had been provided with any of a range of services during the previous six months. Those who had subsequently entered institutions had had above average inputs of the home-help service originally, but so too had those elderly people who agreed that it would be impossible for them to continue to live at home without social services. A marginal productivity analysis (i.e., an analysis of the level of increased output from increased input) revealed that the amount of home-help input made little difference to the eventual probability of admission to an institution, but that it dramatically increased the probability that the elderly person would regard it as essential to their survival in the community (Table 4.8).

It would be dangerous to conclude from this, however, that home help made no difference to the well-being of recipients, as those who have above average inputs of help before entering institutions are likely to be the most frail people if targeting is working effectively.

As well as its direct function of supporting disabled people in the

Table 4.8. Destinational outcomes[1] for a 'typical' recipient of community social services (after Davies *et al.* 1990)

Weekly level of service	Entering institutions (%)	Dead (%)	At home and thinking that social services enabled them to remain so (%)
No home help; no meals-on-wheels	3	4	NA[2]
2 hours home help; no meals-on-wheels	4	5	5
4 hours home help; no meals-on-wheels	5	6	17
8 hours home help; no meals-on-wheels	6	7	61

[1] Predicted from a statistical model.
[2] Not applicable.

community, home helps are also seen as helping with social isolation. Bebbington *et al.* (1986) report three-quarters of clients as valuing the home help's company. It is probably also true that home helps are used to keep an eye on isolated, elderly people felt to be considerably at risk. Although cheaper alternatives exist for this purpose (such as peripatetic wardens and alarm systems), home helps are regarded as more reliable and often in a position to provide an early warning of problems.

4.6. Inter-agency co-ordination

4.6a. Home-help and social-work teams

The home-help service generally operates from accommodation shared with community social-work teams, although the nature of the working relationship between home-help organizers and social workers varies considerably. In some areas, social-work teams may not reflect any client specialization so that organizers have to work with a greater number of social workers who have little focus on working with elderly people. In other areas, there are specialist teams for elderly people, although these teams are rarely integrated with the home-help service.

4.6b. Home-help and health services

The relationship between the home-help and health services, particularly community nursing, has been subject to much attention; gaps and overlaps in service provision are widely recognized to be problematical (Hunter *et al.* 1988). In many areas, there are formal arrangements joint consultation between the local authority and DHA, and joint planning of care and joint finance, but a range of problems limits their effectiveness. These include a lack of co-terminosity between the areas of health and social services, the differential status of health and social services, representatives on joint care-planning teams, and the political pressures brought to bear in the use of joint finance.

With the reduction of residential facilities and the emergence of a client group with considerable personal-care needs, both home-help and nursing services have responded with more flexible roles and the boundary between the services has become blurred. While joint planning and joint working evoke notions of collaboration, the reality of daily work at field level involves differing definitions of needs, pressures of budgetary constraints, staffing restrictions and so forth, which encourage protective self-interest and attempts to offload on to other agencies where possible. A brief look at the performance of the core tasks of case management as revealed in a study of domiciliary services in 10 local authorities serves to demonstrate the nature of joint working between domiciliary nursing and home-care services.

Case finding. Nearly half of the cases in the study sample referred to social services departments were referrals from health personnel; in contrast, only 8 per cent of the sample was referred by social services staff on to health services.

Assessment. In practice there is little inducement for either set of practitioners to carry out broad, problem-based assessments, as the resources required to meet the needs are not always in the control of the practitioner concerned. Organizational constraints led to assessments of disability *for* particular services in many cases.

Care planning and service packaging. In practice, services are co-ordinated within rather than between agencies. The reality of co-ordination involving services outside the social services department could best be described as 'arranging services' or 'liaising' with existing service providers. Care plans are used more frequently by nurses than social services' practitioners, and, while these are left in patients' homes and can be examined by anybody involved, in practice the staff of social services departments are not encouraged to use them.

Monitoring and reassessment. These ensure the ongoing match between needs and services. While NHS patients are reassessed on a regular basis, this is not done systematically by home-help sections of social services departments, although the contact of the home help is said to provide a monitoring service in itself. Liaison between health and social services personnel to facilitate reassessment of need did not match up to the number of elderly people receiving both services simultaneously. Of 177 clients receiving both services, contact was made in less than half the cases and case conferences occurred in only 12 cases over a 6-month period (Davies *et al.* 1990).

4.6c. Home-help and private home-help services

While the publicly provided home-help service (together with community nursing) continues to dominate provision of care in the home, the private sector may become more important in future. Private domestic help to the well-off has always been a feature of British society, but in recent years, many small private home-help agencies, and a few large ones, have been springing up in wealthier areas throughout the country on a for-profit basis. This growth has perhaps been stimulated by the coming on stream of employment-related pension schemes, providing higher incomes in retirement for some elderly people. The private sector provides a range of services from domestic and personal care to private nursing, and their selling point is their flexibility. Initially these agencies seemed to fill gaps in what the traditional, rather inflexible, public service could provide, by working in the evenings and weekends, for instance, or by providing additional hours to suit the client. Now, as public services are forced to target more and more on the most frail and vulnerable clients, the private agencies fill in the vacuum left among the less frail who can afford to pay. This suggests that they supplement and complement the public sector, but they may also sometimes substitute for it, either because the client prefers to pay and therefore be in control, or by arrangement with the public service, which will reimburse the client or pay the private agency itself, or because the public service withdraws when a private one goes into the home (Lawson 1991).

There is evidence that home-help staff feel that their jobs may be threatened, especially in authorities whose political climate prediposes them to the contracting out of services to other providers (Midwinter 1986; Lawson 1991). The Griffiths report (1988) recommends the extension of the use of private-sector providers to promote choice and competition between services, so that the private sector and its relationship to social services departments is likely to become more important over time. As it becomes more common for departments to charge for home-help services or for current charges to rise, it will be interesting to see what choices clients make. However, social services departments currently have no statutory obligation or right to monitor and inspect private domiciliary services.

4.6d. Home help and the voluntary sector

The voluntary sector does not seem yet to be heavily involved in the provision of home-help/home-care services. The voluntary sector was involved in the organization of some home-help schemes in the 1940s but withdrew during the 1950s, lacking the administrative capacity to run the schemes on the required scale (Means and Smith 1985). The Women's Royal Voluntary Service (WRVS) remains active in the organization of many meals-on-wheels schemes to this day, but is financed largely by local authorities. Age Concern, a voluntary organization with groups all over the country, commonly provides day centres and lunch clubs, also with financial support from local authorities, and other voluntary agencies are more involved in sitting/social-contact services (benefiting informal carers as well as elderly clients) and daytime activities, which supplement and complement public services (Lawson 1991).

Generally, home-help organizers are responsible for allocations of meals-on-wheels, or certainly can be, even where direct referrals to WRVS can result in service. Direct links between home helps and other voluntary inputs such as day centres and sitting services are scarce. Voluntary services of this type are usually funded totally or in part by the local authority—by grant, contract, or other means. The Griffiths report (1988) recommends that social services departments should help maximize voluntary-sector activity, again to provide choice and competition. (NB: The 'voluntary sector' includes unpaid volunteers as well as funded organizations with paid staff. The latter may charge for services but are run on a non-profit basis.)

4.7. Managing the service

How is the service managed? Is there a clear direction in which the service is going? Does the service have a clear idea of what it is trying to do, or is it merely reactive to whatever demands happen to be put most powerfully?

Section 2.3 outlined successive government policy documents in the 1980s which indicated the need for clearer service objectives and better management, and suggested ways of achieving this. A survey conducted in 1988 in four social services departments indicated that changes are being introduced that pick up some of the points raised in the Audit Commission (1986) regarding, for instance, locally integrated services and team-work; the Griffiths report (1988) regarding, for instance, more flexible care packaging, joint planning and cost consciousness; and the SSI reports on the home-help service (1987, 1988), which stress the importance of turning plans into action, improving the performance of case management tasks, improving budget management, and strengthening front-line management. Table 4.9 indicates a range of changes that are taking place (Lawson 1989).

There is still along way to go in resolving the problems of poor targeting and inefficiency indicated in earlier sections, but the home-help service,

Table 4.9. Rationales for choice of change of action

Management objectives	Examples of action to achieve objectives
Targeting on the most frail people; increasing intensity and reducing cover	Develop clear criteria of eligibility and build into assessment and review instrumentation
Improve (quality of, access to, use of) information and introduce budget-management systems	Training in the new ideas and use of instrumentation; introduce new technology and systems
Manipulate charging procedures to generate income and deter better off and less frail people applying for care	Devolve budgets to give accountability with responsibility
Indentifying economies of scale to reduce costs	Introduce bulk shopping and pension collection
Develop more community-based alternatives rather than residential care; get the balance right	Target residential places only on the most frail; screen admissions to residential care; try and find community-based alternatives; transfer resources from residential to community care; more flexible and varied use of residential places
Improve the performance of the core tasks of case management in order to meet need effectively and prevent admission to residential care, and speed up discharge	Introduce clear procedures and practice guidelines together with supporting instrumentation; training and staff development; reduce organizers' work-load to free them for case management tasks, e.g. by computerizing administration; improve supervision of home helps; adjust home helps in teams; expand the role of home helps into home care; introduce multidisciplinary working arrangements
Improve the flexibility of services in order to match resources to needs: this requires flexibility of type, timing, and amount of service	New forms of service, e.g., mobile day care; mixing the supply of care (use of alternative providers); new working arrangements to give more flexible hours covering 24 hours and 7 days; training and staff development; integrate residential, day, and domciliary care, structurally, geographically, and by opening residential places for respite care
Develop a more client-oriented approach	Involving user representatives in advisory bodies; negotiating care packages with clients and informal carers

Table 4.9. (*contd.*)

Management objectives	Examples of action to achieve objectives
Support informal carers	Train/orientate home-care staff in the needs of informal carers for support; add a specific allocation of funds to the home-care budget for use in supporting carers; include assessment of informal carer needs in assessment instrumentation; develop special projects targeted at meeting informal carers' needs
Improve joint working arrangements to allow co-ordinated care and prevent overlaps	Social services department and District Health Authorities working towards joint boundaries at local levels; developing joint strategies and policies; integrating services on a local level; piloting Kent Community Care Model; multidisciplinary assessment panels, care packaging forums, etc.

and services for elderly people as a whole, are being given more managerial and policy attention than ever before.

Furthermore, there are now indications that the 'new managerialism' of the private and public sectors in the UK, which involves an increased emphasis on managers and management, is beginning to affect local authorities (Stewart 1986). *Managing Tomorrow*, a recent pamphlet produced by the Local Government Training Board (1988), discusses the failure of traditional styles of management to cope with the rigours of the changing political, social, and economic environments. It proposes new management themes such as 'thinking total', responsiveness to the citizen and customer, strategic management and policy direction, human-resource management, organizational innovation, and performance review.

5. WAYS FORWARD

5.1. Summary of issues that require attention

The previous sections have emphasized a number of key problems in relation to home-help services for elderly people.

Targeting (i.e., matching resource inputs to needs) is poor: there is an inequitable and inefficient distribution of resources so that those with greatest needs don't necessarily receive most service—the distribution varies from area to area; and services tend to be spread thinly rather than being concentrated on the most frail people at risk of admission to institutional care.

Reasons for poor targeting include poor assessment, inflexible allocations of standard services, and little reassessment; in other words, poor performance of core tasks of case management.

There is poor co-ordination of care provided by different agencies (and by different services within one agency); this problem will become more acute as private and voluntary agencies are encouraged to play a greater role (Griffiths 1988).

The level of outcomes from increased inputs appears to be low, although this may be due, for instance, to the fact that people receiving the most services are the most frail and therefore more likely to enter institutional care.

While the rhetoric is that home helps are moving away from domestic work and towards personal care, the reality is that this change is occurring slowly, and patchily.

There is poor management overall, including lack of clear policies and objectives, and problems in turning policies into action.

The key role of informal carers, who provide the bulk of care at present, is being recognized, and effective ways of supporting and sharing their task need to be identified.

More resources are required for the home-help service if it is to meet expanding needs.

5.2. Some ways forward

As the chapter suggests, the above issues are being addressed in a number of ways, and understanding of the needs of elderly people and their informal carers, and how to tackle them, is gradually improving. The following are some ways forward.

5.2a. Improve the performance of case-management tasks

Experiments in community-care are based on the recognition that a complex service system and great variety in the need-related circumstances of individuals make the effective performance of core tasks of case management a prerequisite for equity and efficiency. Most aspects of equity and efficiency are primarily influenced by the performance of the core tasks, not by service management *per se*, given the framework of services on offer. This applies directly to targeting and indirectly to low outputs from increased inputs (i.e., low marginal productivities). Case management has become a slogan with much shoddy and muddled assertion and argument. In particular, some of it jumps immediately to the concentration of responsibility for the tasks without an assessment of context, and then gets hung up on quite minor contextual factors. However, there seems now to be an acceptance of the thesis that nearly all increases in resources have been applied to extending service provision—increasing its variety, improving its quality, and raising the terms and conditions of the providing staff—and hardly any to creating the capacity to match resources to needs by securing the more effective performance of the core case-management tasks (Challis and Davies 1986; Davies and Challis 1986; Davies and Missiakoulis 1987).

Effective performance of core case-management tasks is deeply contra-cultural. Arrangements and processes are dominated by agency and occupational territorialism, expectations, competencies, and values. Particularly for the heavy users of both community health and social services, good arrangements for case management are as hard to maintain as they are to set up—a point missed in the more optimistic, new managerialist argument. Our observation is that the arrangements are more often than not perverted or strangled. One device is to separate and so protect the new approach by placing it in an independent organization, although this can create problems such as elitism at a later stage.

Gap filling is one of the most important core tasks of case management. Only flexible resources used by case managers to fill gaps can compensate for the failure to develop a personal-care service locally or provide care out of hours, and for the rigidity of the procedures required to pay out even the most modest of expenditures. Wagner (1988) and others specifically argue that case managers should have budgets which they can use flexibly. Case managers should also have information about the costs of services, and an appropriate span of resources charged against the budget allowing their decisions to guide suppliers (Davies *et al.* 1987). This model, piloted in the Thanet (Kent) Community Care Project, is being replicated in various parts of the country. Table 4.10 shows some results of the project.

5.2b. Raise the ratio of investment to direct provision

The contrast between the outcome of community-care experiments and the standard provision and innovation shows that there must be rapid technical progress for some years. In such circumstances, industries make a high ratio of investment to other production costs. This means investment in people: training and the development of competencies; evaluated experiments in the creation of the structural requirements to create environments which allow people to work most effectively. The investment must above all be in people. But we must not neglect artifacts such as off-the-shelf information systems. A comparison between our warm and woolly world of social care and some geriatric practice and some areas of clinical psychology suggests that we should develop sets of off-the-peg models comprising structures, expectations, and assumptive worlds, skills and

Table 4.10. Some results of the Thanet Community Care Project (from Davies and Challis 1986)

Location after one year
- halved probability of death
- doubled probability of survival
- doubled probability of living at home
- maintained first year differences for four years

'Client state'
- improved clients' perception of morale
- improved functional capacities (ADL)[1]
- removed shortfalls in care

Informal carer welfare
- reduced perceived strain
- prolonged and maintained inputs

Costs
- reduced costs to social-care agency
- diverted health care demand to acute treatment without raising costs
- reduced 'marginal costs' of outcomes to social-care and health agencies ('joint supply')

artifacts. People moving into key positions find it easier to look for a fit between the problems and possibilities of a context and a model and then adapt a clearly defined model than to reinvent the wheel, the engine, brakes, coachwork and everything else, all at the same time. This is the logic of the PSSRU's strategy for developing its community-care approach; with its variants of the basic model adapted to client group and context, all described in ways which make application easier.

5.2c. Develop arrangements for personal care

The need to secure the provision of personal care is widely acknowledged. Increasing intensity enables the development of personal care, but in itself is not enough. One study (Victor and Vetter 1988) illustrates how the increase in time inputs from a conventional home-help service was not accompanied by the provision of personal care to a sufficient degree. This contributed to the failure of the innovation. They entitled their paper 'Rearranging the deckchairs on the *Titanic*'.

5.2d. Improve the co-ordination of services provided by different agencies

The provision of personal care can be made either by the health or social services. Davies *et al.* (1990) show that it is becoming increasingly important to secure good field co-ordination of community health and social services. They also show that for many, community health and social care is an episode sandwiched between frequent stays in acute wards of hospitals. Here the case management is needed through time if humane as well as efficient judgements are to be made about patients with needs that cross agency boundaries (Gavett *et al.* 1985). There may not be an organizational solution uniquely correct for all areas; however, the development of organizational frameworks to encourage medical and paramedical inputs is vital. Financial inducements through community-care development grants for such programmes may help.

5.2e. Develop the capacity of the locally responsible agency to develop and implement trade and industry policies

The guiding metaphors traditional in social care are inappropriate for the next century. The statutory agencies will no longer monopolize the supply and financing of long-term care but will co-ordinate provision from a number of sources (Griffiths 1988). They may well find it extremely difficult to find a framework which produces good outcomes for clients and which does not present huge organizational problems.

Most social services departments lack the analytical capacity to see the implications of the new contexts. They are aware of the speed with which market opportunities can develop and be seized. However, they are often conservative, even in the areas nearest to their experience. For instance, in the post-Griffiths mixed economy of financing and provision, quite different arrangements are required if the traditional providers are to compete with new entrants from the private sector. One aspect found in the USA is that the traditional providers find it too difficult to adapt to the new challenges. They therefore lose out initially and are cut adrift by their parent organization, which would otherwise face financial or political embarrassment. Some eventually make it but the market meanwhile becomes dominated by the new entrants, who have debased quality by replacing it with price competition

This runs counter to the ambitions of thoughtful British directors of social services, who would like to define their market at the end of the range where assured quality control is most vital, while also allowing competition.

However, it is interesting to note the experience of the British NHS, which has been contracting out domestic, laundry, and catering services since 1983. In the early stages of competitive tendering, private contractors were winning 60 to 80 per cent of all NHS contracts. That situation has been reversed, with in-house teams now holding 80 per cent of all NHS contracts (Joint NHS Privatisation Research Unit 1988). Many DHAs managed to get their act together and improve services under threat of competition; will social services departments be able to do the same?

6. CONCLUSION

These are exciting times for the academic as well as for the provider of services, and the implications of the adoption of case management as the key to future provision (Griffiths 1988) suggest that academic attention must switch from the services themselves to the systems and approaches of organizations in providing these services. This is also an era in the UK when the responsibility of individuals and 'communities' for providing their own welfare is being extended, while state provision retreats to a co-ordinative function (Griffiths 1988).

In response to these changes, the Domiciliary Care Project at the PSSRU is currently engaged in shifting the focus from the social services department to the consumers of services. The Project is developing a new perspective complementary to our production of welfare approach (POW); this we entitle the social production of welfare, SPOW for short (Netten and Davies 1990; Qureshi, Challis, and Davies 1989). This is intended to develop an understanding of individuals within their social networks, and the relative contributions to the welfare of the consumer's household. We pursue such an understanding through an analysis of the production of commodities necessary for personal well-being; personal care, domestic care, nutrition, security, and social interaction. This work will provide analyses of the relations between social services departments and carers, developing conceptual argument about the role of carers in the social production of welfare. It will examine opportunity costs to carers, the nature of stress, and the impact of services on these. The findings are published in *Community Services and the Social Production of Welfare* (PSSRU Domiciliary Care Project 1992).

REFERENCES

Arber, S., Gilbert, N., and Evandrou, M. (1988). Gender, household composition and receipt of domiciliary services by the elderly disabled. *Journal of Social Policy*, **17,** 153–77.

Audit Commission (1985). *Managing social services for the elderly more effectively.* HMSO, London.

Audit Commission (1986). *Making a reality of community care.* HMSO, London.

Bebbington, A. C. and Davies, B. P. (1983). Equity and efficiency in the allocation of the personal social services. *Journal of Social Policy*, **12,** 246–52.

Bebbington, A. C., Charnley, H. M., Davies, B. P., Ferlie, E. B., Hughes, M. D., and Twigg, J. (1986). *The domiciliary care project: meeting the needs of the elderly*, Interim Report to DHSS, August 1986, Discussion Paper 456. Personal Social Services Research Unit, University of Kent, Canterbury.

Bebbington, A. C. with Moennadin, R. (1989). *Target efficiency of the home help service in 1985*, Discussion Paper 619. Personal Social Services Research Unit, University of Kent, Canterbury.

Central Statistical Office (1987). *Economic trends*. HMSO, London.

Challis, D. and Davies, B. (1986). *Case management in community care*. Gower, Aldershot.

Chartered Institute of Public Finance and Accountancy (1987). *Personal social services statistics: actuals 1985/6*. CIPFA, London.

Clarke, L. (1984). *Domiciliary services for the elderly*. Croom Helm, London.

Davies, B. P. (1967). *Research evidence of the committee on local authority, and allied personal social services (The Seebohm Report)*, Note 4—The Effect of Authority Organisation on Spending and Provision. HMSO, London.

Davies, B. P. (1968). *Social needs and resources in local services*, Michael Joseph, London.

Davies, B. P. (1981). Strategic goals and piecemeal innovations; adjusting to the new balance of needs and resources. In *A new look at the personal social services* (ed. E. M. Goldberg and S. Hatch) Policy Studies Institute, London.

Davies, B. P. and Challis, D. J. (1986). *Matching resources to needs in community care*. Gower, Aldershot.

Davies, B. P. and Missiakoulis, S. M. (1987). Heineken and matching processes in the Thanet Community Care Project. *British Journal of Social Work,* **17,** (suppl.), 55–78.

Davies, B. P., Darton, R. A., and Goddard, M. (1987). *The effects of alternative targeting criteria and margin levels for the opportunity costs to the SSD of care in local authority homes 1987*, Discussion Paper 484. Personal Social Services Research Unit, University of Kent, Canterbury.

Davies, B. P. *et al.* (1990). *Resources, needs and outcomes in community-based care*. Gower, Aldershot.

Dexter, M. and Harbert, W. (1983). *The home help service*. Tavistock, London.

Gavett, W. J., Drucker, W. B., McCrum, M. S., and Dickinson, J. C. (1985). *A study of high cost inpatients in Strong Memorial Hospital: Final Report*. University of Rochester School of Medicine, Rochester, NY.

Goldberg, E. M. and Connelly, N. (1981). *Evaluative research in social care*. PSI, London.

Gorbach, P. and Sinclair, I. (1981). *Pressure on health and social services for the elderly*. National Institute for Social Work, London.

Griffiths, R. (1988). *Community care: an agenda for action*. HMSO, London.

Hedley, R. and Norman, A. (1982). *Key issues in the home help service*. Centre for Policy on Ageing, London.

Hunter, D. J., McKeganey, N. P., and MacPherson, I. A. (1988). *Care of the elderly: policy and practice*. Aberdeen University Press, Aberdeen.

Joint NHS Privatisation Research Unit (October 1988). *Second round tendering: in-house successes*, Special briefing. Joint NHS Privatisation Research Unit, London.

Lawson, R. (1989). *Change and its management in community social services for elderly people*. Discussion Paper 621. Personal Social Services Research Unit, University of Kent, Canterbury.

Lawson, R. (1991). Interorganisational partnerships in the provision of home care for elderly people, Discussion Paper 626. Personal Social Services Research Unit, University of Kent, Canterbury (in press).

Levin, E., Sinclair, I., and Gorbach, P. (1986). The effectiveness of the home help service with confused old people and their families. *Research, Policy, Planning*, **3,** 1–7.

Clarke, M. and Stewart, J. (1988). *Managing tomorrow.* Local Government Training Board, Bristol.

Means, R. and Smith, R. (1985). *The development of welfare services for elderly people.* Croom Helm, London.

Midwinter, E. (1986). *Caring for cash: the issue of private domiciliary care.* Centre for Policy on Ageing, London.

Ministry of Health (1946). *National Health Service Act.* HMSO, London.

Ministry of Health (1944). *Circular 179/44.* HMSO, London.

Ministry of Health (1947). *Circular 118/47.* HMSO, London.

National Joint Council for Local Authorities' Services (Manual Workers) (1985). *National guidelines for job description and pay structures for home care workers.* NJCLAS, London.

Netten. A. and Davies, B. D. (1990). The social production of welfare and consumption of social services. *Journal of Public Policy*, **10,** 331–47.

OPCS (1988). *General Household Survey 1985.* HMSO, London.

Personal Social Services Research Unit Domiciliary Care Project (1992). *Community services and the social production of welfare.* PSSRU, University of Kent, Canterbury.

Qureshi, H., Challis, D. J., and Davies, B. P. (1989). *Helpers in case-managed community care.* Gower, Aldershot.

Seebohm Committee (1968). *Report of the committee as local authority and allied personal social services.* Cmnd 3703. HMSO, London.

Social Services Inspectorate (1987). *From home help to home care: an analysis of policy, resourcing and service management.* DHSS, London.

Social Services Inspectorate (1988). *Managing policy change in home help services.* DHSS, London.

Stewart, J. (1986). *The new management of local government.* Allen & Unwin, London.

Tobin, S. and Liebermann, M. (1976). *Last home for the aged.* Jossey-Bass, San Francisco.

Townsend, P. and Davidson, N. (1982). *Inequalities in health: the Black Report.* Penguin, Harmondsworth.

Townsend, P. and Wedderburn, D. (1965). *The aged in the welfare state.* Welwyn.

Victor, V. R. and Vetter, N. J. (1988). Rearranging the deckchairs on the *Titanic*: failure of an augmented home help scheme after discharge to reduce the length of stay in hospital. *Archives of Gerontology and Geriatrics*, **7,** 83–91.

Wagner, G. (1988). *Residential care: a positive choice.* HMSO, London.

5

Home-care services in France

Jean-Claude Henrard, Joël Ankri, and Marie-Claude Isnard

1. Historical development of the *maintien à domicile* of elderly people
2. Existing home-care services for elderly people
   2.1. Home-help services
   2.2. Home-nursing services for elderly people
   2.3. Other services
3. Informal support
4. Co-ordination
5. Conclusion

Notes

References

For nearly 30 years, politicians have all been proclaiming the importance of maintaining elderly people in their own homes, by quoting from numerous official reports produced by experts and important civil servants. Behind this happy unanimity, what are the aims, implicit or not, of *maintien à domicile*, and what means are available to achieve them? How do they fit in with the social and health services and with the support given by the person's family, which is rarely mentioned? Does the central plan of action—services for home help and for help with personal care—answer the needs of the population it serves?

In an attempt to answer these questions, this chapter will examine the historical development of the *maintien à domicile* of elderly people, the existing system and its relation to other measures, and the fragmentary data available on its operation.

1. HISTORICAL DEVELOPMENT OF *MAINTIEN A DOMICILE*

In France the definition of social policy and the responsibility for its implementation fall principally to the state. The policy is formulated through official reports and declarations by the political authority responsible and is formalized in statutory texts. Briefly running through the successive formulations and their formalization makes it possible to draw out the different aims assigned to services for maintaining people in their homes and thereby the maintenance of the home itself.

The first home helps date back to the 1920s, when certain private associations suggested the provision of people who could assist or temporarily replace a mother who was unable to cope with her family responsibilities. Under the Vichy regime, the family was one of the basic values of the 'national revolution'. A law passed in March 1942 made the teaching of domestic science compulsory for young girls. Household advisors were created; they were employed by social centres and family allowance offices (created in 1932). After the war, the concept of family workers was created. These people helped to maintain household and family activities, helping or replacing mothers, or frail and disabled elderly people.

Until the 1960s, there were not really any specific policies for older people. The only policy was that of assistance for the poor, many of whom were elderly people, in the form of regular provision of assistance in cash or in kind. At this time the majority of elderly people lived with their families. However, some charitable associations developed from the help schemes for isolated and elderly sick people, the financing being ensured by *départemental* social aid and then by the primary sickness benefit funds, with which agreements were signed (1958–1960). At this time, sickness insurance and old-age insurance, as part of the general security system, were financed by a common fund. A complementary benefit was added to the care provided by doctors and medical auxiliaries in the form of home help for domestic chores and personal care. The home help was then considered to be an auxiliary to the nurse and the primary aim of their intervention was to 'avoid the hospitalization' of a sick elderly person who was not too seriously ill.

In 1960, the Commission for the Study of the Problems of Old Age was created, chaired by one of the founders of Social Security, P. Laroque. Instituted at the beginning of the Fifth Republic, which was characterized by the reinforcing of the role of the state, this Commission reported in 1962. Its report set out the foundation for a social policy on old age, centring on maintaining people in their own homes.

The notion of the autonomous, actively participating, 'third age' replaced that of old age. If elderly people were to live independently in their own homes, the public powers had to develop a series of measures and services for acting on housing problems, proposing social activities, and offering help with household chores and with health care for those whose lives were less autonomous as a result of being ill. This package was intended to ensure globally 'the social integration of elderly people' and 'avoid the admission to institutions' of those less autonomous. So, while the home helps remained the auxiliaries of the nurse in some cases, in which they were paid by sickness benefit, in others they could intervene without medical justification if it was to avoid admission to an institution, and they were then paid by the old-age insurance schemes (with a limit of 30 hours a month for a single person and 48 hours for a couple).

In 1967, old-age insurance was separated from sickness benefit, and home help is now financed purely by old-age insurance, apart from social welfare for the poor.

The proposals put forward by the Laroque report (Commission for the Study of the Problems of Old Age 1962) were only to see a significant development, with specific programmes for elderly people, in the course of the sixth and seventh five-year plans for economic and social development (1970–1974 and 1975–1979). The programme completed as part of the seventh plan intended to prevent 100 000 elderly people from having to enter institutions through the development of services for 300 elderly people in 322 sectors (State Ministry of Social Affairs 1972). Results were confined to the development of clubs, restaurants, and home-help services (for example, 7000 clubs, 2000 restaurants, and 1800 home-help services were created outside the areas of the plan between 1970 and 1975). To the previous objectives, the priority action programme of the seventh plan added the social participation of retired people and the improvement of the home which became compulsory for each of the areas created. To solve the difficulties of co-ordination, the state provided training grants for the managers of the area programmes. Here again, however, the action of the state was confined to the *'pump priming' grants*, the financing was shared (between the state, the benefit offices, and the local communities) and the responsibility for the choice of services was left to the local authorities. Because of the local financial crises, they tended to choose the cheapest services reaching a maximum number of people (Guillemard 1986, p. 396): clubs (there were to be as many as 15 000); cultural and physical activities; information campaigns. These campaigns were behind home helps (for whom financing was becoming a problem) but far in advance of the services for health care at home, which the regional sickness benefit offices hesitated to finance, particularly because of the opposition of the independent nurses. These services were only legally registered by the state in 1978.

The preparation of the eighth plan (1981–85) gave rise to the report *Vieillir Demain* (Growing Old in the Future), which clearly underlined that the aim of *maintien à domicile* had not been achieved (General Planning Commissariat 1982, p. 270). This report stressed the importance of continuing relationships between generations, even though various surveys had shown that the number of elderly parents living separately from their married children was increasing. It was suggested that keeping elderly people in a family environment should be facilitated and that a complementary relationship between relief by professionals and relief by volunteers and families should be developed. In 1981, a specific ministerial structure for elderly people was created, which aimed to implement the proposed policy. The nursing-care services for elderly people in their homes were regulated, which facilitated their rapid expansion. These services were intended to 'help the family or the neighbourhood' to take in a dependent elderly person and look after them in their day-to-day life, which might involve some nursing care. They should 'avoid separation through hospitalization' (or 'encourage the return home' if necessary) or 'admission to an institution'. These services should be understood to be at the neighbourhood level, integrated into the general scheme of taking responsibility for elderly people; the co-ordinators were responsible for facilitating the institutional links between the different services, and between the services and the residential institutions.

After 1983, the development of these services was curbed, the major aim being to reduce social expenditure. The stress was then put on the neighbourhood services (solidarities), where it was difficult to see whether the aim was to strengthen the ties between the generations (the minister responsible for the elderly action was, for six months, responsible for family action) or to control social expenditure. In 1986, this ambiguity reappeared in the circular on the alternatives to hospitalization (Ministry of Social Affairs and National Solidarity 1986*a*) where, faced with hospital expenses and over-provision of short stay beds, the minister suggested the development of alternatives, notably to the hospitalization with little medical justification of certain elderly people. The intention was to shift financial and personnel resources to socio-medical institutions and intermediary forms of care (already suggested in 1982) like day hospitals and nursing services, so facilitating the 'maintenance of contact with the family'.

This policy did not see daylight with the change of political majority in 1986. To 'facilitate the maintenance at home of elderly people and the employment of people with few qualifications', measures were taken which bypassed the traditional home-help services and facilitated the creation of intermediary associations whose purpose was to provide private cleaners for elderly people and which exempted people over 70 who used the service from paying social contributions. However, a new angle on dependent elderly people was suggested in the Braun report (Braun later became the Minister for Elderly People), which reaffirms the priority of *soutien à domicile* (Braun and Stourm 1982, p. 182). It proposed to facilitate maintenance in the family (by various fiscal measures), placement in a foster family, and development of co-ordinated nursing and care in the home, to be reinforced by financial means for difficult cases. These proposals show that nearly 30 years after the Laroque report, 'maintenance in the home' had not given rise to the implementation of a co-ordinated global policy. Successive surveys show an increase in the number of people living in institutions, partly linked to the quantitative insufficiency of means of help at home (see Appendix 6, Table 1).

This brief review of the major reports and statutory texts on policies for elderly people shows that the objectives sought under the heading of 'maintenance in the home' have varied in the course of time and according to the person in charge. For example, there could be opposition between the person responsible for social action and the ministers in charge of the administration of compulsory insurance. The representatives of the health professionals have not been very concerned with home-care measures except when these measures threatened to take away part of their potential clientele. Thus, for example, independent nursing staff resented the change whereby the responsibility for co-ordinating nursing care at home was entrusted to a salaried nursing manager. Home-help services, for a long time, have only been concerned with home help in the strictest sense and their associations have remained very marginal as regards the development of policies for elderly people (Gaullier 1986). The National Union of Associations for Care and Services in the Home, which is the most important organization, has become aware of its role (1984 Congress) as partner and creator of a socio-medical policy in conjunction with financing bodies and locally elected representatives.

The population itself has never acted on the problems of maintenance in the home. The preparation for the National Conference on the Retired and the Elderly (November 1982–March 1983) allowed associations and representative bodies to reaffirm:

- their desire for social integration;
- the necessity for implementing an urban policy aiming to bring the different generations closer and to support families looking after a dependent elderly person; to create as wide and as complete a variety as possible of home-help services, functioning in an adaptable and evolutionary manner in order to meet the different levels of need and capable of ensuring the continuity of care even if the person's dependence becomes total (Secretary of State for Elderly People 1983).

The implementation of such a policy, as we have argued, has only been partially successful.

2. EXISTING HOME-CARE SERVICES FOR ELDERLY PEOPLE

The existing services intended for elderly people, or used by them, are numerous. The following list considers only those most typical, according to the types of activity for which elderly people receive help, with a view to international comparison.

- Everyday domestic tasks (home-making, house repairs, administrative tasks).
- Personal care (hygiene and mobility).
- Technical care (nurses, chiropody, etc.).
- Supervision (keeping an eye on the person, alarm system, etc.).
- Socialization (provide company, social stimulation, etc.).

To this can be added housing improvements (restoration, installation of modern conveniences, etc.).

These activities are more or less well catered for by one or several types of service. Some services provide help with several of these activities, others with just one. Some services are not specifically intended for elderly people but are freely available to them; others are for their sole use.

Services may go to the home—whether the home be individual or collective (sheltered housing, for example)—or they may be in the locality and accessible to elderly people (for example, meals might be brought to the home or eaten in a luncheon club). The concepts of home and of services for maintenance at home need to be defined. We shall limit them to the individual home and to services which go to the home (Appendix 6, Table 2). Homes and services are rapidly evolving, with the development of some intermediary structures between individual homes and collective housing that ensure services on site and can also call upon other services.

Two services are particularly relevant because of their specificity and the activities which they provide: home-help services and home-nursing services for elderly people.

2.1. Home-help services

2.1a. Organization and funding

The collective agreement applying since 1 July 1983 to the staff of these services defines the duties of the home help: to carry out physical, social, and moral work contributing to the maintenance at home of elderly people.

The oldest services have been in existence for nearly 35 years. Their purpose is to provide help with domestic chores for people who are completely incapable of carrying them out because of their state of health. The request is made by doctor's prescription (or by a local social worker), establishing the number of hours needed. Two sectors are responsible for these services, each with their own type of client, funders, and legal status.

The first is the public sector: there is a statutory provision for people of

65 years or more needing help because they live alone or with a person who cannot carry out the day-to-day maintenance of the house, and whose income is less than a certain level. It is financed by *départemental* social welfare and provided by municipalities. It is part of the compulsory assistance for the poor. The conditions of life and the resources are assessed by a social worker. The minimum ceiling for resources[1] is fixed by the state, each *département* having the option of setting a higher ceiling. The maximum number of hours of help which a person can receive is 30 a month. Given that it is a social welfare payment, part of the amount spent can be recoverd on the total net assets of inheritance in excess of 250 000 fr. The *obligation alimentaire*[2] was withdrawn in 1977.

The second is the private sector: provisions are ensured by associations financed by old-age insurances and complementary pension schemes for those of their affiliated members having a higher level of resources than the social assistance ceilings. Each system for the elderly and each funding scheme freely determines its own social action, which results in great diversity in awarding home help, according to the funder involved. In the case of the general system for salaried workers, the conditions regarding age and family commitments are identical to those for social assistance; the conditions for the resources reach a ceiling of roughly twice the amount of social welfare. Occasionally it is possible to disregard one ceiling. The maximum number of hours is 30 per month, with the option of special dispensation. The finances available for distribution to the beneficiaries vary according to the resources, from 5.30 frs to 43 frs.

Where the local authority does not have a home-help service, or when it is insufficient, the elderly person can get an allowance to buy in help (the sum granted corresponds to a maximum of 60 per cent of what it would actually cost).

For 1986, the distribution of beneficiaries, of the number of hours granted and the related expenses is given in Table 3 in the Appendix 6. The important thing to note is that the eligible population is not known, as the number of people meeting the required level of resources is not known. Nevertheless, it is reasonable to assume that home help was received by 6.9 per cent of those aged 65+ and by 11.4 per cent of those aged 75 or over (in 1985).

There are major regional variations concerning the number of beneficiaries, and the development over time (Appendix 6, Table 4). These variations are not easily interpreted. They suggest that the resources of the retired people and the particular local funding arrangements are more important than the disabilities of the elderly people.

In 1986, there were about 100 000 home helps, corresponding to about 40 000 full-time equivalents, as the majority worked part-time. This corresponds to a total of 5.7 per 1000 of people aged 65 or over.

2.1b. Staffing and tasks performed (Attias Donfut and Rozenkier 1981)
Home helpers are usually middle-aged women (half are between 45 and 60 years old). As we have just seen, they usually work part-time. Half of them have worked previously in a non-skilled manual job or in an office job. About a third are younger and have never had a job before. Their training is minimal, there are no statutory training requirements. A minority have taken specific training—subsidized by the Ministry for Solidarity—at a higher general level of training; such people are generally older, employed by the large municipalities, and have been in the post for more than two years.

A survey undertaken by the 'general regime' of Old Age Insurance (National Office for Old Age Insurance for Salaried Workers; CNAVTS) shows the following. Home helps basically do housework (particularly sweeping or hoovering—90 per cent of cases; cleaning furniture—75 per cent of cases; making the bed—50 per cent of cases; washing up—30 per cent of cases). Very often home helps carry out tasks which the elderly people could easily do themselves. They also help the elderly person maintain a relationship with the community, particularly by doing the shopping (27 per cent of cases), and, indeed, by household administration (7 per cent of cases). In a minority of cases, the home helps take over the preparation of the meals (9 per cent of cases) and of personal care, particularly washing (5 per cent) and taking a bath or shower (3 per cent).

Several problems emerge from this survey. The nature of the help given by the professionals varies. These variations are linked to the ambiguity concerning the role of the home help, underlined by the General Inspectorate of Social Affairs (IGAS) (1976) in its 1976 annual report, which finds that the use of material help as psychological help with isolation increases confusion. For the IGAS, the disability of the person should be the main criterion for the distribution of the service and the psychological aspect a secondary criterion. It is not right that, using the pretext of the psychological role of the home help, some services should not allow them to clean windows or wash floors. The previously mentioned definition of the role of the home help, in the context of the collective convention signed in 1983, does not clarify this ambiguity.

2.1c. Who benefits?
The origin of the request is, in a third of cases, a doctor, and, for a further third, a local council social worker. In three-quarters of cases, the reason is a health problem. The percentage of beneficiaries increases with the increase in age (Appendix 6, Table 6).

People who are incapacitated physically and have problems in the carrying out of household chores are seven times more likely to receive a home help than those who are not, particularly if they live alone (Curtis and Bucquet 1987). In the survey by the CNAVTS (Attias Donfut and Rozenkier 1981), people living alone represent 71 per cent of beneficiaries (out of 30 per cent of the population aged 65 or over). However, a scale of disability was constructed empirically from the results of a multivariate analysis of some variables of functional ability. This showed that the majority of beneficiaries (57 per cent) have little or no disability and that the very 'bad' cases represent about 6 per cent. Three out of four beneficiaries are women (60 per cent of the general elderly population) and the women are older than the men (average age of women, 79 years; average age of men, 76 years). The duration of care is greater than 60 months in 17 per cent of cases, and greater than 36 months in 18 per cent of cases. No data exist regarding the eventual discontinuation of the service provision.

The question of 'target efficiency' can be looked at from two perspectives: first, by looking at the proportion of those in need of home help who actually receive it (horizontal target efficiency); and secondly, by measuring the proportion of those in need among all recipients of home help (vertical target efficiency) (Bebbington and Davies 1983).

Three regional enquiries concerning the health of people of 65 or over carried out by a team from INSERM (Colvez *et al.* 1985) give an 'epidemiological' definition of home-help needs. The target group is composed of people living alone (or with others but not receiving help from within the household) *and* having a physical disability and/or unable to carry out housework.

By this definition of need, only 35 per cent of those in need actually receive home help, and of those receiving home help only 60 per cent need this service. Such findings raise questions about the distribution criteria of such a service, and about the factors responsible for such poor functioning: poor information; difficulties of access to the service; quantitative insufficiency; poor use of existing services due to imprecise distribution criteria and professional discretionary power (Henrard 1987).

The home-help service has seen a steady increase in the number of beneficiaries, the aggregate volume of hours of service, and expenditure. thus, in 1973, there were 115 000 beneficiaries of 18.4 million hours, and in 1985 there were 500 000 beneficiaries of 65 million hours; spending increased from 92.7 million fr. to 3.7 billion fr. In the same way, it is apparent that the average number of hours per beneficiary has diminished significantly, from 160 hours to 129 hours annually. This is because the decision makers recommended an increase in the number of beneficiaries, but the financial means have not followed suit since 1976. As far as the 'general regime' of Old Age Insurance is concerned, for example, the agreements between the regional offices and the associations of home-help services favour the awarding of help to people who need less than 15 hours of help per month. This is partly due to increased costs that followed the upgrading of the profession in 1983, as formalized by the collective convention, whereby it receives better training and higher salaries.

Table 5 in Appendix 6 shows the development in the distribution of the number of hours of home help received between 1977 and 1987 by those funded by the general old-age insurance scheme. There is a very noticeable increase in the percentage of beneficiaries receiving less than 2 hours per week, and only 8000 people benefited from significant help in 1987. This figure could be multiplied by two if the number of beneficiaries from other funding sources were included. It can thus be seen that the people with severe disabilities needing significant help rarely benefit from home help.

2.2. Home-nursing services for elderly people

2.2a. Organization, funding, and staffing

Although foreseen in the law of June 1975 relating to social and socio-medical institutions, regulations were not specified until six years later, in May 1981. Home-nursing services were recognized as one of the priorities of the minister responsible for the elderly, who defined the objectives and the operating conditions in a circular in October 1981 (Ministry of National Solidarity 1981). The objective assigned to them is to prevent, postpone, or shorten stays in hospital and in socio-medical establishments (governed by the hospital or social sector). Their principal function is to give nursing *and* personal care (by carrying out specific care that enables people to perform basic tasks of daily living). The care should be more continuous and better co-ordinated than that provided on a fee-for-service basis.

This service can be created and run by a public or private body: for example, by a social service centre of a municipal authority, a health centre or municipal nursing-care centre, a public or private retirement home, or a home-help association. Authorization to provide services under this law is given by the prefect (who is the state representative at the departmental level) after advice from the consultative regional board for social and medico-social institutions.

Home nursing is provided on medical prescription. Sickness insurance provides all the financing. The service functions on the basis of a provisional budget comprising a number of provisional days multiplied by an average daily allocation. The latter cannot be higher than the ceiling fixed jointly by the ministers responsible for health and social security, who are also responsible for the budget. This daily allocation was 116 fr. in 1987.

Home nursing theoretically functions for 12 hours a day. A salaried nurse co-ordinates and organizes the various interventions. The nurses employed can by salaried or be private, independent workers, in which case they reach an agreement with the managing body and have paid holidays. It is compulsory for auxiliary nurses to be salaried. More often than not, these professionals have not received specific training.

In 1984 there were 650 services employing 1400 salaried nurses and 3500 care assistants. More than 3500 independent nurses had reached an agreement with a care service. These services disposed of 22 200 'places' (bed equivalents; Ministry of Social Affairs and National Solidarity 1986*b*), corresponding to about 55 000 periods of care for 45 000 people. In 1987, there were 780 services and 28 200 'places', corresponding to about 57 000 beneficiaries and 70 000 periods of care, at a cost of 908 million fr. financed by sickness insurance schemes (nearly two-thirds by the general scheme).

In 1984 there were major geographical disparities. About a third of the *départements* had a capacity of less than 3.5 'places' for 1000 inhabitants of 75 years or over. Twelve *départements* benefited from a capacity of more than 10 'places' for 1000 people of 75 or over—the national average being 5.9 'places' for 1000 people of 75 or over. In 1986, the national average increased to 8 'places' for 1000 people of 75 or over.

As regards staffing of these services, the rates were 0.7 per thousand people aged 65 or over, and more than 1.4 per thousand people aged 75 and over in 1984.

2.2b. Who benefits?

The eligible population is theoretically those aged 60 years or over for whom nursing care at home has been prescribed by a doctor. The prescription depends on knowledge of the existence of the service by both the elderly people and their families, and by the doctors. It depends equally on the existence and availability of services. Need in itself does not therefore guarantee service provision. If it is estimated that about 500 000 people alone are dependent just for the activities of everyday life, then about 10 per cent benefit from the service, which necessarily implies that independent nurses, and especially the informal support of family and the neighbourhood, play a predominant role (Henrard 1987). The distribution of the rates of beneficiaries, according to age, is given in Appendix 6, Table 6. This clearly shows an increase with age, but also shows a relatively stable rate of meeting needs, the need for help increasing in frequency with age.

The functions most frequently carried out concern help with the activities of daily life: for example, 98 per cent of people receive help with washing, five to six times a week. Help with mobility and the prevention of pressure sores is given to two out of three people, about six times a week. Real nursing duties are only necessary for one person out of six (dressing of wounds, injections), indeed considerably less for some duties (intravenous feeding, washing and/or changing bladder catheters), about five times a week.

The average age of the population cared for is 81 years (79.5 years for men; 82 years for women); 80 per cent are over 74 years old. Some 90, 66 and 30 per cent of the beneficiaries of this service receive, respectively, daily help for two, three or all four basic activities of daily living (getting up, washing, getting dressed, eating); 43 per cent of the people suffer from incontinence and 40 per cent have psychiatric problems ranging from slight disorientation to senile dementia. On regrouping the problems of physical dependence, incontinence, and psychiatric disturbance, three groups emerge, according to their severity:

10 per cent are cases requiring only very little help with basic activities but having psychiatric problems or being incontinent;

54 per cent are more serious cases requiring partial help for all or some of the basic activities (28 per cent of them have psychiatric problems);

36 per cent are very limited in their abilities and need total help with all the basic activities (60 per cent have psychiatric problems).

Among those people receiving help, a quarter live alone, a third with their partner, and a third with a younger person. However, these data do not provide any information on the degree of social and family support.

The number of visits made by the service increases with the difficulty of the case, from an average of 7.6 visits to the least dependent to 10.3 to the most difficult cases.

Two-thirds of those receiving help cease to need help during the year, for 18 per cent this interruption is due to death, for 35 per cent to the deterioration of the condition requiring hospitalization, and, for 14 per cent, to recovery.

As a whole the study of the nursing services clearly shows that these provide care for a physically dependent population, about 40 per cent of which suffers from psychiatric problems and more than 40 per cent from incontinence. The beneficiaries appear to be well targeted. Links with other services and informal support will be considered below.

2.3. Other services

2.3a. Supervision

Two types of service can be identified, as follows.

A telephone alarm system. This has been organized by the general council in several *départements*, the implementation and management of which is usually conferred on a co-operative association of several local, municipal, or associative partners. The financing of the operation is jointly ensured by the *département* and the local authorities, and occasionally by the region when it concerns investment in the development of a telephone exchange. The scheme includes either a *départemental* telephone exchange linked to the public telephone network, or local listening centres at emergency services such as the fire brigade or establishments for elderly people. The telephone exchange or the listening centres, when called by the subscribing elderly person (to whom several types of alarms are available), mobilize volunteers in the neighbourhood. Those interested pay a subscription for the service.

Home carers. This function is not financed at the moment. When independent nurses offer this service, sickness insurance reimburses part of the expense on a poorly contracted basis; when it is for people who are seriously ill, some complementary retirement funds are willing to share the cost of night care, which is by staff who are usually not well qualified, and who are employed by associations or on their behalf. The bulk, if not all of the cost, rests on the elderly person or their family.

2.3b. Technical care

Apart from help provided by the home-nursing services, much technical help is given by medical auxiliaries working independently. It is known that care from auxiliaries increases with age. Their interventions are three and a half times more frequent among those over 79 years than in the general population (13.5 times a year rather than 4 times a year).

2.3c. Socialization

Apart from the clubs said to be for the 'third age' and the organization of travel, socialization in the home is not well developed in France. There are certainly organizations that send volunteers to visit isolated elderly people, but they vary in numbers. They are often from religious or Friendly societies. Some clubs, particularly those in rural districts, use volunteer visitors.

2.3d. Domestic tasks

Apart from home-help services, there are services for bringing meals to the home or ensuring more occasional help (helping out with small jobs, for example). These services are provided by the municipalities' local authority or by non-profit organizations, in which case they are subsidized by the municipality. They are more or less financed by the users, depending on their resources.

2.3e. Housing action

Because maintenance at home assumes there is a sufficiently comfortable house, programmes for home renovation have been made possible by premiums or subsidies from the state (Ministry for Social Affairs and/or Housing Ministry) or by retirement funds to the elderly owner-occupier, or by management (housing) associations, regrouped in the National

Federation for the Protection, Improvement, Preservation and Transformation of the Home. In each case, the beneficiary must have resources below a certain ceiling. The grant is awarded to make the house conform to the minimal norms of habitation and to save energy, to install modern conveniences, and adapt it to the needs of those physically handicapped. About 45 000 houses benefit from this annual programme.

2.3f. Cash payments

Some elderly people can benefit from social welfare payments, either those intended specifically for the elderly population or those for the disabled population (including elderly people). They are all means tested. They are financed by income tax. Thus the state finances basic allowances at home. The *département* finances allowances to cover home-help services when these services are insufficient in number; it also finances the third-person allowance for the disabled. The technical decision for its allocation is under the jurisdiction of COTOREP (Départemental Technical Commission for Vocational Rehabilitation and Guidance). The allowances are paid by the municipal social-service centre.

A housing allowance, which is means tested, can be allocated to an elderly person—or to a family with whom they live—by the Family Allowance Office. They allow the payment of a higher rent than the personal resources would make possible. Four billion and seven hundred million francs have been allocated by the Family Allowance Office to about 710 000 elderly beneficiaries.

2.3g. Financial incentives for families

Tax payers who take in a person of 75 or over can deduct from their gross income the benefits in kind which they provide up to a limit fixed at 14 000 fr. per elderly person cared for (the elderly person must not have resources above a certain ceiling). The situation is the same for tax payers who are relieved of the *obligation alimentaire* by taking in under their roof an older relative in need. Tax payers caring for a disabled person living with them are entitled to a tax reduction.

2.3h. Family placement

A law to facilitate long-term care in a family of one or two disabled people or dependent elderly people was passed in July 1989.

3. INFORMAL SUPPORT

Because of the growing number of older people living apart from their married children, because women are becoming more and more professionally active, and because the geographical mobility of the generations is increasing, it is often concluded that the ties between the generations are weakening. The increase in numbers of very elderly people in the decades to come is therefore felt to be catastrophic by funding agencies who think that all help for dependent elderly people must be provided by professionals.

In fact, living apart does not mean the absence of family support. Some demographers talk about 'cohabitation in the neighbourhood or nearby' (Roussel and Bourguignon 1976). We have already discussed the importance of informal help, given the poor supply of professional services.

Several recent studies confirm the importance of this support. Help in kind through services or temporary provision of a home during a crisis (widowhood, accident, illness, convalescence), for formerly retired people from the Paris region, was more frequent in 1986 than 10 years previously (Cribier 1989). The appearance of incapacities leads to a tightening of the family network, which provides an important social support in, for example, a rural population in the *Midi Pyrenees* region (Grand *et al.* 1989).

Three regional studies (Gauthier and Colvez 1989) (Appendix 6, Tables 7 and 8) show the importance of family help for elderly people confined to bed or armchair, and for people with one or several disabilities. The help becomes more frequent as the dependence becomes more severe.

A further study (Frossard and Ennuyer 1988), in two regions, of people receiving home-nursing care shows that informal support, particularly from the family, is predominant whatever the degree of dependence and even though the volume of help provided varies according to who provides the information (elderly person or principal helper).

So, all the studies show the importance of informal support, particularly for people severely dependent, and especially the importance of family support, particularly from women, whether spouses or daughters. More qualitative studies show that there is no standard behaviour and that the relationship between the helper and the helped is complex, being associated with objective factors (degree of dependence, duration of help, socio-economic situation of the helper) and subjective factors (sense of duty, moral rather than physical suffering, family conflicts) (Favrot 1986; Frossard and Ennuyer 1988). The situation also varies between rural districts, urban districts, and cities. Finally, the contribution of the professionals in relation to family support is complex and this dimension is rarely taken into account in France, where administrative and professional discourse is dominant.

4. CO-ORDINATION

A particularly complex problem is hidden behind this term. Even all the social actors—decision-makers, professionals, volunteers, and elderly people—support the idea of co-ordinating the policies and services intended for elderly people, the levels at which this should apply are rarely detailed (Henrard *et al.* 1989, p. 154).

Four levels must be clearly distinguished:

- the level of formal national policies in the statutory texts;
- the level of planning and programming of resources;
- the level of links between the service organizations;
- the final, individual level of co-ordination of various services for complex cases.

The first of these comes up against the bureaucracy of all the ministerial departments. Each office carves up the social field into target groups with corresponding, specialized allowances that satisfy the needs as defined in terms of norms and conditions of distribution, and each office manages its client population by specifying standardized regulations. In doing this, each is in competition with the other administrative offices responsible for the same population. Even though there is a minister responsible for elderly people, it seems impossible to impose or even negotiate a co-ordinated global policy to enable, for example, the redistribution of funds and personnel from the hospital sector into proper services for maintaining people at home.

The second level suffers from the distribution of powers between the state and the *départements* embodied in the decentralization laws of July 1983 and January 1986. The state is responsible for health planning at the regional level; the *départements* are responsible for their own planning of services, and for social and socio-medical institutions. This hardly facilitates joint planning between health and social care.

The third level concerns the institutional links between the services. At the time of the creation of the sectors of the programme for priority action as part of the seventh plan, some efforts were made, as we have shown, but they came up against the multiplicity of funders and management bodies. Only some local experiences have succeeded in creating lasting links between the parties involved.

Finally, the individual level was the object of the creation of co-ordinators in 1981. Their funding, initially subsidized by the state for a short period, was not taken over by local financing, so that most of the posts have been withdrawn.

On the whole, nobody is capable of mobilizing the different intervenors necessary to resolve complex cases, due to lack of budgetary flexibility and co-operation between the different professionals, the volunteers, and the informal helpers.

5. CONCLUSION

Le maintien à domicile, considered to be a priority by the public powers for nearly 30 years, has not seen the development expected. The fragmentation of responsibilities at all levels, the priority attached, since 1978, to the control of social expenditure, and the ignoring of the role of informal support have reduced this policy to some limited, 'pump priming' programmes. The recent decentralization of social action, particularly for elderly people, has aggravated the dichotomy between the health sector and the social sector.

Today the picture is one of numerous intervenors distributed very unequally within the whole area. The home-help service, the most important by far, remains a service for people whose resources are below a certain ceiling; the meeting of needs and the targeting of the beneficiary population are far from perfect. The home-nursing services cannot develop except through redeployment of the resources of the public hospital sector, which would raise much opposition.

As long as there is no one person responsible for the local policy, as long as the funders refuse to amalgamate the sums which they allot to a common fund, and as long as institutional links remain problematical, there is no hope of a real service for maintaining people at home, functioning 24 hours a day, 365 days a year, integrating all the providers; it is important that home help should become a service like all the rest, with better specified criteria for allocation.

Finally, it is essential that a complementary relationship should develop between professionals, volunteers, and informal helpers. The highly decentralized training and information could contribute to breaking down the stereotypes regarding the ties between generations, and the necessary professional response to dependent elderly people.

NOTES

[1] Social assistance ceiling: 2802 fr. per month for one person, on 1 January 1988; ceiling of 'general regime' of old-age insurance: 5920 fr. per month; minimum guaranteed wage: 4860 fr. per month on 1 June 1988.

[2] Obligation of family members to provide basic-needs maintenance.

REFERENCES

Attias Donfut, C. and Rozenkier, A. (1981). *Etudes et recherche. Vieillir chez soi* I: Les bénéficiares. National Office for Old Age Insurance for Salaried Workers, Paris.

Bebbington, A. and Davies, B. (1983). Equity and efficiency in the allocation of personal social services. *Journal of Social Policy*, **12,** 309–30.

Braun, T. and Stourm, M. (1988). *Dependent elderly people*. Ministry of Social Affairs and Employment, Documentation Francaise, Paris.

Colvez, A., Varnoux, N., and Bucquet, D. (1985). *Différences régionales de l'état de santé des personnes agées vivant à domicile*. INSERM Report U 164, Paris.

Commission for the Study of the Problems of Old Age (1962). *Politique de la vieillesse* (The Laroque report). Documentation Francaise, Paris.

Cribier, F. (1989). Les vieux parents et leurs enfants. *Gérontologie et Societé*, **48,** 35–50.

Curtis, S. and Bucquet, D. (1987). Characteristics of elderly people receiving home help in three regions of France. *Revue Epidemiologie et Santé Publique*, **35,** 318–22.

Favrot, G. (1986). L'activité de soins dans le système d'activité familial—facteurs d'insertion et de rejet. Ministry of Social Affairs, Paris.

Frossard, M. and Ennuyer, B. (1988). Travail familial, solidarité de voisinage et maintien à domicile des personnes agées. *Cahiers de l'Ecole Nationale de la Santé Publique*, **3,** 1–19.

Gaullier, X. (1986). Quel avenir pour le maintien à domicile des personnes agées? *Revue Francaise des Affaires Sociales,* **40,** 9–31.

Gauthier, A. and Colvex, A. (1989). Les enquêtes régionales sur l'etat de santé des personnes agées realisées en France entre 1978 et 1988. *Cahiers Statistiques Solidarité Santé* (Paris), **16,** 37–50.

General Inspectorate of Social Affairs (1976). *Les dépenses sociales: fonction vieillesse*, Annual Report 2, pp. 131–282. Paris.

General Planning Commissariat (1982). *Vieillir demain* (The Lion report). Documentation Francaise, Paris.

Grand, A. *et al.* (1989). La famille dans le support social des personnes agées. *Gerontologie et Societé*, **48,** 51–8.

Guillemard, A. M. (1986). *Le declin du social-formation et crise des politiques de la vieillesse*. Presses Universitaires de France, Paris.

Henrard, J. C. (1987). Blocage des filières de soins. *Revue Epidemiologie et Santé Publique*, **35,** 298–308.

Henrard, J. C., Ankri, J., Cassou, B., and Law-Koune, J. D. (1989). *Le système francais de soins et aides aux personnes agées—description et analyse de son fonctionnement*. CTNERHI–PUF, Paris.

Ministry of National Solidarity, Ministry for Health, Secretary of State for Elderly People (1981). *Personnes agées. Soins infirmiers à domicile*, Official bulletin, special section 81/43.

Ministry of Social Affairs and National Solidarity (1986*a*). *Circulaire No. 86–14*, 7 March, Paris.

Ministry of Social Affairs and National Solidarity (1986*b*). Les services de soins infirmiers à domicile pour personnes agées, caractéristiques, activités, clientèles. *Solidarité, Santé, Cahiers Statistiques*, **8** (Feb), 87.

Ministry of Solidarity, Health and Social Protection (1988). Elderly people in France. Some statistics. *Informations Rapides SESI,* **125,** 1–17.

National Office for Old Age Insurance for Salaried Workers (1978). *Action sanitaire et social. Aide ménagère à domicile. 1977 statistics*. Paris.

National Office for Old Age Insurance for Salaried Workers (1988). *Action sanitaire et social. Aide ménagère á domicile. 1987 statistics.* Paris.

Roussel, L. and Bourguignon, O. (1976). La famille après le mariage des enfants. *Cahiers de l'INED*, **78,** 1–268.
Secretary of State for Elderly people (1983). *National conference on the retired and elderly people*. French Health Education Committee, Paris.
State Ministry of Social Affairs (1972). *Circulaire No. 5 A.S.* 1st Feb. Paris.

6

Home-care services in the Federal Republic of Germany

Margret Dieck and Vjenka Garms-Homolová

6.1. Development of home-care services and policies for older people
1. The hierarchy of services and of service systems
2. The history of home-care services
3. The role of health insurance
4. The role of social welfare provision
5. Bridging the health and social-services systems: provisions for home care for frail people
6. The rationale behind service priorities, service hierarchies, and the inclusion or exclusion of elderly people
7. Organization and finance of formal home-care services
8. The extent of service provision

6.2. Allocation of home care in one federal state: a case study from Berlin (West)
1. The structure of the study
2. The functional capacity and structure of informal support as criteria of need for home-help services
   2.1. The distribution of the criteria of need
   2.2. The need for external support
3. Service provision in Berlin
   3.1. Claim entitlement and financing
   3.2. The main organizational form: the community-care centre
   3.3. The extent of provision
   3.4. Internal organization
4. Allocation and claim mechanisms
   4.1. The service from the provider's perspective
   4.2. The viewpoint of the referral agencies
   4.3. Home care and home help from the user's perspective

Notes

References

6.1 DEVELOPMENT OF HOME-CARE SERVICES AND POLICIES FOR OLDER PEOPLE

1. THE HIERARCHY OF SERVICES AND OF SERVICE SYSTEMS

There are three basic elements of community nursing:

(1) specialized nursing (*Behandlungspflege*)—nursing as support for medical treatment (e.g., injections, bandaging, insertion of catheters, treatment of pressure wounds);
(2) basic nursing (*Grundpflege*)—basic personal care: making of bed, appropriate body position, bathing, basic health monitoring like taking temperature, etc.;
(3) home help (*Haushaltshilfe*)—home making, running of household.

Within today's health services, this hierarchy of services is abundantly clear. Thus, as far as *health insurance* coverage is concerned, only the need of specialized nursing allows for provision of basic nursing as well as home help, if required. This is because nursing services at home are defined as adjuncts to medical treatment within health insurance, i.e., within the service system that offers either services in kind or full-cost insurance coverage for those deemed ill. Nursing services alone are not provided by health insurance but only if medical treatment is needed. However, within the means-tested, *social welfare* system, nursing services and home help can be provided to frail elderly people, even if they are not undergoing medical treatment.

From 1991, a new nursing service for the frail is provided by health insurance. It too is a 'pure' nursing service, plus home help if necessary. However, as such service is not part of medically oriented treatment, it is clearly limited (by the number of hours of delivery as well as by costs incurred by health insurance).

A schematic plan (Table 6.1) of the temporal development of types of home-care services in the Federal Republic of Germany (FRG) traces definitions as well as combinations of service in both the health insurance and the social welfare system of delivery. It lists types of home nursing or home care from (i) to (v) and types of home help from (a) to (f), and illustrates the various legal regulations.

2. THE HISTORY OF HOME-CARE SERVICES

The roots of the organized home-care services of today are in the traditional, comprehensive community care which was mainly offered by the parishes

Table 6.1. The development of types of home-care services[1] in the FRG

Year	Health insurance		Social welfare	
	Service delivery		Service coverage	
1911	Home nursing (i) encompassing help and supervision at home instead of hospital treatment as a discretionary service (*Hauspflege: Hilfe und Wartung*)			
1961 (1962)[2]			Home nursing (ii) encompassing supervision and care at home, provided either in kind or as cash reimbursement for informal carers (*Häusliche Pflege: Wartung und Pflege*)	Help in the running of the household (a) if no informal helper can take over and upkeep of the household is deemed necessary (*Weiterführung des Haushalts*)
1973 (1974)	Home nursing (i)	Home help (b) if patient or spouse cannot run the household during illness, no other household member can take over and a child under 8 years is in the household (*Haushaltshilfe*)		
1977 (1978)	Nursing care (iii) encompassing specialized nursing and possibly basic nursing instead of hospital treatment as a statutory service and as a service ensuring effects of medical treatment as a discretionary service. Provided in case no household members deliver service (*Häusliche Krankenpflege*)	Home-help (b)		

1981 (1982)	Nursing care (iii), now also to be provided by other nursing staff than registered nurses and nursing aides—e.g., by old people's nurses as well	Home help (b) and on a discretionary basis home help (c), which is not restricted to the condition of the child in the household and opens the possibility of reimbursing home help for an older person as well (*Haushaltshilfe*)	
1988 (1989)	Nursing care (iv) encompassing specialized nursing and possibly basic nursing as well as home-maker services (f), in general for a maximum of 4 weeks. Home-maker services include provision of meals, cleaning of rooms, laundry, shopping. Nursing care is provided as a statutory service instead of hospital treatment, as a discretionary service to ensure effects of medical treatment. Provided in case no household member can deliver service. (*Häusliche Krankenpflege—Behandlungspflege, Grundpflege, hauswirtschaftliche Versorgung*)	Home help (d) if patient is responsible for the running of the household and is prevented due to illness, no other household member can take over and a child under 8 years is in the household. Home help (e) also relates to prevention of the patient to run his/her household, but is not restricted to the condition of a child in the household. This service is discretionary (*Haushaltshilfe*)	
1988 (1991)			Home-nursing (v) for the very frail, encompassing basic nursing and home-maker services (f), limited to a maximum of 1 hour per service and 25 services per month (*Häusliche Pflegehilfe für Schwerpflegebedürftige—Grundpflege, hauswirtschaftliche Versorgung*)[3]

[1] Starting point is traditional home-care services, i.e., comprehensive community care developed within the social services, not closely defined but encompassing, in case of need, nursing care as well as home-help. Such service is provided if no household member or family member can render the service needed, mainly at the discretion of community nurses.

[2] The first year reported relates to the year in which the legislation was passed, the year in brackets relates to the year in which the legal provisions came into force.

[3] This service is covered by health insurance, but (in deviation from the general rule) by means of cost coverage, not service delivery in kind.

as part of charity, but was also always understood by the churches, both Protestant and Catholic, to be a branch of missionary work within the country. Community nurses employed by the political unit, the municipality, were rare and, in fact, continue to be so.

Aside from the churches, citizens themselves organized home-care services by means of self-help (i.e., members of a self-help organization were served by it in case of need) or as an expression of charity. These initiatives were taken because the poor laws did not provide for these services.

Both origins of home-care services continue to have an impact, for out of these roots have grown the six non-profit welfare organizations of today, who continue to run home-care and home-nursing services, so far in an almost exclusive position of market dominance.

Here and there the traditional type of community-care service still survives, although now it is largely limited to basic nursing, at a minimal level, and home help—without the former element of professional and specialized nursing that formed part of community care. This type of home care has continued to exist in Berlin (*Hauspflege*); it persists in other parts of the FRG as a type of social service. Since 1982, new legislation has provided an opportunity for remuneration of these services, now defined mainly as home-help services, by health insurance companies on a discretionary basis.

3. THE ROLE OF HEALTH INSURANCE

Statutory and nation-wide health insurance for the working population came into effect at the beginning of 1884. The elderly were not included in health insurance until 1941, i.e., after a considerable time lag. In 1911 the original pillars of the health services—ambulant medical services, medication and other products for health support, and hospital treatment—were extended to include home care. This step was taken with hesitation, on the following grounds: first, it was not clear whether provision of home care would be an effective means of reducing pension payments for invalidity; and secondly, the precondition of a service that was available in all regions could not be fulfilled by the home-care organizations, which were poorly developed and poorly financed. Nevertheless, home nursing (type i) was introduced as a discretionary service of health insurance, to be offered as a *substitute for hospital treatment*, i.e., as a means of filling the gaps which still existed in hospital provision in certain regions. In the thinking of that time, medical progress was bound to hospitals and they were therefore given priority. Even now, home nursing is mainly provided as a substitute for hospital treatment. In addition to this, the health insurance companies can, on a voluntary basis, fund services at home for people undergoing medical treatment in order to ensure its (positive) effects. This regulation has been in force since 1977 (Krankenversicherungs-Kostendämpfungsgesetz 1977); Marburger 1981; Poske 1986).

A *raison d'être* for the home-help services provided and financed by statutory health insurance was the provision of a service *for mothers and infants*. This historical root is still to be found in today's regulations (see Table 6.1; types b and d). Originally, home-making services were provided as an addendum to ambulant nursing services to households where there was a child under the age of 8 years or a handicapped child, and where no other household member was able to provide the care needed. This narrow regulation excluded ill elderly people as possible recipients of the home-making service, until a new law ('Krankenhaus-Kostendämpfungsgesetz' 1981) opened up for the additional discretionary services of health insurance organizations in 1982 (home-help types c and later e).

Finally, it must be mentioned that home care is provided on the basis of 'statutory insurance in case of accidents encountered in connection with gainful employment'. Since 1926, home-care provision within that branch of insurance had not been restricted as an alternative to hospital treatment. It could be provided for people who only needed nursing care not medical treatment. Because accidents could lead to long-term impairment, home care provided by family members could also be encouraged by payment of small lump sums to meet part of the additional expenses to the household. Basically, these stipulations remain unchanged today. Elderly people are not the target group, although they are at the same time not excluded from service provision.

4. THE ROLE OF SOCIAL WELFARE PROVISION

Before the new social welfare legislation in 1961 (Bundessozialhilfegesetz 1961), home care did not form part of the range of services provided routinely within poor-law regulations. The new concept of social welfare led to the introduction of home nursing (type ii) for persons not able to care for themselves because of handicaps or illness. Social welfare administrations may pay lump sums to clients in order to cover additional costs to the household; they may finance the contributions of the main carer to his/her own statutory pension insurance; or they may cover the costs of organized, formal, home care (*Häusliche Pflege*).

Provision is also made within social welfare legislation for services that ensure the running of the household of a person who cannot undertake all aspects of housework themselves. Included are services for members of the household that concern their personal needs, i.e., this service is defined rather widely in order to cover any situation of need for home-help services—even including aspects of home-care (home-help type a). There is, however, an intended restriction on the time span; this service is not provided indefinitely. But, in practice, restrictive time limits seem not to be imposed on clients (Brandt 1988).

In 1984, the social welfare legislation (Haushaltsbegleitgesetz 1984), emphasized that priority should be given to services for people in their own homes rather than in institutions. The reason given by parliament was that services provided at home are at the same time more humane, more appropriate and, last but not least, less costly.

Social welfare payments as well as services are always *means tested* in Germany. This test not only concerns the welfare recipient but also the family members, who are by civil law obliged to provide support within certain limits. For the elderly this means that their sons or daughters, if earning their own living or having capital (even a rather modest amount) will have to be means tested and may have to pay for the upkeep of their parents. Means testing is a strong deterrent to utilization of organized services as opposed to informal care, quite apart from the actual financial burden. Three states (Berlin, Bremen, and Rhineland–Palatine) have introduced allowances allocated on the basis of disability rather than of financial means (see below).

5. BRIDGING THE HEALTH AND SOCIAL-SERVICES SYSTEMS: PROVISIONS FOR HOME CARE FOR FRAIL PEOPLE

The health insurance reform of 1988 has introduced a home-nursing service (type v) combined with a home-making service (type f) geared to the very frail living at home. In fact, this can be taken to be a kind of revival of traditional community-care services, as basic nursing and home care are again closely linked in one service for clients who do not clearly fit into the service system directed towards the (acutely) ill. This new arrangement was introduced in January 1991, so it is not yet possible to assess its full impact.

Within the legislation are decreed clear restrictions on service delivery as to time (a maximum of 1 hour per service), the number of services (a maximum of 25 services per month), and total costs (a maximum of DM 750 per month). This is exceptional, for services are normally rendered in kind by health insurance. The 'normal' (in kind) procedure continues to be in force for nursing care and home help offered to ill people in need of medical treatment (nursing care type iv, and home help types d and e).

6. THE RATIONALE BEHIND SERVICE PRIORITIES, SERVICE HIERARCHIES, AND THE INCLUSION OR EXCLUSION OF ELDERLY PEOPLE

Within statutory health insurance, home care (type i) was first provided from 1911, although on a discretionary and restricted basis (as an alternative to hospital treatment). This service included home making as well as nursing care (basic and specialized). Elderly people were, in general, excluded on the assumption that they would be likely to need not medical treatment but primarily, through frailty, nursing care.

Between 1973 and 1977 a diversification, accompanied by specialization, took place in health services provision (Leistungsverbesserungsgesetz 1973; Rehabilitationsangleichungsgesetz 1974; Krankenversicherungs-Kostendämpfungsgesetz 1977). In 1973, nursing care and home-making services were separated. This step allowed for specialization of nursing services, made most explicit in 1977 when it was decreed that such services (basic nursing as well as specialized nursing) were only to be covered by health insurance under condition that they were offered by trained nursing staff (registered nurses, registered nursing aids, children's nurses, but not old peoples' nurses, already well established as a profession) (nursing care type iii). At the same time, provision of nursing care became mandatory as a substitute for hospital treatment; on a discretionary basis, health insurance companies could, in addition, finance nursing care in order to secure the positive effects of medical treatment. This step was taken in response to pressure from municipalities and states, who wished to finance their newly founded 'social stations' (*Sozialstationen*, i.e. community-care centres); see Section 7 below and 6.2, Section 3.2 *et seq.*) as the main agents of community nursing not only through social welfare but also through health insurance. There was an outcry among the organizations catering for elderly people. Because old peoples' nurses were excluded, it was obvious elderly people were not a target group for this new legislation and the services it brought about.

The legal basis of home care for the elderly within health insurance changed in 1982 (Krankenhaus-Kostendämpfungsgesetz 1981). For nursing care (iii), the restriction of services remunerated to the above named professions was abandoned. Now all nursing professions as well as other persons able to offer the necessary services could be financed. And the already mentioned change concerning home-making services took place, so that health insurance companies could now, in their own right, decide to provide support to others than the small and closely defined group who receive a mandatory service. At last, home-making services were, under restricted conditions, offered to elderly people as well, or to households that looked after an elderly frail person (home help type c). (This legislative change later led to the incorporation of home-care services, up to then run separately, into the 'social stations' of Berlin).

Health-care services in general rely on need attested by a medical doctor and they are given in kind (with the exception of sickness benefits). Home care, since the very beginning of its introduction into health-care legislation, is quite another matter. The principle of *subsidiarity* is important here: services or financial support for nursing or home making are only provided if no other member of the household can do so. The old *hierarchy* remains as far as health legislation is concerned: specialized nursing is provided as an addendum to medical treatment; basic nursing as an addendum to specialized nursing; home-making services (except to replace sick mothers and housewives) as an addendum to specialized nursing. And within the home-care and home-nursing services we encounter the principle of subsidiarity in so far as formal care is only provided if informal services are not available. This principle is most strongly upheld in welfare legislation, where responsibility for such services originally developed.

Two aspects of this hierarchy are worth noting, because they are fundamental to the German system of health and social care. First, the linking of home-nursing and home-making services to medical treatment, which until now has been a basic principle guiding health insurance cover. This means that frail elderly people in need of care, but not in need of medical treatment, are excluded from provision within health insurance. If they and their nearest relatives (children or parents) have no financial means, social welfare provision will step in. This dominance of medical treatment over nursing and social support, which effectively excludes chronically frail people from a right to services, has been much criticized and debated. Different government commissions have been at work, draft legislation has been presented in parliament, but, for reasons of cost, no major change has been made. It is possible, however, that the ground is now cleared for change: the new health reform of 1988, which took effect from 1991, has introduced the concept of home care (albeit of limited amounts) for frail and severely impaired people (who do not necessarily need medical treatment). It is too soon to judge the possible impact of this reform. It does seem, however, that it will no longer be possible to argue reasons of *principle* for excluding frail people, and as such this piece of legislation may turn out to be more significant than was perhaps intended, although its effectiveness will depend on the willingness to provide finance.

The second aspect of the hierarchy concerns the stress on family obligation. This has always been on the agenda in the debates about both health insurance and social welfare legislation. When home-making services were first covered by health insurance in 1973, this included help or financial support for relatives providing care. This was changed in 1977, after protests from the insurance organizations and the medical profession that family members had a moral obligation (*sittliche Verpflichtung*) to help each other. Similarly, the duty of children to provide for their parents is emphasized within social welfare legislation. Thus monetary support can be enforced by law but personal services cannot. The principle of subsidiarity works in the following way: if there is informal service provision, no formal services are offered; if formal services are needed, then, in the first instance, the family has to pay for them (except for services covered by insurance), and only if the family is unable to pay do the formal providers step in.

During this long period of rearranging home-nursing and home-making services within health insurance, and, in fact, within the adjacent legislation, which extends over the 1970s and 1980s, social welfare regulations in the field have remained unchanged and undebated. What has, however, been a constant point of discussion is the financial load that municipalities have to carry in order to meet the costs of nursing care, mainly within institutions.

7. ORGANIZATION AND FINANCE OF FORMAL HOME-CARE SERVICES

As described above, the field is dominated by non-profit making, charitable organizations. Up to 1970, services were mainly provided by community-nursing organizations closely linked to the churches, and by nurses employed by the parishes themselves. There were also some voluntary organizations outside the church. Because of a lack of personnel, the situation became rather alarming, as shown by information from the Catholic, non-profit, welfare organization (*Deutscher Caritasverband*): between 1957 and 1970 the number of home-care organizations fell by 24 per cent; the available nursing staff (mainly nuns) decreased by 41 per cent; the average age of community nurses was 58 years (Dieck 1979, p. 124).

Such is the background to efforts by different states of the FRG to create new organizational forms within which home care would be made available. Instead of mainly 'one or two women's organizations', which expected total commitment for little pay from their staff, these new organizations employed 'worldly' people. They aimed to improve working conditions, and the co-ordination and supply of services. This was the time of the conception of the so-called social stations, first in the state of Rhineland-Palatine in 1970. (Berlin, the last state to introduce social stations, started its programme in 1982.) One main reason for their success in comparison with other organizations since 1970 lies in the financial promotion programmes designed by different states, and also in the access to increased finance from health insurance bodies. A service which formerly had been offered free of charge (community nursing) was now more and more effectively oriented towards schedules of fees, to be reimbursed by health insurance, by the patients, or by social welfare. This orientation came from the schedules already operating for ambulant medical services.

The network of finance running to different organizations in different regions of the FRG is rather intricate. It is not that other organizations than social stations are excluded from it, but it is safe to say the social stations are well in the middle of this web.

In recent years, a growing number of nurses have decided to work freelance in this market or have joined newly developed, for-profit, nursing organizations. Home-makers' services are, in any case, mostly privately organized and financed, if not provided by the informal care system. The market of home-care and nursing services continues to be dominated by non-profit welfare organizations. In the early 1970s, they controlled between 70 and 80 per cent of the market (Dieck 1979, p. 121). Today, all the social stations in Berlin are run by non-profit welfare organizations. In Northrhine-Westphalia in 1988, nearly all home-care and community-nursing organizations were run by non-profit welfare organizations, and very few were run by municipal organizations.

The sources of finance vary greatly but the following examples go some way to explaining the present situation.

The Protestant church and its welfare organization (*Diakonisches Werk*) investigated the finances of its community-nursing organizations (a total of 2923) in 1967, i.e., before organizational reform was implemented. The finance came from the sources shown in Table 6.2 (Thermann 1970): We can compare this information with data from Northrhine-Westfalia in 1983 and 1987 (Table 6.3); all types of home-care and nursing-care organizations are taken into account (Bäcker *et al.* 1989, p. 283). Service organizers

Table 6.2. Sources of finance in 2923 community-nursing organizations in 1967

Source	Percentage contribution
Contributions by the church/of service organizer	58
Payments by help recipients	14
Subsidies from municipalities	11
Charitable contributions	10
Pension insurance	4
Social welfare administrations	3
Health insurance	1

Table 6.3. Sources of finance in home-care and home-nursing organizations in Northrhine-Westphalia, 1983 and 1987

Source	Percentage contribution	
	1983	1987
Health insurance	27	38
Contribution by service organizer	22	12
Subsidies from municipalities	18	14
Subsidies from the state	11	9
Payments by help recipients	12	13
Social welfare administrations	10	8
Other sources	–	7

organizers have managed increasingly to withdraw their own revenue from service financing. The municipalities and the states, and also social welfare budgets, have become more important as sources of revenue. Nothing much has changed for the recipients of help. Most striking is the increase in finance from health insurance. Here are the effects of the legislative changes of 1977 and 1982, which facilitated access by the elderly population to services remunerated by health insurance. If trends demonstrated in Northrhine-Westphalia continue, home care and nursing care will, in the future, become increasingly a service of the health system as opposed to their development within the social services system.

8. THE EXTENT OF SERVICE PROVISION

Service provision for elderly people living in their own homes and not in institutions (and these are 95 per cent of the 65+ age group) continues to be a family task in Germany. The main carers are the spouse (wife or husband) as well as the daughters and, to a lesser extent, daughters-in-law and sons. Neighbours and friends will help with errands and some household chores, but will normally refrain from nursing care. The same is true for voluntary workers.

It is estimated that in 1976 to 1978, when Socialdata investigated the nursing and home-making needs of the population of the FRG, we had the following proportions of elderly, impaired/frail people dependent on help and service in their everyday life at home (Brög *et al.* 1980): population aged 65+ years, 18 per cent; population aged 65 to 79 years, 12 per cent; population aged 80 and over, 53 per cent. Based on this investigation, according to which some 1.5 per cent of those aged 65+ received organized support services at home, we calculate an average coverage of not more than 3 per cent today. Provided that these figures come near to reality, then 15 per cent of the 65+ age group living at home is cared for solely within the informal system, whilst 3 per cent receives formal and informal care.

No reliable comparisons can be made for estimating the growth and development of services over time. According to the findings of different investigations carried out in the 1970s, elderly people already constituted 80 to 90 per cent of the clients of some community services (Dieck 1979, p. 134). What has changed is the composition of the service or, perhaps more precisely, the labels attached to services provided, because of changes in finance and the time accorded to one unit of service.

Another approach to the question of service provision is based on the numbers of (full-time equivalent) nursing staff per 1000 of the population aged 65+. A recent compilation of data gives figures (Table 6.4) for 1986 (Baum *et al.* 1989). Such ratios give no information on the percentage or

Table 6.4. The number of (full-time equivalent) nurses per 1000 of the elderly population aged 65+ years in various cities

Berlin	5.4	Dortmund	2.4
Hamburg	2.9	Stuttgart	3.0
Munich	2.3	Düsseldorf	1.4
Cologne	1.5	Bremen	1.6
Essen	1.5	Duisburg	3.5
Frankfurt	2.2	Hannover	2.8

number of elderly people receiving home-nursing services, because the distribution of services to different groups of recipients is unknown. However reliable or unreliable the reported ratios may be, they can be contrasted with the planning figures from the mid-1970s. At that time, indices for planned coverage by the nursing service varied between 0.2 and 0.3 per 1000 of the total population (Dieck 1979, p. 135). In 1986, the ratio reached is reported to amount to 0.4 per 1000 of the total population, or to 2.4 per 1000 of the population aged 65+, i.e., the indices once planned have been surpassed, on average, some 10 years later.

Because of the difficulties in estimating service coverage, it will become clear that general data on the type of service distributed and the age of recipients are not forthcoming. The near total neglect of statistical evidence of community-service coverage seems to indicate the lack of importance attached to such services, whatever the rhetoric may be.

Home-making services, separate from nursing care, are a topic in themselves. Since Blume (1968) compiled his findings from various investigations into the living conditions of elderly people, it has remained a well-proven fact that housework is one of the problem areas for many living alone or as a couple, and that about 10 per cent of households with a head aged 65+ report unmet needs in this respect. In more recent studies, the comparable percentages vary greatly, and further figures are not presented here. It is obvious, however, that household support tends to be needed primarily for more strenuous work such as hanging curtains, cleaning windows, cleaning staircases and pavements, wiping floors, changing beds, etc. If such strenuous work is not done by a family member or a friend or neighbour, which would be normal, then home helps tend to be hired privately. In fact, pure home-making services are seldom offered by social stations today. They are, if in existence, the realm of traditional organizations operating in the field, dedicated to the concept of home care (see above). Interestingly enough, most studies of the living conditions of elderly people do not take the trouble to differentiate between self-organized home-making services and those offered by social services.

We do know from a number of studies that the willingness of elderly people and/or their families to take in organized nursing services is not generally very great. This attitude is based on norms concerning filial duty, and it may well be enhanced by the conditions under which community nursing care is offered: clients do not always know what to expect or how much the service might cost them. Rejection of help from outside the household and family or the closer circle of neighbours and friends seems even stronger with regard to home-making services. In a study by Münster (1980) only half of the elderly people who reported difficulties with household chores were interested in additional help. In Baden-Württemberg the elderly people who were deemed in need of home-making services but were not receiving any argued they did not wish to burden anyone, or that they were just managing, or that they did not have the necessary financial means (Ministerium für Arbeit, Gesundheit und Sozialordnung 1983). A study from Berlin (Kuhlmeyer 1974) suggested that many elderly people, although in need of help, were unwilling to accept a stranger into their house, even if they could pay for this help themselves.

6.2 ALLOCATION OF HOME CARE IN ONE FEDERAL STATE: A CASE STUDY FROM BERLIN (WEST)

1. THE STRUCTURE OF THE STUDY

This case study[1] shows that the introduction of community-based services brings about changes which are not always improvements, and that even the improvements reached remain limited if the services offered are not matched to needs, i.e., if they fail to cover the necessary range with the necessary continuity and flexibility, and, moreover, if they function selectively and without co-ordination. The study focuses on home care and home help, the services which combine the management of the household with social and personal support. As already argued, in the FRG and the federal state of Berlin (West), the region of this case study, these services do not command any priority. They are largely provided as secondary services to back up nursing care and are neither well enough developed nor satisfactorily organized. These services are placed on the fringe of both health care and social services—a position which, given the strict separation between these, proves time and again to be a precarious one. In some respects, claim entitlement is governed by the criteria of the health-care system (the health insurance institutions), despite the fact that the service, and especially the need in question, is at odds with these criteria.

This case study of domiciliary care in one 'city state' in the FRG has three parts. The first is an estimation of care needs from the personal characteristics of 70- to 90-year-old inhabitants, which takes due account of the potential for help of the informal support network. The study pays only scant attention to the extent to which use is actually made of the organized services.

The second part concentrates on the following questions:

- Which services are available in the area of the study?
- What is the nature of formal claim entitlements?
- How are home care and home help allocated in this region?

The third, explorative part examines allocation and claim mechanisms, and the corresponding routines from the perspectives of the service providers, the relevant 'gate-keepers', and the users.

2. THE FUNCTIONAL CAPACITY AND STRUCTURE OF INFORMAL SUPPORT AS CRITERIA OF NEED FOR HOME HELP

Our approach to the need[2] for home help/home care is based on two different dimensions: first, the need arising from restricted functional capacities for coping with the activities of daily living; and secondly, the lack of informal support. Proceeding from the notion of criteria of cumulative need, this part presents some findings on the extent of the need for home help/home care. The assessment is based on data that have been compiled within the framework of a survey[3] of the metropolitan population born between 1897 and 1916.

2.1. The distribution of the criteria of need

Gerontological studies measure functional status by means of so-called scales of activity of daily living (the ADL index). Our survey draws on two instruments. First, the index developed by Katz *et al.* (1963), with 14 items all relating to elementary activities, e.g., 'to walk between rooms', 'to get in and out of bed', etc. Secondly, the index of 'instrumental ADL' with eight items (Lawton and Brody 1969), which has activities like 'to go shopping for groceries or clothes', 'to handle money', etc. Our data are based on self-assessments by the respondents. The classification scheme is based on help needed and difficulties in performing the tasks. The items are rated on a 4-point scale: 'without difficulty', 'with difficulty but without help', 'not unaided', and 'not possible'.

We first made a summary assessment of functional capacities to get a general idea of the order of magnitude of need. We then examined the functional abilities for individual activities to find sub-groups among the aged population whose functional capacities were diminished in certain areas. Such an analysis provides indications of the type of help required. Both approaches are adopted in the following.

1. An index has been constructed (Appendix 7, Fig. 1) for the summary assessment of functional ability. The results show that functional disabilities increase with age, and are most frequent among women, especially among those aged 85 years or more. Ninety per cent of 70- to 74-year-old men but only 40 per cent of the 85- to 89-year-old men had no difficulty in performing the activities of daily living concerned. Within these age groups the proportion of fully capable women shrinks from 80 to 26 per cent, respectively. The proportion with multiple impairment of activities is 7 per cent of the 70- to 74-year-old men and women, but 42 per cent of the 85- to 89-year-old men, and as much as 52 per cent of the women at this age.

2. Our second step of assessment aimed at the activities of daily living that may cause particular problems. A number of basic activities, e.g., dressing, eating, going to bed, were handled without difficulty by the large majority of respondents, even by the oldest amongst them. For activities that demand greater physical strength and/or more mobility (e.g., carrying heavy loads, cutting toe-nails), the impact of age was clearly apparent, especially among men, but the deterioration seemed to start at an earlier age in women: in the 70- to 74-year-old group, a higher percentage of women than men reported being unable to carry out such 'difficult' activities. For activities involving mobility outside the home (going for a walk, coping with stairs, etc.), the reduction in functional capacities was only clearly noticeable among our oldest respondents (men and women of 85 years and over).

An increasing number of the activities required for maintaining independence became problematical with advancing age. The need for support in the 'younger' cohorts of old people mainly concerned activities requiring muscular strength. A need for help with light housework and daily housekeeping was identifiable mainly amongst the oldest respondents. Generally speaking, the need for support as identified by the criterion of functional capacity was clearly related to the age and sex of the population.

3. *Household structure and marital status*. Next we turned to the structure of social relationships and the availability of people whose help could compensate for the old person's deficiency in coping with the activities of daily living. Here especially household structure and marital status were considered. In the main, we found only two types of households: the single-person household and the so-called marital household (see Garms-Homolová and Hütter 1988*a,b*). The majority of women lived in single-person households. Only between 20 and 25 per cent of men lived alone, except for the oldest group, where the figure was 40 per cent. Marital status was the main determinant of this structure: to be widowed, unmarried, divorced, and separated meant largely to live in a single-person household; the married old people, mostly men, lived in two-person households and were, once in need of help, in a position to ask for basic support. As we have reported elsewhere, care giving by the spouse is of fundamental importance. Only a small minority of married men and women did not have any care-givers in the event of illness. But among unmarried people, the proportion without care-givers was significantly higher: 32 per cent of the unmarried men and 47 per cent of the unmarried women. Increasing age was also associated with a general reduction in the informal social network available. Here too sex-specific effects were evident: in each age group, more women than men had no children and, except for the oldest age groups, it was more often women who had no siblings.

As regards use of services, this was associated with levels of functional ability—the more the disabilities, the greater the use of community services. But this use was also relatively greater amongst women, which suggests that the availability of informal support is important.

2.2. The need for external support

In order to identify the need for support, we selected activities of daily living from the ADL index that could be covered by services provided within the framework of home help/home care. These are: strenuous housework (e.g., cleaning windows), carrying heavy loads, light housework (e.g., washing dishes), shopping for food and clothing.

In establishing the level of need for help, the following alternative responses served as the criterion: 'I am unable to do this unaided' or 'I am unable to do this at all'. On this basis the following classification was made:

- No need for help: all four activities can be carried out unaided.
- Some need for help (low level): strenuous housework and/or carrying heavy loads is only possible, if at all, with help.
- Distinct need for help (high level): light housework and/or shopping only possible, if at all, with help (strenuous work cannot be carried out).

This classification serves as a basis for estimating the levels of support needed. Whereas strenuous housework only has to be done occasionally, perhaps once a week, light housework has to be done virtually daily. Table 1 in Appendix 7 shows that need for help increases with age, and that women need help at an earlier age than men. The higher impairment rate among the cohorts of younger old women clearly results from activities which call for physical strength.

This distribution of the need for help cannot be equated with the need for organized services. Although the basis is the impairment of functional capacities, the resulting need for organized services is linked to a second, necessary condition: that the help required cannot be provided by other members of the household. These considerations led to the construction of a second index, which made it possible to focus more on the need for external support by organized services. The decisive criterion is whether or not people live alone. On this basis a new scale was constructed:

- no need for external support;
- low level of need for external support;
- high level of need for external support.

Table 2 in Appendix 7 shows that for all age groups the need for external support was considerably higher for women than for men. There were women in all age groups with a high level of need for external support, whereas only the oldest group of men had such levels of need. More than a quarter of women over 85 years of age had a high level of need for external support (compared with only 11 per cent of men).

The indices constructed here undoubtedly mirror extremes of need, with the general need for support based exclusively on functional capacities demarcating the upper limit, and that concerned with the specific need for external support representing the lower limit, which assumes a well-functioning, informal support network. This assumption is problematical for two reasons. First, in the population group surveyed here, multi-person households were usually married couples, where both members were of advanced age and where the functional abilities of both were at best threatened with impairment. The death of one spouse leaves a gap which is difficult to fill. Abrupt changes in need must therefore be expected, which almost overnight can transform a minimum need for external support into the above-mentioned high level of need.

Both extremes in need assessment are contrasted in graphic form (Appendix 7, Fig. 2). The increase in the levels is charted out for the different age cohorts, this information at the same time indicating the amount of latent need, which is marked by the possibility of loss of the spouse, and which increases in the higher age groups and differs first and foremost by gender. Women of all age groups under review had a lower level of informal support available. On the upper rim of the figure, we see the low level of need for external support, which, in the best case, could be satisfied by sons and daughters, other relatives, neighbours, friends, etc. Their willingness to do so, however, cannot be predetermined. Nevertheless, this basis weakens progressively with increasing age as the number of relevant social relationships decreases through deaths among the close relatives and friends around the very old person. The most problematical group is older women who live alone and who are economically weak. Compared with men or other women who do not live alone, they had the lowest net household income and were the least likely of all the groups under review here to be able to afford services against payment. This group ought to be the prime target for service provision.

3. SERVICE PROVISION IN BERLIN

Service provision in the FRG and Berlin was outlined above. To summarize briefly, there are:

(1) nursing services—
    (a) specialized nursing;
    (b) basic nursing;
(2) Home care—basic personal care and home making, and 'home help'—home-making services.

Our analysis focuses on the services under (2), although for reasons we shall next explain, one cannot understand their operation without considering nursing services.

3.1. Claim entitlement and financing

Home care and home help were formally created to help persons with impaired functional abilities to cope with everyday living. The limitations of these services, however, become evident if one examines the criteria of entitlement, financing, and allocation. The problems which emerge here curtail substantially the scope of the care provision. Some of these problems are examined in the following.

3.1a. The allocation of home care/home help depends on home nursing

Until recently the costs of home care/home help were only paid by the health insurance institution as statutory payments in conjunction with nursing (para. 185b, Section 4, Reich Insurance Code) (Reichsversicherungsordnung [RVO] 1986). This coupling has by no means been divorced by the new law (para. 37, *Gesundheitsreformgesetz* [GRG] 1988, 1989). 'Home help' is still part of home nursing. Additionally the health insurance institution can reimburse the costs incurred by their members who have children under 8 years of age (para. 38[2] GRG 1988, 1989). This new law emphasizes the fact that illness is the decisive criterion for the granting of home care and home help as a statutory payment by the health insurance institution. If patients do not require medical treatment but only care, they cannot claim reimbursement of the costs by the health insurance institution. A very old patient is automatically suspected of not being ill but dependent on care, and consequently the cost reimbursement can be stopped at any time.

3.1b. Service orientation instead of patient orientation

The purpose of providing home help/home care is to prevent or shorten a stay in hospital, to guarantee the necessary medical and care provision, and to ensure continued household management. Home help can also be granted as a 'corollary' to nursing if hospitalization is necessary but impracticable, or when out-patient medical treatment presupposes such help. These criteria clearly show that the 'need' for these services has little to do with the 'personal need' of the patients, i.e., with their functional impairments in coping with day-to-day living and running their homes. Instead, it is the requirements of the care system which are of primary importance. In principle, thus, these services can be used to regulate the duration of hospitalization and ensure a balance between in-patient hospital care on the one hand and community medical care on the other.

3.1c. Dependence on household structure and the informal network

As in the case of nursing, the health insurance institutions only cover the costs of home help/home care if the services cannot be provided by persons living in the patient's household (paras. 37 and 38, GRG 1988, 1989). Care-givers who are related to the patient by blood or marriage (up to second degree) are not entitled to any reimbursement. Reimbursement of travel costs and loss of earnings are a discretionary matter and remain specific to each individual case. But, in principle, being limited in time, these services call for supplementary services from the informal social network. The number of hours of care required per day and week is determined by the social worker at the community centre. The maximum claim period is four weeks; exceptionally the time can be prolonged. The medical service of the health insurance institution examines if the requirement is for longer or not. In many cases it is not possible to ensure continuity of funding and discontinuities arise long before the end of the claim period is called into question. As mentioned already in 6.1, from January 1991, a change came into force. It will improve the situation at least of the people heavily dependent on care and of their relatives. The term 'heavily dependent on care' in this context means that the person 'is helpless and continuously needing intense help for all regularly recurring activities' (para. 53[1], GRG 1988, 1989). These persons—so-called *Schwerpflegebedürftige*—get help for management of the household lasting up to 1 hour per visit and up to 25 visits per month. Yet the costs which the health insurance institution will reimburse must not exceed DM 750 per case (para. 55[1], GRG 1988, 1989). Since 1 January 1989, it has also been possible to get so-called *Urlaubspflege*—care during the holidays of the informal helpers. This provision covers up to four weeks and 1800 DM (para. 56, GRG 1988, 1989).

3.1d. Criteria for receiving support from social assistance

If the health insurance institution is not willing to pay for home care/home help, funding may be forthcoming from the social assistance institutions under the provisions of the Federal Social Assistance Act (BSHG, para. 68; BSHG Care assistance, para. 69; Home care, para. 70; Maintenance of the home). This type of funding, however, is only granted after a means test and can therefore also have financial implications for close relatives.

3.1e. High costs

In the event that no claim can be made on the health insurance institution and the person in need of home care/home help does not qualify for social assistance, he or she has to pay privately for the services required. The rate is currently being revised in connection with a number of quality requirements, especially improving the staff's qualifications. (Abgeordnetenhaus von Berlin 1990) At present, private service providers occasionally have lower rates. An army of unskilled people (foreigners and immigrant Germans from Eastern-bloc countries) offers unqualified service (housekeeping) at considerably lower rates.

For a particular group of people, which includes the blind and the severely sight-impaired, the deaf, and the totally dependent, an entitlement to care is offered, in Berlin, by way of partial compensation under the terms of the Care Benefits Act. This benefit is not affected by the individual's income. It is intended to cover partly the additional costs incurred by the special nature of the affliction. The amount awarded depends on the degree of disability or dependence[4] and is therefore oriented towards the individual concerned. The degree of disability or dependence is determined by medical examination. In order to qualify for the higher grades of care benefit, a recognized, extraordinary, care need is required.[5] The benefit granted under the terms of this legislation takes the form of both monetary and non-monetary awards. The latter include an entitlement to up to 48 nursing visits per year and, in addition, help may be claimed for keeping the home running if the care-giver is absent. The above-mentioned benefits are curtailed if the person in need can enforce statutory claims arising from such need for care elsewhere, or if he or she is an in-patient for more than one month. This regulation is valid only in the city state of Berlin. A federal law came into force on 1 January 1991. The health insurance institution may pay DM 400 per month instead of the reimbursement for home help, when applied for by a person heavily dependent on care (para. 57[1] GRG 1988, 1989).

3.1f. Selectivity and discontinuity

The features of claim entitlement and allocation show that home help/home care is available only to a limited group of persons and that the make-up of such groups also differs, depending on the funding institution. This selectivity results in discontinuity in care provision: if one and the same person needs such services for a long time, he/she has to enforce his/her claim against a succession of different financing institutions. This always implies a process of 'redefinition', which can prove to be time consuming, and also involves uncertainty and even interruptions in care provision.

3.1g. Dependence on 'gate-keepers'

Various experts have to be called upon in connection with the redefinition process: the general practitioner, the hospital as an institution, the hospital physicians, and the medical examiner appointed by the insurance institution concerned. These experts, all medical professionals, have various assessment criteria for distinguishing between 'sickness' and 'health',[6] but have no specific criteria for assessing a person's ability to cope with the requirements of everyday life, the main yardsticks for determining a need for home care/home help. The general practitioner and also the hospital physician serve simultaneously as treatment experts and assessors, a dual function which can lead to conflicts of role and of interest. There is a constant danger that the interests of the physician or the hospital as an institution will prevail over the patient's need for care when the decision is made to discharge the patient or to help him/her in hospital. As already pointed out, there is a strong possibility that claim entitlement will be manipulated to become a mechanism for regulating care provision.

3.2. The main organizational form: the community-care centre

The year 1981 brought the establishment of the first so-called *Sozialstationen* (community-care centres) in Berlin, which aimed to offer a 'community-based concept of social services' covering service provision in the whole area of Berlin (West) (see Hornemann 1986). This intention was accompanied by another, that of accelerating the reduction in hospital beds. From 1982 on, this new type of organization was then introduced on a wider scale, and the development is still continuing. Today the services are available throughout the entire city. The main guiding principle is that of proximity to the individual. Indeed, this is reduced to a question of location rather than encompassing the spirit of a particular care concept (Trojan and Waller 1980; Tietze *et al.* 1981; Garms-Homolová and Schaeffer 1983). Each community centre is responsible for an area determined by the administration. In a few cases, two or more areas overlap, so that care is provided for patients falling within the competence of another centre.

The community centres are run by the welfare organizations. In some cases they work as independent associations. The funding of community-care centres takes the form of grants from the Berlin Senate towards personnel, material costs, and fees for services rendered. Some investments are made from the welfare organization's own resources.

This new organization was created to serve as a co-ordination point for help and social contact, and for the provision of services to ensure that people can remain in their home environments. It is also intended to offer counselling and assistance to the disabled and liaise with the informal network. The main services offered by the community centres are home nursing, home care/home help, family care (starting), meals-on-wheels, counselling and networking, and mobilizing informal help.

3.3. The extent of provision

As indicated above, there is generally very little information available on the extent of provision.

By 1990, there were 70 community centres in Berlin (West). In 1986 only 56 centres existed. They provided nursing for 6063 patients per week (sample survey from 27 October to 2 November 1986), with a total of 42 036 visits totalling 36 453 hours of care. In the same year they also provided 2.9 million hours of home care/home help (Senator für Gesundheit und Soziales, no year of publication). These figures do not indicate how many elderly people received services. As regards nursing, Berlin seems to be better off than any other city in Germany (see p. 130). As regards the proportion of elderly people receiving home nursing/home care, our own study found that 10 per cent of those aged 70 years and over received some home service during one year. No distinction was made between home nursing, home care or home help, simply because the elderly people themselves were not able to make this distinction. The distribution was strongly associated with age and sex; see Appendix 7, Table 3.

Looking at the distribution of services in relation to our three need categories defined above, the picture shown by Table 6.5 emerges. This does not say anything about the amount of help received. But even without this information, it is quite clear that there is a considerable amount of uncovered need. Fifty-seven per cent of those with a high level of need did not receive any home-care services during the year studied.

Table 6.5. Recipients of home care by need[1]

	% receiving some home-care[2] service in one year			
	No need	Slight need	High need	Total
No	95	87	57	90
Yes	5	13	43	10

[1] For definition, see p. 134 *et seq.*, 'need for external support'.
[2] Includes home nursing, home care and home help.

3.4. Internal organization

Affiliation to a larger welfare organization has a decisive impact on the profile of the various community centres. The community centres run by the ecclesiastical welfare organizations are generally a branch of the church's community work. From the outset, therefore, they have had roots in the local neighbourhood, established modes of operation, and a profound understanding of community care. New institutions, which mostly are still in the consolidation phase, have often only a weak affiliation to a welfare organization. They have to compensate for their lack of tradition and establish their own community base. This absorbs energy, calls for a strong staff commitment, and puts a great deal of stress on the staff. Still other types of community centre have a centralized structure, with an authoritarian style of management and a strong hierarchy downwards. But however different the traditions and modes of operation, many community centres are still wrestling with the problems arising from the fact that they are still in their infancy. Today there is also a vastly increasing number of private-sector providers. Their operations are market-oriented and guided by financial considerations, rather than any principle of geographical proximity to the individual. Consequently, their activities are not necessarily limited to a particular geographical area. However, they do tend to operate within certain boundaries, but these are much wider than those served by the community-care centres.

The staffing differs between community centres. For example, the number of staff employed ranges from 12 to over 100. The exact figures are impossible to ascertain, because of the wide range of employment arrangements involved—permanently employed, full-time and part-time staff plus, in most cases, a large number of personnel working on a fee basis. The high rate of fluctuation in staff has decisive implications for the organization and the work atmosphere. Often staff working on a fee basis only report back once a month to settle their accounts. They therefore do not know the centre or its patients very well. A further group of staff should be mentioned: the relatively broad-based network of voluntary personnel who have traditionally done community work.[7] No less diverse is the range of qualifications, which extends from graduate social workers and registered nurses to untrained personnel. The social workers are responsible for social counselling, the co-ordination of voluntary staff, and to some extent cost-accounting aspects.[8] The home-help/home-care services are mostly staffed by contract personnel with relatively minor qualifications. Private-sector providers and a few ecclesiastical institutions use identical staff for nursing and home help.[9] Domiciliary nursing belongs to one division, home care/home help to a different one. Their accounting is also mostly kept separate. In ideal circumstances, the divisional manager assesses the need by making contact with the patient in his/her home or the hospital. The manager then clarifies the financial aspects of the care, refers the patient to complementary services, and assigns the patient a nurse or helper. Some community centres try to ensure continuity; if possible the patient always has the same nurse. Other centres prefer staff rotation or group care-giving: the patient is confronted with a varying number of different faces. The reasons for this differ. They depend on the availability of personnel, but also on the conviction that such changes compensate for a lack of social contacts. The private-sector care providers and some ecclesiastical institutions have a different approach: each member of staff is responsible for a number of individual patients and covers both types, nursing and home help.

Some community centres do not provide the services until it is clear that the costs of the individual case will be covered. Others take action immediately and accept the financial risk involved. They also continue to provide their services even during the interruption of the flow of funds and try to cover their costs retrospectively. Other community centres interrupt their services because they do not accept the financial risk. Such discontinuities can only be bridged by the patient paying for the services during the interim or trying to find some form of compensatory solution which, as is shown later, usually takes the form of admission to in-patient care.

4. ALLOCATION AND CLAIM MECHANISMS

4.1. The service from the provider's perspective

The term 'provider' means, in this context, the staff of the community care centres (*Sozialstationen*): nurses, home-care assistants, and home helps.[10] We examine the way in which home care/help operates, and also the problems confronting the care providers in their day-to-day routines.

Even today, this service has to battle with a great number of difficulties. First and foremost amongst them are undoubtedly the problems of consolidation, acceptance, and information. The staff of other health and social institutions are still not properly aware of the range of services offered by the community-care centres. Six to seven years after these centres were first introduced, their staff still encounter not only ignorance but also a resistance to information—primarily on the part of general practitioners and hospital physicians (the most important partners for co-operation), many of whom simply close their eyes to the very existence of the services offered and to the way in which community-care centres operate.[11] The consequence is poor co-ordination and ineffectiveness of the out-patient institutions. For the service providers and the staff of the community-care centres, this problem implies a heavier work-load. They usually have to prepare the ground locally before they can really start their work.

A quite different problem is the shift in the focus of activities of the community-care centres. Originally intended as institutions for acute nursing and short-term intervention in the care or domestic field, these centres have today become, *de facto*, long-term care facilities.[12] It was only at the outset that the centres were used by a clientele who corresponded to the officially intended profile and who only needed short-term support. Very soon, quite a different clientele was demanding their services: elderly patients in need of long-term care. The average age of the clients is estimated by the staff to be 75 years and more. The problems which these patients face are usually complex and, besides calling for considerable and widespread co-ordination, imply a range of previously unanticipated tasks. The work involved overstretches the capabilities of the community-care centres. So far, they have looked for solutions within the institution itself. One strategy has been to acquire a mixed case-load that always includes a number of so-called lighter cases who are easier to care for. The lighter cases are then used more or less as compensatory material to spread the organizational and financial load. All community-care centres, though to different degrees, are facing a financial crisis, which they are trying to overcome by applying the principles of business management. This takes place at the expense of the staff. They have to overstretch themselves and also provide services that, in their opinion, do not focus on the patients and their needs but have to give priority to the continued existence of the institution.

The staff, therefore, feel unable to cope with the patients' misery. Despite a strong sense of commitment they can only rarely aspire to a type of patient care which does justice to their ideals; they only seldom experience job satisfaction and generally feel let down by the charity organization to which the care centre belongs and sometimes even by their centre itself.[13] 'It's a lonely job' is the general opinion of the staff, irrespective of whether they are employed in the home-nursing or home-help service. The situation is even more acute for casual staff and volunteers, as they do not even have the opportunity to discuss their problems with colleagues.

This problem is becoming more intense because of the expansion on the market of private-sector providers. Being from the outset business-oriented, the private-care centres are viewed by the community-care centres as threatening competitors, especially as far as the lighter cases are concerned. The community-care centres accuse the private providers of choosing the 'easy cases' and leaving them with the problem cases—the derelict, difficult, and confused patients. Also, when patients look like becoming cases requiring long-term care, private providers seem to be particularly keen to hand them over to the community-care centres. There is evidence here of a tendency to get rid of certain patients by shunting them elsewhere, a practice which can also be found in the hospital sector (see Garms-Homolová and Schaeffer 1989). The private providers counter the criticism by accusing the community-care centres of being inflexible. In hospitals, many social services departments prefer private service suppliers as these are always ready to take over patients, even at weekends. Some conservative general practitioners also prefer to work with private services, as they see the community centres as the beginning of socialist medicine. There is also strong competition between the various community-care centres which belong to different charity organizations. The diverse operating conditions enable some centres to supply a broader range of services (for example, the centres run by the churches) whilst others are constrained by their budgets.

A number of other problems dominate the everyday work of the service providers:

1. *Poor service co-ordination*. Early contact with the prospective patient in a hospital or a home is not a practicable proposition. The duty super-

visor is often only familiar with the case records and allocates patients to a nurse on the basis of these. The actual condition of the patient and his/her care requirements therefore remain unknown until the first job has to be done.

2. *Poor timing*. Hospitals tend to discharge patients at midday on Fridays in order to simplify the work schedule for weekends. The Friday discharge routine, however convenient it may be for the hospitals, is very inconvenient for the community-care centres, and because it clashes with their weekly work schedule (also the duty roster for the weekend has already been drawn up beforc Friday noon). Thus patient contact usually begins by telephone and the situation has to be clarified at a distance. Any further contact and care depend entirely on the staff's sense of commitment. At worst, nothing is arranged before Monday—that is unless the staff 'weaken' and give up their off-duty time in order to go shopping for the patient and try to bridge the care gap on their own initiative until the beginning of the week.

3. *Restricting job definition*. Only seldom can the members of staff work in strict accordance with their job description. Usually, there are a number of other tasks to be carried out before the real work can commence—tasks which are grossly under-rated in the tariff lists of the health insurance institutions, e.g., the mobilization of back-up support. Yet organized service is only effective if the patient's informal social network can be mobilized and co-ordinated.

4. *General practitioners' unwillingness to co-operate*. This is an obstacle encountered at various points in day-to-day routines, for example when care needs to be continued, for which a prescription from the doctor is required. General practitioners, the community-care centre staff complain, do not act on their own initiative; they need to 'chase up' the practitioner and do the necessary motivational work. Staff have to plead on behalf of the patient so that the general practitioner is willing to sign a prescription. The staff usually try to get round their problems by directing the patients to those general practitioners who are known to be co-operative. This, however, can result in conflicts with doctors in general, and may involve the risk that the few co-operative practitioners are reprimanded by the insurance organizations for over-prescribing.

5. *Arbitrary and increasingly bureaucratic care allocation*. As a rule, allocation is determined by institutional and financial considerations. The community-care centres thus have clients who are not in need, yet are entitled to all services, while others urgently require services but are not entitled at all. For financial and other reasons, the community-care centres are not in a position to adjust the service that they supply to the needs of their clients. The care personnel are daily confronted with real need but

have to work to orders and avoid any activity that cannot be covered by the medical card. If payment for an individual patient is not guaranteed, the care centre operates at its own financial risk. The greater the centre's financial difficulties, the more frequently are the staff instructed to do only what is absolutely necessary.

On the other hand, older patients are sometimes referred to certain services without it being verified whether they really need or even want them. The member of staff arrives to find that the patient has a well-functioning, informal, social support network, and that organized services are not required. But care is still provided, even in such cases, because of the inflexibility of the funding arrangements, with the health insurance institution paying for the services allocated irrespective of all other considerations, but on the other hand not paying more if the services needed are more than those allocated. Increasingly bureaucratic arrangements for allocation are leading to such action routines: 'The patient is becoming ever less important, the bureaucracy ever more important'—this is the unanimous view of staff of community-care centres, who complain of the general preponderance of bureaucratic considerations in the centres' work.

6. *Training standards.* Quite different problems arise from the low training standards found among the staff, or more specifically among the home-care assistants, whose previous training is at best only scant and who are neither trained specifically to deal with patients nor prepared for working with old people.[14] They do not know how 'a patient has to be done' (Bittner 1981) and often allow themselves to be treated or even abused as 'domestics'. This lack of training is a particularly serious shortcoming when the care is long term: many home-care assistants become too involved in their case. Their lack of objectivity and detachment generally results in problems and conflicts.

4.2. The viewpoint of the referral agencies

Home-help and home-care services can be obtained via various channels. If the health insurance institution is to fund the service, the allocation has to be made on the basis of a physician's prescription.[15] Usually, the patient's first contact is after discharge from hospital. The priority concern of the social services department at the discharging hospital is therefore that of finding a suitable care provider, while clarification of the funding has only secondary importance. This department, however, can only take action if a certificate has been issued by the hospital physician in charge of the case attesting a need for home nursing/home care. As already discussed, this task often causes difficulties for physicians as they are not at all trained to assess nursing and home-help needs. To overcome the problem the health authority has introduced a 'transfer form', which first of all contains a hospital nurse's opinion of the patient. Such information has to bridge the gap between the hospital and the domiciliary service. It is expected that a stronger involvement of the hospital nursing staff will also motivate the medical staff to prescribe home care/home nursing more often than they did in the past.

A second, relatively seldom used channel is via a general practitioner. Data collected in seven community-care centres by the health authority show that this was used in 14.5 per cent of all cases (Liedke and Wanjura 1988). As a matter of principle, the general practitioner's prescription has to be available before the service can be claimed, a requirement which leads to interruptions in care or at least considerable uncertainty as to whether or not the service will be continued. If the patient has no such insurance cover or is assessed as being in need not of treatment but instead of care, the home-care/home-help services cannot be funded by the health insurance but only by social welfare provision, which is limited to the poorest groups.

The following section examines the problems of allocation as seen by the allocating agencies.

4.2a. General practitioners

Community-care centres could be of crucial importance to the work of general practitioners as the majority of the practitioners' clientele are elderly or aged patients, usually with multiple chronic disorders. In practice, however, the practitioners do not see centres in this light. Their primary interest is in the management of their practices, and they are exclusively concerned with medical treatment. Consideration of the non-medical management of care as a field of concern to physicians—this is a concept which meets with incredulity on the part of general practitioners in this country, who still show very little interest in such less lucrative matters.

General practitioners are aware of the existence of the community-care centres and some of their services, but have no specific knowledge of the full range of potential services. A similarly superficial view is held of the importance of these services for medical care and for the concept of continuing care of the elderly.

It is only when imminent hospital admission is to be averted for one of their patients that general practitioners start to consider community-based services. But their knowledge is far from sufficient for co-operating constructively with the community-based services, which are viewed as informal support measures that have no direct importance to medical care. The physicians tend to regard the care and the social services as inferior services to fall back on as a substitute when the informal social network fails. In the view of general practitioners, this informal network is the real, natural, and indeed ideal provider of such services. Here, as elsewhere in the care system, it is a 'patronizing indifference' on the part of the general practitioners which governs their attitude towards co-operation (Bollinger and Hohl 1981). The work of the community-care centre is never fully appreciated as being a valid professional contribution in its own right.

4.2b. Hospital physicians

Hospital physicians[16] have formal authorization to judge and make a binding assessment of patients and their condition, with special emphasis being placed on assessment of the 'disease' (understood here to mean an irregularity in the physical or mental condition; see Schaefer and Blohmke 1978) and the 'need for curative treatment'. These criteria are decisive prerequisites for home-help and home-care services to be recognized as the statutory responsibility of the health insurance institutions.

The 'average' hospital physician has no intimate knowledge of community-oriented care and of corresponding facilities. All the hospital physicians interviewed were aware of the existence of the care centres and some of their basic activities, but only a few were able to name several care centres in their district or the hospital catchment area, and even fewer knew which centre co-operated with their hospital. Generally, hospital physicians have no insight into the operational realities and practical work of the community-based services. Consequently, their evaluation of services delivered to the home are based largely on assumptions which are beset with contradictions. The establishment of community-care centres is regarded by all hospital physicians as having been a positive measure. In the words of one doctor: 'Because of them we are able to get the patients discharged immediately.' However, the performance potential of the community-care centres is considered to be too limited because physicians estimate their elderly patients' needs as very extensive (Garms-Homolová 1989). It is not primarily the discontinuity of the care that hospital physicians saw fit to comment on—some even emphasized that after discharge, patients can return to their former care assistants. On the contrary, they criticize various time aspects of service provision (too short, too infrequent, too inflexible) and also the unsound financial basis of the services.

Being regarded as secondary services to support home nursing, the home-help/home-care services are allocated only in connection with home nursing. Eligibility for home nursing is therefore a prerequisite for obtaining home help/home care, which are often the services really required. In many cases, according to the physicians, old people are admitted to hospital in order to be entitled to home help/home care. This practice reveals one of the major problems facing this and also other fields of care for elderly people. In order to obtain one service, others which are not really necessary also have to be claimed. This, however, results in an increase in financial and staffing inputs, although one of the advantages anticipated from community-based services when they were introduced was cost saving. A second problem is that this practice is increasingly leading to the 'relabelling' of patients and their conditions. 'A bit of rewording has to be done' so that the desired service can be secured. The need for 'white lies' is something which can be found wherever needs exist that do not 'count' in the eyes of the administration, e.g., the need to extend a hospital stay (Garms-Homolová 1990).

Hospital physicians see the main disadvantage of services delivered to the home as their time limitations. Another issue criticized by hospital physicians is the lack of interest shown by general practitioners, who are not believed to give adequate attention to very old patients and to support the work of the community-care centres.

Although hospital physicians believe that the gaps in care should be filled in primarily by helpers from the informal social network, they usually have no confidence in the supportive strength of today's urban families. For this reason, too, many physicians prefer to refer people to a nursing home, in particular to avoid them being re-admitted to hospital.

4.2c. Hospital social-service departments

Hospital social-service departments[17] serve as 'gate-keepers' providing access to services, i.e., identifying a suitable provider, establishing contact, arranging for (initial) funding, and possibly also preparing the patient's relatives and other members of the social circle for his or her discharge.

Rather like hospital physicians, the staff of hospital social-service departments likewise report that the advent of community-care centres has facilitated and speeded up discharge procedures considerably. The range of patients for whom discharge home becomes a possibility has broadened since the community-based services came into existence. Even severely disabled patients can now return to their own homes using several of the centre's range of services.

Often it is possible to arrange that after return from hospital the patient is placed in the care of the same 'nurse'. But in the greater number of cases the staff of the social-service department complain of service discontinuity and constant fluctuation in personnel: 'One never knows which woman to expect. . .'.

Considerably more difficult for the staff of hospital social-service departments is a case which the health insurance institution alleges to be merely a 'care case'. The patient is not seen as requiring clinical treatment and therefore he/she has to be discharged from hospital as quickly as possible. At the time of discharge, however, there is no certainty that home care can be funded. An application for coverage by social welfare must be accompanied by proof that the health insurance will not cover the cost. This places the hospital staff in an impossible position. On the one hand they have to try to avert a rejection of liability by the health insurance institution because the patient might have to be detained in hospital when no funding for the home care is found to be available; on the other hand, they require such a rejection in order to obtain funding elsewhere. Disruptions in home care/home help cannot be precluded at this point. Only a few centres are at present still able to start providing care in the absence of guaranteed funding. Where it is not guaranteed, the patient is regarded as fee-paying, a status which may incur considerable costs for the patient and possibly also for relatives.

4.3. Home care and home help from the user's perspective

Most users are not able to distinguish beween home-help, home-care, and home-nursing services.[18] At best they differentiate between the type of activity carried out, and between individuals; occasionally they know which agency is providing the service. Only in exceptional cases can very aged clients give an account of the way in which they obtained their home-help/home-care assistant, what forms had to be filled in, and how the costs are covered. It is equally difficult for them to understand how the system functions, and to judge the quantity and quality of the services they receive.

Most clients of the home-help/home-care service require long-term care, often stretching over several years. During this time the care provided suffers from discontinuities and disruptions, and these result in an accumulation of problems. Over this course the patient's relationship with the informal social network is being destroyed and pathological structures develop to fill the void. Our analysis shows that the patient's career, measured as a negative trajectory ('decline trajectory' in Schütze 1981), follows an ever steeper and more rapid downward curve.

The most striking problems are caused by the limitations of the service. Individual 'needs' cannot generally be met from either the qualitative or the quantitative viewpoint. The result is increasing self-neglect and decrepitude, and often admission to in-patient care. Such problems occur with particular severity when the scope of the services is suddenly reduced because of a shift in funding. As the home help/home care cannot make up the resulting gaps, the transitional measures are either to employ a paid cleaner or leave the work to the informal circle of helpers. However, many elderly patients do not have the necessary financial resources. Usually they are not strong enough to make the necessary arrangements, and they therefore try to muddle through by themselves. The first consequence is a loss of the functions that had previously been mobilized and rehabilitated:

patients who have been discharged from hospital as 'walking cases' become bed-ridden again.

Such a regression is only one result of the discontinuity in care provision. Our case analyses show a large number of types of discontinuity and disruptions with a correspondingly wide range of causes and consequences, as follows.

1. Disruptions resulting from *a switch in the care-providing institution*: if the source of funding for the care alters, there is usually a change of agency providing the care and employing the carers—this often resulting in conflicts between different providers.

2. Disruptions resulting from *the division of labour*: quite often the aged patient is cared for by a whole corps of people whose tasks and activities are poorly co-ordinated, sometimes even totally uncoordinated. And no one considers himself or herself to be responsible for subjectively perceived needs.

3. Disruptions resulting from *staff rotation*: for example, each weekday may bring a different care assistant providing home care at a different time.[19] This leads to disorientation of the patients, because they have no opportunity to consolidate a relationship with at least one carer. And whereas on the one hand they treat such helpers as domestics, on the other they are not able to demand from them the work to which they are entitled.

4. Disruptions resulting from *work organization practices* at the community-care centres: staff leave-periods and public holidays are especially liable to cause disruptions—services are drastically cut, appointments are not kept, regular working hours not adhered to, and different care assistants or temporary replacements become the order of the day. The aged clients find it very difficult to cope with such 'hard times'. Furthermore, the home-help/home-care assistants generally do not come at a time which fits in with the daily routine of the patients. Work organization schemes and duty rosters, however, cannot be arranged to allow for optimally individualized scheduling of service. To the clients, the organizational constraints are incomprehensible and their own care assistant's duty schedule a mystery.

5. Disruptions resulting from *staff fluctuation*: the home-care/home-help services are provided by various categories of personnel, the largest amongst these being staff paid by the hour and volunteers not bound to the care centre by any formal and permanent employment relationship. Such casual staff only stay for a short time, changing jobs frequently and sometimes swapping 'cases' amongst themselves, so that the patient is regularly confronted by different care assistants. There is no time to communicate. This is an especially serious problem because, for the

needy, these 'short-term' helpers are their only means of establishing and/or maintaining contact with the outside world.

With temporary staff, casual staff, mainstream drop-outs and, more recently, even people who are themselves 'cases for the authorities',[20] the service providers are now falling back on potentially problematical helpers. On being confronted with such people the original social network may abandon the patient; for example, previously helpful neighbours may 'not want to be involved any more'. Moreover, such helpers do not have the necessary stamina, and are mentally and physically unequal to the task.

There are clear indications that the home-help/home-care services are most effective when the need for them is limited in terms of time input and scope, and when standard, routine procedures suffice. If the client needing care has the advantage of well-functioning, informal social network, it is generally possible to avert the symptoms of insufficient care. The situation is similar when care is only needed for a short time. However, very old people usually require quite different services: long-term care, continuous and comprehensive care—a type of provision to which the existing services are not geared. The permanent inadequacy of the care has long-term consequences: among others the psychological deprivation of the client and a deterioration of the client–helper relationship. The special dynamics of such long-term care relationships are a subject which has not yet been given adequate attention. It would appear that these dynamics have implications which seem to be virtually indistinguishable from the effects long since recognized and referred to as the hospitalization syndrome.

NOTES

[1] This report is based on the study 'Care of the elderly—needs and barriers' carried out at the Freie Universität of Berlin, FRG. The research grant is provided by the Deutsche Forschungsgemeinschaft. The first section draws on data collected within the framework of sub-project 1 of this study—a survey of a random sample of 427 persons born between 1897 and 1916, and presently living in inner-city districts of the metropolitan area of Berlin (West). Persons in institutions and foreign citizens were not questioned (Garms-Homolová and Hütter 1988*a,b*). The second and third sections are based on data compiled in the course of the sub-project 2. Here an analysis of old patients'/clients' trajectories has been made, especially focusing on the processes of care allocation (Garms-Homolová *et al.* 1984, 1987).

[2] The term 'need' has a multitude of meanings. In this section of the report we are concerned with subjectively perceived deficiencies and with possibilities of the network of informal relationships to compensate for such deficiencies. Other aspects of 'need', e.g., those which result from the system of values of the existing society, are not considered within this report. But in Section 2 the term represents the meaning attached to it by politicians and by the system of social security. In the

third section we analyse the discrepancy between the professionals' interpretation of the term on the one hand and, on the other, the users' understanding of it.

[3] See note 1.

[4] Under the terms of the Care Benefits Act only those persons count as 'helpless' who need considerable and lasting nursing and help with the activities of daily living. In particular, dressing and undressing, feeding, care of the body, physical exercise and mental stimulation belong to such activities.

[5] An 'extraordinary' need for care is the decisive criterion of the entitlement to the higher degree of care benefits. The term 'extraordinary need' means, that as a consequence of the suffering of the helpless person, the continuous presence of a care-giver or continuous care giving is required.

[6] They conform to the biomedical model of illness. Yet this model is not suitable as a basis for assessing the functional abilities required in the course of day-to-day life (World Health Organization 1980; Mishler *et al.* 1981).

[7] Admittedly, this practice is not without its critics. The staff of the community centres complain that many tasks are carried out by inadequately trained persons and that this is an unacceptable way of attempting to overcome the grave financial problems that afflict most centres: voluntary workers merely receive reimbursement for their expenses.

[8] Among the private-sector institutions, which have recently also taken to employing social workers, the duties of these are largely confined to referral and cost management.

[9] This is linked with the special cost-regulating situation described before, but is further legitimized by private-sector providers: 'Anyone who considers himself to be above clearing up mess does not even need to apply to work for us.' These therefore invoke ethical and personality-specific arguments in order to legitimize this mix of functions.

[10] The empirical basis is represented by semi-structured interviews with the staff of the community-care centres and private-sector care providers. Interviews carried out within the framework of case inquiries have also been taken into account in this context.

[11] The social workers in hospitals also criticize the physicians' unwillingness to co-operate (Schaeffer 1989).

[12] The care of the chronically ill is included into the concept of care by the community centres. However, the meaning of chronic illness is different in this context, referring only to single, acute episodes which have to be treated by medical and nursing staff. Difficulties arise from lasting conditions of illness, as the community-care centres do not have adequate financial means and staffing for care in such cases. Similar problems dominate the whole system of health services, which are no longer adequate to deal with long-term illnesses and with the particular developments of functional conditions that often occurr within the oldest old population (Garms-Homolová and Schaeffer 1983).

[13] Such development could be observed in the other health institutions as well.

[14] There is no particular education to approve the qualification in this field.

[15] The contractors are the health insurance institutions on the one hand and the main charity organizations on the other. According to a contract dated back to 26 May 1986.

[16] The data basis is semi-structured interviews with 20 physicians of different specialties, working in general hospitals.

[17] We are referring to interviews with social workers in social services departments located in general hospitals. Eighteen social workers were interviewed individually; seven groups of social workers were also interviewed.

[18] This part of the report is based on case analysis. The data were collected over 18 months. During this time we 'escorted' the very old patients on their way out of the acute hospital and continuously across the services offered by the system of health care (see Garms-Homolová *et al.* 1984, 1987).

[19] The very old respondents usually had the greatest difficulties in categorizing the helpers and assistants. 'On weekends', one old lady reported, 'a male nurse visits me, Molly comes on Mondays, Tuesdays and Thursdays, someone different on Friday, and Sabine comes each evening.'

[20] We are witnessing a development in which 'the clients' (persons dependent on social welfare, unemployed, etc.) are engaged by the charity organization to care for the very old patients and for persons in need of assistance. The social distress and social problems of one group are used as an instrument to solve social problems of another group.

REFERENCES

Abgeordnetenhaus von Berlin (1990). Beschlussempfehlung des Auschusses für Gesundheit und Soziales v. 26. Sept. 1990 zum Gesetz zur Förderung der ambulauten gesundheits- und sozialpflegerischen Dienste (Sozialstationengesetz Sorstag), Druchsache 11/1190, 1–4.

Bäcker, G., Dieck, M., Naegele, G., and Tews, H.-P. (1989). *Ältere menschen in Nordrhein-Westfalen. Wissenschaftliches Gutachten zur Lage der älteren Menschen und zur Altenpolitik in Nordrhein-Westfalen zur Vorbereitung des Zweiten Landesaltenplans.* Ministerium für Arbeit, Gesundheit und Soziales des Landes Nordrhein-Westfalen, Düsseldorf.

Baum, C., Koch, M. and Seeger, M. (1989). *Vergleichbare Strukturdaten des Sozial- und Gesundheitswesens ausgewählter Grossstädte der Bundesrepublik*, p. 22. Senator für Gesundheit und Soziales Berlin, Berlin.

Blume, O. (1968). *Möglichkeiten und Grenzen der Altenhilfe.* Tübingen.

Bittner, U. (1981). Ein Klient wird 'gemacht'. In *Psyche in schlechter Gesellschaft. Zur Krise klinisch-psychologischer Tätigkeit* (ed. E. v. Kardoff and E. Koenen). Urban & Schwarzenberg Psychologie, München.

Bollinger, H. and Hohl, S. (1981). *Sozialarbeiterinnen und Ärzte im Krankenhaus. Eine Studie zum beruflichen Alltag.* Campus, Frankfurt/Main.

Brandt, H. (1988). Haushaltshilfen für alte Menschen. Hilfbedarf, Leistungsrecht und Stellenwert. *Mitteilungen zur Altenhilfe*, **25**, part 1, 12–17; part 2, 13–23.

Brög, W., Häberle, G-F, Mettler-Meibom, B., and Schellhass, U. (1980). Anzahl und Situation zu Hause lebender Pflegedürftiger. Ermittlung der Repräsentativdaten und Situtionsgruppenanalyse. *Schriftenreihe des Bundesministers für Jugend, Familie und Gesundheit.* Socialdata, Stuttgart/Berlin/Köln/Mainz.

Dieck, M. (1979). *Wohnen und Wohnumfeld älterer Menschen in der Bundesrepublik.* Heidelberg.

Garms-Homolová, V. (1989). Discharge from hospital: professional criteria of need and provision. *Journal of Aging Studies,* **3,** 355–67.

Garms-Homolová, V. (1990). Chronisch kranke Hochbetagte im Medizinbetrieb.

In *Chronische Krankheit ohne Rezepte, Argument Sonderband 'Kritische Medizin'*, AS 182. Argument-Verlag, Hamburg.
Garms-Homolová, V. and Hütter, U. (1988*a*). *Between ample sufficiency and fragility: resources in advanced age*. Berichte der Arbeitsgruppe Gesundheitsanalysen und soziale Konzepte Nr. 2. Freie Universität, Berlin.
Garms-Homolová, V. and Hütter, U. (1988*b*). *Siebzig- bis Neunzigjährige in der Großstadt. Differentielle Betrachtung ihrer Lebenssituation*. Berichte der Arbeitsgruppe Gesundheitsanalysen und soziale Konzepte, Nr. 1. Freie Universität, Berlin.
Garms-Homolová, V. and Schaeffer, D. (1983). Auf dem Wege zur gemeindenahen Versorgung: Kontaktladen 'Gesundheit älterer Menschen'. Argument-Sonderband AS 77: *Alternative Medizin*, pp. 164–75. Argument, Berlin.
Garms-Homolová, V. und Schaeffer, D. (1989). Bewältigung chronischer Erkrankungen im institutionellen Kontext. *Zeitschrift für Geronto-Psychologie und Psychiatrie*, **2,** 126–35.
Garms-Homolová, V., Hütter, U., and Schaeffer, D. (1984). Versorgung alter Menschen: Bedarf und Barrieren. Design eines Forschungsprojektes. Unpublished manuscript. Freie Universität, Berlin.
Garms-Homolova, V., Hütter, U., Müller, R., and Schaeffer, D. (1987). Versorgung alter Menschen—Bedarf und Barrieren (Care Delivery Systems for the Elderly). Zwischenbericht im Verbundprojekt 'Vergleichende Untersuchung der Sozial- und Gesundheitsdienste für ältere Menschen'. Unpublished manuscript. Freie Universität, Berlin.
Gesetz über Pflegeleistungen (Pflege. G.) in der Fassung, vom 14 Juli 1986, Gesetz- und Verordnungblatt S. 1106, 1987, S. 1064.
Gesetz zur Änderung des Gesetztes über Pflegeleistungen, vom 8 Dezember 1988; Gesetz- und Verordnungblatt für Berlin, 44. Jahrgang, Nr. 70, 21 Dezember 1988, 2262.
Gesetz zur Strukturreform im Gesundheitswesen (Gesundheits-Reformgesetz-GRG) vom 20 Dezember 1988 (BG BI. I S2477), Gesetz- und Verordnungsblatt für Berlin 74, 31 Dezember 1989, pp. 2450–2579.
Hornemann, G. (1986). *Sozialstationen in Berlin. Ihre Vorgeschichte und Entstehung. Eine Dokumentation*, p. 59. Tintenfass, Rheinbach.
Katz, S., Ford, A. B., Moskowitz, R. W., Jackson, B. A., and Jaffe, M. W. (1963). Studies of Illness in the Aged: The Index of ADL—A Standardized Measure of Biological and Psychosocial Function. *Journal of American Medical Association*, 185, pp. 914–919.
Kuhlmeyer, E. (1974). *Dokumentation der Lebenssituation über 65jähriger Bürger in Berlin*. Senator für Arbeit und Soziales, Berlin.
Lawton, M. P. and Brody, E. M. (1969). Assessment of older people: self-maintaining and instrumental activities of daily living. *The Gerontologist*, **9,** 179–86.
Liedke, D. and Wanjura, M. (1988). Project: Beratungspflege, Part 1. Discussion paper, unpublished manuscript. Senator für Gesundheit und Soziales, Berlin.
Marburger, H. (1981). Die Haushaltshilfe—eine bedeutsame Leistung aller Sozialversicherungsträger. *Soziale Arbeit,* **30,** 62–8.
Ministerium für Arbeit, Gesundheit und Sozialordnung Baden-Württemberg (1983). *Die Lebenssituation älterer Menschen. Ergebnisse einer Repräsentativerhebung in Baden-Württemberg*. Stuttgart.

Mishler, E. G. *et al.* (1981). *Social context of health, illness and patient care.* Press Syndicate, Cambridge.

Münster (1980). *Studie zur Situation der älteren Bürger in Münster 1989, Beiträge zur Stadtforschung, Stadtentwicklung, Stadtplanung 5/1980.* Oberstadtdirektor der Stadt Münster und EMNID, Münster.

Poske, D. (1986). Integration und Diversifikation gesetzlicher Haupflegeleistungen im Sozialrecht. *Zeitschrift für Sozialhilfe/Sozialgesetzbuch,* **25,** 17–26.

Reichsversicherungsordnung (RVO) (1986). Sozialgesetzbuch, 12. Auflage, Stand 01.01.1986. Wirtschaftsverlag Bachem, Köln.

Senator für Gesundheit und Soziales (undated). *Die Berliner Sozialstationen.* Angebot und Entwicklung. Senator für Gesundheit und Soziales—Referat Presse und Öffentlichkeitsarbeit, Berlin.

Schaeffer, D. (1989). Formen der Kooperation zwischen den Krankenhausärzten und den Sozialdiensten. *Medizin Mensch Gesellschaft,* **14,** 45–59.

Schaefer, H. and Blohmke, M. (1978). *Sozialmedizin. Einführung in die Ergebnisse und Probleme der Medizinsoziologie und Sozialmedizin.* Thieme, Stuttgart.

Schütze, F. (1981). Prozesstrukturen des Lebenslaufs. In *Biographie in handlungswissenschaftlicher Perspektive. Kolloquium am SFZ der Universität Erlangen* (ed. J. Matthes, A. Pfeifenberg, and M. Stosberg), pp. 67–156. Verlag der Nürnberger Forschungsvereinigung e.V., Nürnberg.

Therman, G. (1970). Auswertung der Finanzerhebung für Gemeindepflegestationen. *Die Innere Mission,* **60,** 501–5.

Tietze, K. W., Garms-Homolová, V., Korporal, J., and Zink, A. (1981). Was bedeutet die Deklaration von Alma Ata für die primäre Gesundheitsversorgung in der Bundesrepublik Deutschland? *Bundesgesundheitsblatt,* **24,** 121–6.

Trojan, A. and Waller, H. (ed.) (1980). *Gemeindebezogene Gesundheitsversorgung. Einführung in neue Versorgungsmodelle.* Urban & Schwarzenberg, München.

World Health Organization (1980). *International classification of impairments, disabilities, and handicaps. A manual of classification relating to the consequences of disease.* WHO, Geneva.

7

Home-care services in Israel

Haim Factor, Brenda Morgenstin, and Denise Naon

1. Introduction
   1.1. Demographic and socio-economic trends
   2.2. The network of services for the elderly: an overview
2. The development of home-help services
   2.1. Historical Overview
   2.2. The CLTCI law
3. Provision of services today
   3.1. The range of services for older people
   3.2. Home-delivered services
4. Issues in the delivery of adequate services
   4.1. Organizational issues
   4.2. The adequacy of the services currently provided
   4.3. The possibility of substituting for institutional services through the development of community services
5. Assessment and discussion of key issues
   5.1. The personal-care/home-making mix
   5.2. The impact of entitlements on the demand for services
   5.3. Universal access and entitlement versus restricted access and budget constraints
   5.4. Entitlements and the dynamics of finance for home care
   5.5. Cash versus benefits in kind
   5.6. Eligibility assessment
   5.7. Translating disability into benefit level and service needs
   5.8. Centralization versus decentralization of service provision
6. Summary

Notes

Acknowledgements

References

1. INTRODUCTION

1.1. Demographic and socio-economic trends

Compared with Western countries, Israel is a unique feature on the map of ageing. While life expectancy in Israel matches the peak levels of Western Europe, birth rates in Israel are much higher. While Israel is considerably younger than most European countries, the elderly population itself is quite old and ageing rapidly.

Between 1950 and 1985, the elderly population grew from 3 to 9 per cent of Israel's population. Most relevant to the planning of long-term care service is the growth of the dependent aged. The number of 'old old' (over the age of 75 years) is growing at a remarkable rate—from 58 000 in 1970 to 108 000 in 1980, to an expected 170 000 (40 per cent of all elderly people) by 1990, and 198 000 by 2000 (Appendix 8, Table 1). This increase in the number of old old is very much faster than in Western countries. Moreover, the number of elderly people over the age of 85, the most vulnerable age group for disability, will have increased by almost 100 per cent during the 1980s, and will continue to grow rapidly until the end of the century. A rise in the percentage of women among the elderly population and a change in its ethnic composition are also contributing to an increase in disability. As a result, the number of functionally disabled (in terms of activity of daily living (ADL)) elderly people will rise from some 31 500 in 1980 to 44 800 in 1990 and to an estimated 55 900 in 2000, with a corresponding need for expansion in institutional and community services (Appendix 8, Table 2).

Israel's elderly population also has much ethnic and socio-economic heterogeneity, resulting from the different characteristics of the populations that came in each separate wave of immigration. There are two very different groups. First, the veteran elderly, i.e., 'old-comers', are a well-established group, with resources and close connections to the centres of power; they are generally quite able to provide for their own needs. In contrast, the second group of more recent immigrants generally arrived without economic resources and have not lived in Israel long enough to integrate fully into many areas of life. For example, many of these elderly people never worked in Israel, while others worked but did not accumulate full pension rights or other forms of savings. This group, therefore, is often dependent on public support. The absence of savings or pensions for a large proportion of the elderly population is one factor contributing to extensive poverty among older people, which affects about 25 per cent[1] of them (Achdut and Tamir 1986).

Israel has a two-tiered pension system, comprising a basic, flat-rate, old-age pension provided under the social security system, and a work-related pension provided by various occupational pension funds. Today, about a quarter of the elderly population has almost no other income besides the basic pension from the National Insurance Institute.[2] The proportion of elderly people entitled to work-related pensions and the level of these pensions have increased slightly over time, but no more radical change is expected in the near future. Therefore, the ability of disabled elderly persons to participate in financing the services they require will continue to be limited.

Another major social trend which affects the provision of long-term care is the change in the role of women in the family. The responsibility for providing care for older parents or for a spouse is mostly borne by women in upper middle age and old age. During the past two decades there has been a significant change in the proportion of women aged 55+ entering the workforce—from 18 per cent in 1965 to 26 per cent in 1985 (Morginstin 1988). This rate is expected to rise even further during the coming years, and has several implications. Care-givers who are also employed outside the home may be more limited in the amount of help they can personally provide, but may be in a better financial position to purchase care for their own family's needs or that of the elderly parent.

2.2. The network of services for the elderly: an overview

Responsibility for services for the aged is shared by numerous governmental, public, and voluntary agencies. The main government agencies involved in caring for the elderly population are the Ministry of Health, the Ministry of Labor and Social Affairs, and the National Insurance Institute. The principal public organizations that are responsible for the development of services for the aged are the General Sick Fund (Israel's major provider of health care) and ESHEL, the Association for Planning and Development of Services for the Aged in Israel.

The various agencies operate within a clearly defined but complex division of financial responsibility, based on the type of service required and the client's level of disability, classified along the continuum of dependency, from dependency in instrumental (I)ADL (semi-independent) to moderate dependency in ADL (frail) and severe dependency or cognitive impairment (severely dependent).

The Ministry of Labor and Social Affairs is responsible for institutionalization and personal-care services for semi-independent and frail elderly people, the provision of home-making services and special transportation (for example, for medical care) to all classifications of disabled people, and the operation of frameworks for day care and sheltered housing. The Ministry operates through a network of local social-welfare bureaux that provide these kinds of services on a discretionary basis within closed budgetary constraints and are administrated by the local authorities. Most local offices have social workers who specialize in the care of the elderly.

The Ministry of Health is responsible for the institutionalization of severely dependent and mentally frail elderly people, the operation of mental-health clinics, and the development of preventive public health services in the family-health clinics. Services are provided through a network of regional public offices.

At present, Israel has no programme of compulsory health insurance covering the entire population. While medical care is the formal responsibility of the Ministry of Health, most of the medical care received by the elderly, as for most of the population, is provided by voluntary sick funds. These funds are organized through insurance and they finance the full range of health services (hospitalization, rehabilitation, and primary care). The largest is the General Sick Fund founded by the Histadrut, Israel's largest labour union. It insures about three-quarters of the total population, and 95 per cent of the elderly population. The General Sick Fund is organized primarily through a national network of 1200 neighbourhood clinics, which integrate medical, nursing, and paramedical staff. In addition, there are regional continuing-care units which are specifically responsible for supervising and facilitating the care of the chronically ill and dependent elderly patients within the clinics. The sick funds also provide personal care to those who are fully insured, and institutionalization for some elderly people with complex nursing needs.

The National Insurance Institute, under the Community Long-Term Care Insurance (CLTCI) law (see below) provides long-term care services to seriously disabled, chronically ill, elderly people living in the community; its basis is social insurance principles and legal entitlement. In addition to specifically defined personal-care and home-making services, provided through personal entitlement, the CLTCI law provides funds for service development within the community and in institutional settings.

The relationship between central government and the local authorities is no less complex. In principle, the Ministry of Labor and Social Affairs is responsible for the planning and organization of community services for the aged. In practice, however, the services are administered and implemented by the local authorities through the local welfare bureaux, and the Ministry is of assistance only in a professional supervisory capacity. The initiative for the development of the services rests, to a large extent, with the local authorities. These authorities are not all equally aware of the problems of elderly people in their communities or do not have equal access to the resources necessary to establish and maintain such services. This contributes to variations in the type, extent, and quality of the services provided by the different local authorities.

Despite the numerous agencies involved in providing assistance, a study conducted in 1984, before the implementation of the recent CLTCI law, showed that public agencies provided personal care to only 14 per cent of elderly dependent (in terms of ADL) persons residing in the community, and home-making to about 9 per cent of those limited in household management (Morginstin 1984). Most of the care was provided by the family. The significant contribution of the families and the burden which provision of care often entails has been documented by an extensive study of dependent elderly people awaiting institutionalization and receiving home care (Habib *et al.* 1986). This found that 55 per cent of the primary, informal care-givers suffered from overburdening, despite the receipt of home-care services, and one-third reported that they had reached their limits and could not continue to provide the same amount of care. The recognition that existing services need to be significantly expanded, both in the amount of help provided per case, and in the coverage of the target population has served as a major impetus for the development of community services in recent years.

2. THE DEVELOPMENT OF HOME-HELP SERVICES

2.1. Historical overview

In the early years of the State, the elderly were a very small percentage of the population. Still, mass immigration posed difficult challenges because of the needs of older immigrants who had lost their families in the Holocaust and often required medical and nursing care from the day of their arrival. This challenge was primarily taken up by voluntary organizations, among which were the American Jewish Joint Distribution Committee. This organization established a social service agency, Malben, which over a few years in the early 1950s built over 5000 beds in institutions and nursing homes for the aged. Local authorities and other voluntary organizations, such as the Organization of Immigrants from Central Europe and the General Sick Fund, also erected special residences for the aged.

However, during the late 1950s and the early 1960s, Malben gradually reduced the scope of its involvement with institutions, and in 1975 transferred its network of institutions to the Ministry of Health. This occurred partly because Malben's policy was to set up programmes, ascertain their effectiveness, and then turn them over to the relevant governmental bodies, and partly in response to greater awareness of the need to develop community services.

The most important among such community services were alternative housing solutions and home-making services for the elderly. Parallel to these, clubs and day-care centres were opened. Because these services were being developed, Malben was able to initiate, in the 1960s, a reassessment of its institutionalized elderly clients, with the aim of assisting those who were interested and functionally able to return to the community. Thus a total of 1000 residents left the institutions.

Over time there was a gradual transfer of functions from voluntary organizations to the state, similar to the process that was carried out in institutional services. The Division of Aging within the Ministry of Labor and Social Affairs was established, and this began a programme of home care for moderately disabled elderly people, while the Ministry of Health, through its regional health offices, began a programme of home care for the severely disabled. Both these programmes focused on low-income elderly persons and involved fairly severe income tests.

Not until many years later was another important component of the system added with the development of a home-care division by the sick funds, not as an obligatory provision within the health insurance contract but rather on a more discretionary basis.

In 1969, ESHEL was established co-operatively by the Ministries of Labor and Social Affairs, and Health and Finance, and the Israel Joint Distribution Committee. Its purpose was to promote joint planning, implementation and financing of community and institutional services for elderly people, and manpower training.

A major contribution of ESHEL was the introduction of national planning in the field of ageing, resulting in a series of 5-year plans. This approach permitted, for the first time, a rational development of services through regional needs and trends as demonstrated by, for example, need surveys, mapping of existing services, and forecasts of manpower requirements.

It is interesting that some of the services which provide care for the elderly population were originally established to serve the needs of younger people and only gradually evolved into their present function. An important example are the continuing-care units of the General Sick Fund, the country's largest health maintenance organization, which organize and provide home care for disabled people residing at home. These units were first set up in 1973, during the Yom Kippur War, to enable hospitals to release patients, so freeing beds for the many injured soldiers. After the war, these units continued to function and expand, and their major target population rapidly became disabled, elderly, community residents. Another example of such evolution occurred in out-reach screening services. 'Well-baby' clinics, originally established by the Ministry of Health to provide screening and preventive medical care for mothers and their babies, have gradually begun to allocate more positions for nurses to provide preventive health care for the elderly population.

2.2. The CLTCI law

In response to concern about the growing burden of long-term care and the inadequacy of existing programmes, the Israel Parliament enacted, in November 1980, an enabling act creating a Community Long-Term Care Insurance (CLTCI) Branch under the National Insurance Institute to expand the financial resources to cope with the growing need for community services. This policy decision reflected a statutory commitment to assure a basic level of care to one of the most vulnerable population groups, particularly important during a period of reduction in *per capita* spending on health and welfare. In that year, 0.2 per cent of employee contributions to social insurance were allocated to develop a reserve fund for the implementation of the new law. The enactment was completed in April 1986, but CLTCI was not fully implemented until April 1988, when it became possible to apply to the National Insurance Institute for long-term care benefits. The primary aim of the law was to provide long-term care benefits and services through the principles of social insurance: personal entitlement and clearly defined criteria for eligibility. It represented an important shift from budgeted to entitlement programmes of service for elderly people, and from largely selective, income-tested benefits to largely universal ones.

CLTCI in Israel should be viewed as an expansion of social policy for the aged under social insurance. Whereas for the past 15 to 20 years comprehensive measures of income maintenance for the elderly have been developed and refined, this new step reflects a commitment to the statutory allocation of resources for functionally dependent elderly people. The new law was intended to complement rather than replace the existing system of service provision.

Its overall objectives were to reduce unmet needs and the burden of family care-givers, and to enable elderly people to remain in the community and avoid unnecessary institutionalization. It was hoped in some quarters that some of the costs of the law would be offset by reduced institutionalization.

The basic principles underlying CLTCI are:

1. Personal entitlement to services and benefits in the home paid for by contributions from the working population. However, it must be emphasized that the role of these benefits is not to replace but to supplement family care and responsibilities, as the benefit covers only a small part of total needs.

2. Creation of a programme based on decentralized service provision and case co-ordination so as to assure flexibility in the formulation and implementation of individual care plans, but retaining central functions for determining eligibility, reporting, and monitoring based on uniform guidelines and instruments, so as to assure maximum equity under law, as well as maximum control over targeting and budgeting.

3. In addition, a part of the resources is reserved for expansion of the network of available services by allocating funds for development in the community and in institutions, and for manpower training.

The development over time of home-care services and the impact of the new law may be traced by an examination of the development of personal-care and home-maker services. Tables 3 and 4 in Appendix 8 present the changes in the extent of services provided during the last 8 years, during the first stage of implementation and after the full implementation of the law. The number of persons who received personal care grew from 3000 in 1981 to 16 246, covering some 42 per cent of the elderly population in the community at the beginning of 1989; and the average number of weekly hours provided increased from 4.2 to 9.3. The number of persons receiving help in home-making grew between 1981 and 1988 by 29 per cent, and the hours of help provided by 150 per cent from 1984 to 1988 (before the full implementation of the law). The figures for hours of help in personal care include an unknown number of home-making hours because some of the help provided by the personal-care service is, in fact, assistance with basic, home-making activities.

3. PROVISION OF SERVICES TODAY

3.1. The range of services for older people

This section deals with the three main home-delivered services: personal care, home-making and meals. A wider range of services exists, which will not be discussed here. These include (a) institutional services ranging from general and psychiatric hospitals, hospitals for the chronically ill to old-age homes and sheltered housing; (b) community services, which, apart from the services discussed in the following, include laundry services, alarm systems, social visits, transportation facilities, day hospitals, day centres, and clubs.

3.2. Home-delivered services

The following is a brief description of each service, its organization, its target populations, the sources of financing, and the extent of current provision.

3.2a. Non-professional personal care

The nature of the service. The core activities of this service are help in bathing, mobility, dressing, feeding, care of wounds and bandages, administering medications, and general attendance or supervision. Personal-care aids may also take on responsibility for home-making (i.e., laundry, cleaning, cooking, shopping for food), according to the client's needs. However, when the client lives with his or her family, responsibility for home-making is limited primarily to his or her room, but sometimes includes cleaning of the bathroom where incontinence is a problem, and preparation of light meals for the client. The personal-care worker is also expected to maintain ongoing contact with the nurse or social worker responsible for case management and to contribute to the client's general well-being.

The organization of service provision. Personal-care services are now, for the most part, provided through specialized agencies which employ semi-professional, personal-care aids. Over the years, approximately half of the personal-care services financed by the public sector were provided through a large, nationwide, non-profit agency, the Matav Association. The remaining services were provided by workers hired privately by clients and not affiliated to any agency. Recently, with the expansion of services spurred by the new CLTCI law, and with the procedural stipulation that services financed within the framework of that law be provided through a certified agency having legal status, many other agencies have sprung up. These agencies have to be approved by the Ministry of Labor and Social Affairs in order to be contracted to provide services. A recent survey found 55 agencies which provide personal-care services throughout the country: 44 of them are private, profit-making organizations; the rest are non-profit. The Matav Association is still the most important among them, providing services for about half of those receiving care from the public sector. This organization has a well-developed programme of training and supervision, and is frequently contracted to develop similar programmes for other recently established agencies.

The personnel involved in supplying the service. The personnel in this service are mainly women. The Matav Association requires its workers to have at least eight years of education and to pass a 3-month basic course. To date there is no information on the personnel employed by the new agencies that have emerged since the implementation of the CLTCI law.

However, a survey conducted before its implementation indicated that for-profit providers have no organized training programmes (Shuval and Factor 1988). Some of these hire workers who were previously trained and employed by the Matav Association.

The target population, eligibility criteria, and financing. Each of the public agencies participating in the financing of personal-care services has its own criteria of eligibility.

The Ministry of Labor and Social Affairs, acting through the local authorities, provides the financing for personal care to moderately dependent, frail elderly people through a functional assessment. The decision to provide the service is made by the social worker responsible for the client, and is reviewed by the supervisor in the local social services bureau. The elderly person and their family participate in the financing of the service according to a means test. The General Sick Fund finances personal care for the more severely disabled elderly people who are members of the Fund. The decision to provide these services is based on a functional assessment by a nurse from the primary-care clinic and is reviewed by the continuing-care unit. The elderly person and family have to participate in the financing of the service in accordance with their income level.

The National Insurance Institute finances services and a small number of cash benefits according to the following criteria:

1. Men over 65 years and women over 60 years of age who have severe functional disability in ADL or who require constant attention. Eligibility is defined in terms of the degree of functional dependency (mobility in the home, bathing, dressing, feeding, incontinence, and need for supervision). It does not take into account social and environmental factors, or unmet needs. There are two levels of eligibility, according to the degree of dependency as assessed by a public-health nurse from the Ministry of Health in the elderly person's home. The nurse makes an objective measurement of ADL. Each person is given a score based on that assessment. Additional points are awarded to persons living alone who have accrued a minimum of points in ADL dependency and to those requiring constant personal attendance. From the total scores the client is assigned an eligibility level.

2. As the benefit is intended for elderly people living at home, only those not living in nursing homes or nursing wards may apply for it. Those in sheltered housing or old-age homes that are not publicly financed may also apply.

3. Eligibility for benefits is income tested. For single elderly people, only those whose income is over 1.5 times the average wage are ineligible.[3] Actually, fewer than 1 per cent of applicants have been rejected as a result of the income test.

4. There are two levels of benefit, parallel to the two levels of eligibility. The basic benefit is defined at the level of the disability pension from the National Insurance Institute (approximately $250). This is equivalent to approximately 10 to 12 hours of personal care per week. Those who are fully dependent are eligible for a 50 per cent increase in their benefits.

5. The basic entitlement is for a service-in-kind. However, the law has the unique feature that, when services are unavailable and the eligible person is being cared for by a relative living with him or her, he or she is legally entitled to receive a cash benefit of 80 per cent of the benefit for which he or she is eligible, until services become available. This provision reflects a concern with the basic entitlement of the individual under law, even if services are not available.

6. The kinds of provision under CLTCI are carefully delineated in a 'basket of services' which are closely related to direct caring functions. In addition to the most commonly provided service—personal care at home—the benefit can be used to provide adult day-care in day centres, a limited amount of home-making, laundry, and absorbent undergarments for the incontinent.

Beyond the services financed by the public sector, a significant number of disabled elderly also purchase care privately and are often charged higher rates by the home-care agencies. Others find and hire people to provide home care on a purely individual basis. These non-affiliated workers have widely different amounts of training and experience: some have nursing training, but many others may be totally untrained. There is no formal supervision of care in such cases.

The extent of service provision. The National Insurance Institute currently provides approximately 13 700 elderly people with personal-care services in the framework of the CLTCI law, 70 per cent of whom are over 75 years old and 22 per cent over 85 (see Appendix 8, Table 7). Two-thirds of them are women. On average, each receives 10.3 hours of help per week: 71 per cent receive 10 hours or less; and 29 per cent receive about 15 hours per week. The Ministry of Social Affairs provides services to approximately 1800 individuals, and the General Sick Fund to approximately 750 clients. The average number of weekly hours of assistance provided by all programmes is 9.4 (see Appendix 8, Table 5). Of the total of about 17 100 individuals who receive this service from the various public bodies 7020 (41 per cent) receive it from the Matav Association (see Appendix 8, Table 6). A further 830 elderly people purchase the service privately from Matav. Others may purchase the service without public finance from other sources.

3.2b. Home-making services

The nature of the services. In Israel home-making service refers to assistance with household cleaning, and may also include help with laundry, cooking, shopping and other errands.

The organization of the service and personnel. Most home-making services are provided by personnel recruited privately by clients. Until now, there had been no organization providing home-making services. But since the implementation of CLTCI, some of the new agencies employing personal-care aids have begun to organize the employment of home-makers as well.

The target clientele, eligibility criteria, and financing. Home-making services are financed by two separate public-sector agencies. The Ministry of Labor and Social Affairs funds them for elderly people who are physically or mentally incapable of managing their household, live alone or live with a spouse who is also impaired, and have an income below a specified level. Service provision is financed by cash payments made directly to the clients who, with the help of the neighbourhood social worker, find a suitable home help and negotiate the extent of help to be received. Often the payment covers far fewer hours than were formally allocated by the social service bureau.

The National Insurance Institute provides some home-maker services within the framework of CLTCI, but primarily in conjunction with personal care. The new law requires that services be provided through personnel affiliated to an agency that is obliged to provide the number of hours to which clients are entitled.

The extent of service provision. The Ministry of Labor and Social Affairs provides home-making services to approximately 7400 elderly people. There is considerable regional variation in the extent of the service provided, partly because of variations in the characteristics of the elderly population, but also because of budgetary constraints and policy differences among the various municipalities and local councils responsible for the provision of home-making services (see Appendix 8, Table 8).

In addition, many of the recipients of CLTCI provision receive this service jointly with personal care provided in the framework of the new law.

3.2c. Home-delivered meals

The nature of the service. This service provides two forms of meal: (i) hot meals delivered daily, and (ii) meals which are frozen and delivered once a week (7 meals at a time).

The organization of the service. The hot meals are prepared and delivered to the home by local voluntary organizations. The frozen meals are provided by several commercial companies. Referrals for the service are made by the social workers of the local social welfare bureaux.

The target clientele, eligibility criteria, and financing. Elderly people who cannot cook for themselves and who live alone, or with a spouse who is also similarly impaired, are eligible for this service. All clients are required to pay the full price of the products used in the meals (half the total cost of the meal), but the cost of preparation and delivery is subsidized by the Ministry of Labor and Social Affairs in accordance with income level.

The extent of service provision. At present, approximately 3500 elderly people receive home-delivered meals in their two forms (0.9 per cent of the elderly population). Demand is somewhat limited and is lower than the estimated need, partly because of the diverse ethnic groups in Israel, each with its own unique style of cooking, which make it difficult to develop a service that will meet the preferences of all clients.

3.2d. Professional home-nursing visits

The nature of the visits. This service includes giving injections (mainly insulin), taking blood, measuring blood pressure, follow-ups (monitoring), assessment, etc.

The organization of the service and personnel. Home-nursing visits are provided by professional nurses primarily from the General Sick Fund but also by some other, smaller sick funds. This service is not included in the basket of services covered by the CLTCI law.

The target population, eligibility criteria, and financing. The target population includes all the members who are insured in one of the sick funds that operate this service, mainly the General Sick Fund. The recipients of the service are homebound or bedbound people who may suffer from a variety of diseases. No means test is necessary in order to receive the service.

The extent of service provision. In March 1988 about 10 700 elderly patients received professional home-nursing visits provided by the General Sick Fund. These patients constitute three-quarters of the total number of patients visited. The number of visits was 43 000, which means that every elderly patient received 4.0 visits per month on average (see Appendix 8, Table 9). There are regional differences in the number of recipients. In the districts of Jerusalem and Tel Aviv, a smaller percentage of elderly people receives this service than in the southern and central districts. From 1981 to 1988 there has been an increase of 22 per cent in the number of elderly people receiving this service, but a decrease in 23 per cent in the number of visits per patient (see Appendix 8, Table 10) (Shavit and Levinson 1988).

4. ISSUES IN THE DELIVERY OF ADEQUATE SERVICES

4.1. Organizational issues

As noted above, it is not always easy to differentiate between the functions of each organization involved in providing care to the aged population, and duplication or overlapping often occurs. The division of responsibility is particularly complex for non-professional, personal care (Brodsky *et al.* 1988*b*). When the division of responsibility among agencies is based on the client's functional status, as in the case of personal care, responsibility for care is transferred from one agency to another as the client's condition changes. If inter-agency co-ordination is inadequate, these changes often result in discontinuity and unfortunate delays in the care provided. One of the most common problems preventing many elderly people from receiving the services to which they are entitled is the absence of established referral procedures among the various agencies.

Further difficulties arise because the criteria for classifying functional status are ambiguous. In borderline cases it may not be clear which agency should take responsibility for the provision of services.

Before the implementation of the CLTCI, officially the Ministry of Labor and Social Affairs was responsible for the care of the frail elderly clientele, while the Ministry of Health was responsible for the care of the elderly people who required nursing services. The decision as to who was responsible for providing personal care for a specific elderly person was particularly significant because 'frail' elderly people were entitled to fewer hours of personal care per week than severely dependent elderly people.

In a study that examined the provision of personal-care services to the elderly population before the implementation of CLTCI, Dolev *et al.* (1987) found some overlap between the groups receiving services from the different ministries. In terms of level of functional disability, approximately a quarter of those who received services through the Ministry of Labor and Social Affairs in fact met the guidelines for entitlement to services through the Ministry of Health, while a quarter of the elderly people cared for by the Ministry of Health also met the criteria used by the Ministry of Labor and Social Affairs. For both Ministries, more than half of the elderly people receiving care also did not meet fully the Ministries' criteria for service provision. Thus inequity developed, with elderly people of similar disability becoming entitled to unequal amounts of care.

Moreover, the mistaken assumption that the staff of other agencies would provide care may have caused clients to be overlooked by both Ministries. Inter-agency co-ordination is especially important in cases when clients are eligible for services from more than one organization.

The complexity of linkages within the system is further exacerbated by the interdependence of the various agencies for client assessments and the implementation of care plans. The social-welfare bureaux are dependent on information from the sick funds for medical–functional assessments, while nurses involved in providing personal services also require the psycho-social evaluations of social workers for comprehensive assessments of need. Inter-agency co-ordination reduces duplication in assessment tasks.

But, a national study of all of the nurses and social workers involved in providing care for elderly people (Brodsky *et al.* 1986) found that 70 per cent of the workers mentioned at least one problem in obtaining information from other care agencies: difficulties in contacting the agency staff, delays in receiving information, incomplete information, etc. However, despite the division of financial and professional responsibilities among agencies, most professionals feel that they are responsible for providing care to clients over and above the specific services provided by their agency.

The organization of home care in Israel should be understood against the background of the organization of the health and social services. An outstanding feature of the Israeli system is the universal availability of local, primary health-care facilities and social-welfare bureaux. It is thus relatively natural for professionals treating the same clients to establish contact. However, until recently, inter-agency co-operation was primarily the result of individual professional initiatives rather than formal arrangements. This probably explains the great variation in the range and quality of inter-agency contacts for different professionals and agencies (Brodsky *et al.* 1988*b*).

For all these reasons, considerable effort in service planning and development has been devoted to co-ordination between the various agencies. To strengthen and formalize inter-agency ties, a team model is currently being implemented nationally. Operating at the neighbourhood level, each team is composed of the neighbourhood General Sick Fund clinic nurse and the social worker from the local social-welfare bureau. The purpose of the teams is to regularize inter-agency co-ordination by developing a joint care plan for each client, based on a common assessment, and to assume overall responsibility for case management. In recognition of the importance of inter-agency co-operation, under the CLTCI law individual care plans are first formulated by these or other inter-disciplinary teams having direct field contact with eligible persons (Brodsky *et al.* 1988). The plans are then discussed, approved, and implemented by a higher-level local professional committee, as defined by the law.

4.2. The adequacy of the services currently provided

4.2a. Coverage

Extent of coverage as a function of the need for services is defined and measured either in terms of the need for formal services only or of total need for help (formal and informal). Before the implementation of CLTCI, need for services was defined as those unmet needs not being provided by informal sources. The assessment of unmet needs was based on the disability of the client in conjunction with the assessment of the ability of the informal support system to provide care without overburden. The estimate of unmet needs for that period was based on findings from a unique survey of elderly community residents in which public-health nurses made an overall assessment of each person's total need for help, and their unmet needs for formal services (Zilberstein *et al.* 1981).

From this study, and from extrapolation of its findings based on the age, sex, and ethnic composition of the elderly population, estimates were made of the extent of disability in ADL, and of the number of people requiring and receiving formal personal-care service from 1980 through 1988, before the implementation of the new law (Factor *et al.* 1988). In 1980, the number of elderly in need was estimated to be 10 800 and, on average, 8.5 hours of formal personal care were needed per week (see Appendix 8, Table 11). Personal care was actually provided to only 3300 and they received 4.2 hours per week. Thus, the coverage of recipients was 31 per cent, and they received (on average) half of the hours required from formal services. By 1988 (even before the implementation of the new law), the services had increased sharply and therefore unmet needs had decreased. While 14 400 were estimated to be in need of formal care, the system provided services to 9100 elderly people; 8.8 hours of care per week were now provided in contrast with an estimated need of 9.1 hours. Thus, by 1988, coverage rose to 63 per cent of those in need of formal services, and they were provided (on average) with 95 per cent of the required hours of care.

The dramatic increase in the proportion of disabled receiving services in 1988 was due to the National Insurance Institute's release of funds to the organizations already providing services, a preliminary to the eventual implementation of the new law.

Today, the public systen applies a dual approach to the definition of the need for assistance. The law ensures entitlements only for those elderly people who are severely disabled or who have severe cognitive impairment. The population of frail elderly who also frequently require some limited help in personal care, and all of those semi-independent and frail who need help in household management, are not entitled to aid from the new law. For the severely disabled, entitled to benefits under the CLTCI law, the need for assistance is defined universally, determined purely by disability levels, without consideration of the differential ability of families to provide care. For the less severely disabled, not eligible for benefits under the new law, and for those services not covered by that law, the Ministry of Labor and Social Affairs and the General Sick Fund continue to use the selective, discretionary approach as in the past, i.e., where the availability of informal care determines the amount of formal assistance provided.

Thus, a two-tiered system of home care has evolved in Israel. At the first level, CLTCI provides a basic level of care to the severely dependent elderly as a largely universal entitlement. The second level supplements the first selectively by providing, in theory, additional services to those with remaining unmet needs and to those ineligible for CLTCI. It is important to point out that since the new law is now providing care for a largely expanded population of severely disabled, some of the existing organizations have reduced the extent of service delivery very dramatically (see Appendix 8, Tables 3 and 4). There is a suspicion, not as yet fully documented, that the extent of service provision to those not eligible has also dropped below the levels available before the new law was implemented.

No current data are available regarding the number of individuals requiring formal services when these two definitions are taken into account. However, data from the national survey of the elderly in 1985 show that 8.8 per cent of the elderly people residing in the community (34 500 persons) are limited in the activities of daily living (ADL), and require at least one hour of personal help daily, either from the informal or the formal support system. Currently, (March 1989), 17 100 elderly people, or half of the disabled, are receiving personal-care services, mostly via CLTCI (see Appendix 8, Table 12). This is a very significant increase in provision, almost doubling the number of recipients since January 1988.

While we can safely assume that the most severely disabled are receiving a basic level of services under the CLTCI law, we know very little about the extent of unmet needs. However, among those not entitled we suspect that the pattern of unmet needs revealed in earlier surveys largely persists.

More significantly, while the number of recipients has increased dramatically, some of the most severely disabled may also be receiving a lower level of publicly funded services than before, when the system of service allocation was more flexible for meeting needs in-depth. As described above, entitlements under the new law are fixed at two benefit levels (equivalent to approximately 12 or 18 hours of weekly care). Although it was expected that those who are most severely disabled and also have a high proportion of unmet needs would receive additional services from existing organizations, this supplementation is not, in fact, being provided. Data from a study of elderly people receiving home-care services from the public sector (Habib *et al.* 1986, 1988; Dolev *et al.* 1987) indicate that one-third of the severely disabled require more than 18 hours of formal support for personal care and another 4 hours of housekeeping.

4.2b. The basket of services provided

Although a wide range of services has been developed nationally, the new law entitles clients to receive only certain specific services: personal care, day care, home-making, and absorbent undergarments for the incontinent. Those requiring home-delivered meals, physiotherapy or occupational therapy at home, round-the-clock supervision, or home repairs or adaptations, must apply to other agencies. But these services (with the exception of home-delivered meals) are generally limited.

4.2c. Appropriateness of service delivery

Personal-care workers typically only visit a client once a day, usually during the morning, although the client may also require help in the late afternoon or evening and it would be more in the client's interests to split the visit. Moreover, the workers generally do not come at weekends or holidays.

4.3. The possibility of substituting for institutional services through the development of community services

In parallel with the increase in the number of disabled elderly people, institutional services have also expanded rapidly over the years. During the 1980s the number of institutional beds grew by 44 per cent and today there are 18 000 elderly persons residing in long-term care institutions and a further 6000 residents in sheltered housing. However, even this significant increase did not succeed in closing the gaps between the needs of the population for placement and the ability of the system to provide it. This is emphasized by the lengthy waiting-lists for public-sector placement, which provides approximately 10 per cent of the total available beds. For some groups, the lack of beds is particularly acute: for example, for those classified as frail, the waiting may be for two or three years.

Meeting this growing demand for institutional services would require the investment of substantial resources to develop the necessary physical infrastructure, and a continuing commitment of large sums to support ongoing care. An extensive Israeli study (Habib *et al.* 1986, 1988) found that the provision of adequate community care would be possible and less expensive than the cost of institutionalization for a significant proportion of the elderly awaiting placement.

A field demonstration project on a selected group of severely dependent elderly people who had received approval for nursing-home placement showed that the cost of providing services at home in accordance with individual requirements was approximately 70 per cent of the nursing-home cost (Carmeli and Morginstin 1988). Yet, in 1988, even after the large increase in home-care expenditure with the implementation of the CLTCI law, two-thirds of the public budget for long-term care went to institutional services, and only one-third to community-based services (see Appendix 8, Table 13).

The study by Habib *et al.* (1988) also found that, for a significant proportion of the clients at all functional levels, community care would be the appropriate type of service in the opinion of inter-disciplinary teams that reviewed the cases, the practitioners responsible for their care, the clients, and even the family care-givers (see Appendix 8, Fig. 1). A major conclusion of this study, conducted before the new law came into effect, was that many of those waiting for placement applied because adequate community services were not available. Providing all of the services required by this population would have demanded extensive expansion of the services available then.

Furthermore, many acute and rehabilitational hospitals were and continue to be 'backed up' by elderly persons who could benefit from less expensive forms of care—in long-term care institutions or in the community—which are still unavailable. In 1986, 40 per cent of those in rehabilitational hospitals actually required only nursing care and could have been discharged (Korazim and Margulec 1986). By occupying these beds they prevented others who required rehabilitational treatment from receiving it. A better balance among the various care alternatives, as suggested by these studies, might result in cost savings to the public-service system and better care for all of those in need.

Thus, economic considerations, the growing awareness that there are alternatives, and the desire to provide appropriate care for as many people as possible have, during the past decades, led to far greater attention in Israeli long-term care policy to the development of community services and, most importantly, to the legislation of the new CLTCI law. To what extent the services provided in the framework of that law will actually influence the demand for and patterns of institutionalization is currently under study.

5. ASSESSMENT AND DISCUSSION OF KEY ISSUES

5.1. The personal-care/home-making mix

The system of home care for the elderly in Israel has several distinct features that emerge from this analysis. One is the emphasis on the provision of personal care, unlike many other countries, which tend to emphasize home-making services. Personal care is provided at relatively low cost, by semi-professionals not professionals, particularly nurses, as is often done in many other countries. The development of personal care in part reflects the large number of people with such needs in the community in Israel, partly because of the country's low rate of institutionalization. In general we would stress that the extent and nature of institutional care significantly influences the kind of disabled elderly people that remain in the community and, therefore, the challenges to the home-care services. At the same time, the emphasis on personal care may be responsible for some of the organizational problems that have developed within the Israeli system. It has led to a complicated division of responsibility between the health and social services. Whereas the financing of home-making services, until the development of the new CLTCI law, was focused within the social welfare services, the responsibility for personal care was divided between the health services, which were considered responsible for those whose situation was more severe, and the social services, traditionally viewed as responsible for the less disabled. In addition, the development of a semi-professional provider of personal care has also raised questions about the logic of the division of labour between the home-maker and the personal-care aid. There have been various local initiatives that seek to expand the role of the personal-care aid to include home-making chores, thus moving towards an integration of these two roles. Under the influence of the CLTCI law, there is now an even stronger tendency to promote this integration.

Obviously having a single provider of a range of home-care services has its advantages. On the other hand, the issue is a complex one because it is felt that the ability to attract and employ qualified persons in personal-care jobs might be more limited if they are also required to assume what are considered lower status, general home-making responsibilities. The question of the desired degree of specialization or integration of these two functions remains an open one.

5.2. The impact of entitlements on the demand for services

A question of considerable interest which has emerged from the Israeli experience is that of the impact of entitlement on the degree of demand for home-care services. When the availability of these services was limited by budgetary constraints, there were frequent claims, particularly by the General Sick Fund authorities who provided home care for the more severely disabled, that they were responding to all applications even though the amount of help being provided was limited. However, we find that under CLTCI there has been a very significant expansion in the number of elderly people who have applied for assistance, even in the most disabled category, which is the target population of the new law. There are two possible explanations. One is that the professionals in the field had a very biased view of the actual demand for help and that applicants were being discouraged in various ways from applying, so that the potential demand was not realized. The second possibility is that a system in which eligibility is based on principles of entitlement has a major impact on demand. Perhaps of greatest significance is the sense that the right to assistance under a social security programme had been earned by past contributions, although we should remember that, in fact, under the new law, all elderly people were included in the insured population despite the fact that most of them had stopped working well before payments began and therefore never actually made any contributions. An additional although related factor is the lack of stigma generally associated with applications for benefits to the National Insurance Institute. Extensive efforts were made by that Institute to publicize the entitlement to assistance. Widespread use was made of attractive publicity in the various offices of the National Insurance Institute, which are well-frequented by the elderly. Various counselling services were made aware of and distributed information about the law. The law was widely publicized in the newspapers and other written media, and there were even television spots devoted to such information. Another factor is the lack of self-participation in the cost of receiving services under the law.

Several studies are now under way which will help us to understand better the different attitudes of elderly people towards receiving help before and after the new law.

5.3. Universal access and entitlement versus restricted access and budget constraints

As has become apparent from this account, the extent of home-care provision in Israel until the expansion of resources that began with CLTCI was very low and a consensus had developed about the need to expand its availability. At the same time, there was a debate about two opposing strategies for expanding the availability of care (Habib and Factor 1988). One approach emphasized a broad concern with reducing the burden of care. This concern was based on the belief that most families living with a disabled elderly person were in need of some degree of formal support and that it was important to provide this assistance on a non-discretionary, equitable, and entitlement basis of social-insurance principles. The implication of this approach was one of extensive impact and coverage: to make a moderate amount of support widely available rather than enabling more intensive in-depth support to meet needs on a more discretionary basis. The second approach tended to have as its objective an intensive impact in meeting needs. Proponents of this view claimed that as resources were limited and it was not possible to provide for anything approaching universal needs, it would be better to concentrate resources on those having unmet needs. These needs were not only seen in terms of level of disability, but also in relation to the availability and quality of informal care. They would be best met through discretionary rationing among those families interested in and requiring in-depth assistance of this type.

The final decision adopted a more universal approach that would provide a basic level of services within a system of social-insurance principles.

Two cost-containment measures were structured into the programme to ensure some control in anticipation of a widespread uptake of benefit. The amount of resources that could be provided to an eligible individual were limited and clear-cut criteria of eligibility were defined, restricting the eligible population to the most severely disabled, defined more or less as those who need assistance in at least two of the basic ADLs, for example, bathing and feeding. A rigid instrument was introduced, based on the principle of scoring.

A further implication of adopting this universal approach, given the existing budgetary restrictions and the consequent restrictions on eligibility, was that the new law could not and should not replace existing sources of care but rather had to be viewed as a complement to other programmes. As noted above, complementary support would remain essential for several reasons; the new law does not provide enough hours of care to those who are eligible; there is a large ineligible population; and assistance is not always immediate because of administrative procedures, so that immediate, temporary support would still be required from supplementary sources. While coverage of personal-care needs has increased dramatically, the end result was that, at least during the period of transition, the system has become, in some senses, more fragmented in relation to divisions of responsibility for the basic home-care services. The introduction of the law has also led to confusion about the exact role of supplementary sources, and there is considerable concern that the realignment of entitlements within the health and social service system is not adequately making available the supplementary support that the designers of the law had expected.

Beyond expanding the resources available for providing care, the introduction of the law resulted in an overall system based on a dual set of principles: one in which eligibility is unlimited by budgetary considerations and one in which it is limited; one in which there is less flexibility for discretion by professionals and one in which there is more. Under these circumstances, the distinction between eligibility and non-eligibility under CLTCI can be particularly significant to the individual if supplementary support is not available from other sources. As a result, it will be important to examine, as part of the monitoring of the programme, whether there is a tendency among some of those making the professional assessments to include elderly people who perhaps, on strict grounds, would not fully meet the disability criteria. There is a degree of subjectivity involved in assigning persons to the various levels of disability, despite the considerable efforts made to prevent this by standardizing procedures (see Appendix 9).

The creation of a dual system based on a dual set of principles also raises questions about the future development of home-care services. To what extent will future development be based on the expansion of coverage under CLTCI, and to what extent will it be based on reinforcement and enhancement of the ability of the supplementary system to provide services based on budgetary constraints?

A further interesting question is whether the strategy whereby a basic level of care is universally available while a system of supplementary finance and provision is retained on a discretionary basis can be viewed as simply a local solution or as a reasonable compromise between the conflicting concerns and principles which are characteristic of other countries as well.

5.4. Entitlements and the dynamics of finance for home care

Before the development of the new CLTCI programme, one of the major issues of contention was between those who were interested in an entitlement programme, so as to guarantee full access to benefits and to provide more protection over time, and those who wanted to ensure more flexibility and control by the government bureaucracy.

A critical element in the debate over entitlement and budget-restricted programmes was the nature of their long-term dynamics. Entitlement programmes have several built-in features that affect this dynamic.

In talking about approaches to financing, one should distinguish two separate elements. One is whether finance is earmarked for the programme, and the second is whether the benefits are granted by entitlement. While these two will usually go together, this need not be the case.

The availability of earmarked finance (such as in the CLTCI law under social insurance) has several direct implications for the availability of finance over time, and for the flexibility of the system as needs change. First of all, the social security wage-base will generally increase with overall growth in the population and with the level of wages. Thus the programme has a built-in capacity to adjust itself to these factors. This feature characterizes any arrangements for earmarked financing, whether or not accompanied by entitlement on the benefit side.

Entitlement has several other implications. It obviously means that within a given year the budgetary limitations cannot restrict access to benefits. This is in itself an important element. The more complex question is what are the dynamics if a deficit should emerge. Unless the deficit is due only to short-term factors such as a temporary decline in the social security wage-base, there will either have to be an adjustment of the benefit or in contributions. This is in contrast to a budgeted programme in which the adjustment can simply take place in the form of an increase in uncovered needs, growing waiting-lists, and discouraged applicants. Thus an entitlement programme forces the issue of the growth in needs and how it must be addressed in terms of financing and coverage.

A further feature is that an entitlement programme is most likely to favour the preservation of benefits where there is a general cut-back in government expenditure, which may be applied automatically to all discretionary, non-entitlement items. The main reason is that actual decisions about the programme have to be made within a legislative setting. While all government budgets must be formally approved each year by a legislative body, the legislature does not necessarily dwell upon each item. Proposed changes in entitlements would have to become the direct focus of legislative decision making. This also affects the dynamics of the process, and depends on the nature of the legislative system and the orientation of the legislature. In Israel, for example, it is often claimed that the legislature will generally tend to favour increases in finance rather than reductions in social benefits. By contrast, in the case of a budgeted system, a proposal to increase the budget would not be submitted to the legislature without the prior approval of the Finance ministry, which might exercise a veto. It would thus not even come before the legislature unless there was a forceful initiative by one of the advocates of the programme.

On the other hand, where a change is required and advocated in a programme, such as a proposal to raise benefits or modify requirements, legislative procedures would slow down and complicate the process, whereas the regular, budgetary means could be more convenient for implementing change.

Given the dual system that has emerged for financing home care, where some provisions are based on entitlement and some are not, a further question arises. What happens to the non-entitlement component in such a system? Does it tend to be forgotten or neglected; or does it tend to be even more vigilantly preserved as a way of avoiding further expansion of the entitlement programme?

As mentioned earlier, in Israel the immediate response of the system to CLTCI was a cut-back in provisions within other programmes. This response, rather than being to protect and preserve existing programmes, was, of course, due to budgetary pressures. It was also probably due to the tendency of other ministries that are partners in the implementation of the new law to welcome an alternative source of financing rather than considering CLTCI a threat to existing responsibility and control. However, it will be important for future research to examine whether funds 'saved' in other programmes as a result of these cut-backs will be reabsorbed into general reserves or will be reallocated to provide better coverage for social services and populations not entitled to benefits under CLTCI.

5.5. Cash versus benefits in kind

Against the background of debate as to whether cash or in-kind benefits should be provided, CLTCI is a clear statement in favour of in-kind benefits. Offering a cash benefit as a viable option in a flexible programme was seen by its proponents as a means of compensating family care-givers for services, and of enabling elderly people to make independent choices in their acquisition of services. Cash benefits would allow individuals more variety in the services they could choose and the option of hiring persons not affiliated to an agency, or would simply be an additional source of income in place of services (which could then be provided by a family member).

However, as stated earlier, CLTCI specifies that eligibility for cash benefits is restricted to those cases where services are unavailable and where there is a family care-giver living with the eligible persons. Eligible persons living alone cannot receive a cash benefit; however, these persons receive first priority in access to institutions. Cash benefits are only provided temporarily until appropriate services can be developed in a given community.

The underlying assumption of CLTCI is that services are more effective than cash benefits in reducing the real burden of care by sharing caring functions with the informal care-givers. It was also thought that in the long term the provision of services in kind would have a greater impact on stimulating the availability of services, as has in fact occurred. However, when coupled with the stipulation that payments be made only to certified providers, providing home help through agencies means considerable, labour-related, 'overhead' administrative costs, making the service more expensive than it might be if it were provided by privately hired individuals, and perhaps allowing fewer service hours than an individual could obtain on a less formal basis.

5.6. Eligibility assessment

We now turn to issues concerning the organizational structure of CLTCI. There are a number of organizational issues that accompanied the development of home care both outside and within the new law. One issue of interest is who should make the functional assessments that are the basis of determining eligibility. In Israel there is a strong tradition that functional assessment is done by nurses. It would even be considered professionally inappropriate, for example, for a social worker to undertake these evaluations. Therefore, the Ministry of Social Welfare relies on functional assessments by nurses from other organizations in order to allocate the funds available for home care. Correspondingly there is a general tendency to recognize that social assessments are within the professional realm of social workers. This division obviously has broad implications. One is that a comprehensive assessment of an elderly person, almost by definition, requires assessment both by a nurse and by a social worker. Its advantage is in encouraging a comprehensive, team approach, where both these assessments are required, but there are organizational complications and extra input of professional manpower.

A further aspect of this issue was whether the functional assessment should rely primarily on self-reporting by the elderly client and a review of the medical documentation for verification, or whether it should be based on a systematic examination of the elderly person by the nurse. Regulations for CLTCI require an actual examination in the home, according to a manual, where the elderly person is specifically requested, if possible, to attempt to dress, to eat, to get in and out of the shower or bath, and to move around the house. The nurse is expected to look for evidence of incontinence, such as a plastic sheet in the bed or packages of absorbent undergarments. These demands are somewhat controversial and it is not clear to what extent the nurses adhere to them.

A third issue relates to the place in the system of the personnel who would carry out the assessments. There was a major discussion as to whether those involved in providing direct care for the elderly should also make the assessments, or whether independent, public-health nurses, not directly involved in ongoing care should do so. The concern was that those involved in direct care would tend to be too liberal in their assessments of eligibility and would be subject to more intensive pressure from the elderly person and their families. On the other hand, the public-health nurses base their assessments on one visit and do not have the advantage of sequential observation of the elderly client. In the end, this issue was resolved in favour of using the public-health nurses. The resolution of this issue was also related to the degree of centralized responsibility in administering the programme, as discussed below in Section 5.8.

5.7. Translating disability into benefit level and service needs

A particular pattern of dependency in ADL and IADL does not directly translate into the kind and amount of services required by the individual. This kind of decision is generally left open to the discretion of professionals. It involves a number of elements, including practical considerations, such as how much time it takes to bathe a person; value considerations—how often should a person be bathed; and environmental factors, such as the type of bathing facilities in the home. It is also influenced by a range of factors that concern how the service is organized. Is it possible, for example, for a home helper to make frequent short visits, or is there a required minimum time for a home visit? Are there different providers of care with strict role divisions so that more visits are required and more travelling time is lost (see Habib and Naon 1987 for an analysis of these various factors and an attempt to address them in the Israeli context)?

In relation to these difficulties, it has been frequently reported that professionals tend to use various rules for service delivery that do not necessarily adapt a specific care plan to the individual's situation. This is particularly the case when the resources available are very limited in relation to total needs.

A programme based on entitlement according to consistent and universal criteria of eligibility must therefore come to terms with this aspect of the decision-making process. In CLTCI, a scoring system was developed that is supposed consistently to translate disability into eligibility. The determination of whether one is disabled enough to be eligible for benefits, and the division between the two levels of care, are based on the score allocated. Appendix 9 contains the actual functional assessment, and the scoring system and levels of eligibility. This scoring system is certainly a unique effort and achievement in introducing a high degree of consistency in assessment. The rigidity of this type of approach is in the strict categorization of the levels of eligibility, which allows for only three broad categories rather than some continuous indication of the care required. This means that people in different circumstances will receive the same level of support.

The development of this kind of instrument is an attempt to accept the challenge of how to make decision making more effective and how to achieve greater consistency and equity. In CLTCI, having such a defined scale was considered crucial in meeting the need to defend decisions about eligibility within the judicial system.

5.8. Centralization versus decentralization of service provision

A basic issue faced by the home-care system is the extent of reliance on locally available nurses and social workers rather than on more regional and centralized professionals. Within the social service system, the local professional has always served as the key figure in assessment and care planning, his or her decisions requiring approval by a supervisor at a higher level. In the health system, the situation was more complex in that the Ministry of Health administered the service in district health offices; in the General Sick Fund both local nurses and regional extended-care units could initiate assessment and care planning, although the regional offices had to approve the final allocations in all cases. Within the health and social services there has been a strong tendency towards providing autonomy in decision making at the local level.

Within CLTCI, the issue of decentralization took on other dimensions. Because it is a statutory programme of social insurance, there is a very strong emphasis on principles of uniformity and equity, because these are part of the ideology of social insurance and because all decisions made within such systems of entitlement are subject to judicial review in Israel.

There is, in Israel, a very strong tradition of access to appeals, which is part of social insurance legislation, and much use is made of appeals by applicants and beneficiaries in cases such as involve disability insurance.

Because rights are subject to legal review, assessments of eligibility must be based on criteria that will be defendable in that review, and this was a major concern to the National Insurance Institute during planning. As mentioned earlier, this concern influenced the nature of the eligibility criteria themselves, but beyond that there was also a concern that once appropriate criteria had been adopted they would be implemented in the most consistent way possible and with full respect to due process. This led to concern that if assessments were widely dispersed among a large number of local professionals, there was likely to be a much greater variation in the quality of these assessments, both because of the numbers of people involved and because it would be more difficult to provide what is considered to be appropriate training for such a large number of people. It would also be more difficult to be selective and to exert quality control over how well a particular professional was qualified to make these assessments, and to ensure administrative follow-up and control. These were some of the considerations in favour of having assessments done by a smaller number of nurses from the Department of Health only. Similar factors influenced the decision to have a relatively small number of units responsible for care planning, reporting, and service delivery, at a regional rather than a local level. One must keep in mind, of course, that Israel is a small country to begin with, so we are talking about small regions. In the end, the country was divided into 35 major regions, within which the average number of elderly people was about 6000, and an additional, 200, smaller regions.

On the other hand, because the new law provided not cash benefits but services in kind, and because direct payments were to be made to providers rather than to the family or to the elderly person, who would then purchase services and provide receipts, the law required that a specific plan should be worked out for how the funds were to be used, in co-operation with professionals. Given this stipulation, it became clear to those planning the law that these regional committees, which would not be staffed by those directly in contact with the elderly client, could not assume the role of direct care planners in most cases. Therefore, an informal responsibility was placed on the front-line practitioners, through the inter-disciplinary teams that were being developed at the local level, to collect the information needed for planning, to prepare the plan, and to bring the recommendations to the regional committee. Once the care plan has been approved, either the nurse or the social worker from the inter-disciplinary team, depending on the nature of the case, is also given formal responsibility for following up the implementation of the plan.

As a result, although the law refers only to regional committees, the inter-disciplinary teams were given unofficial recognition within the procedures that were adopted to accompany the law, and as a matter of fact provided a strong impetus to the development of these multi-disciplinary units. In some instances, however, there are no front-line practitioners able to deal with the needs of the elderly. The regional committee then assumes this responsibility directly and serves as an important back-up to this function.

This set of arrangements reflects the interrelationship between centralized and more localized administration, and some of the considerations involved on both sides. Also involved is the basic autonomy of the front-line professional and the degree to which it is felt that his or her decisions should be subject to review at higher levels.

6. SUMMARY

In this chapter we have briefly reviewed some of the main features of the provision of home care in Israel, and some of the main issues that have been addresed in the development of the system. As we noted, one critical characteristic influencing the system has been the extent of need for personal care among the elderly living in the community, and the attempt of the system to respond to this and not only to home-making needs.

We have attempted to illustrate how there are a number of critical dimensions in the design of home-care systems that have important elements of interaction. The adoption of an entitlement approach had a strong influence on other decisions that were made about coverage, the level of care that can be provided, centralization and decentralization, the nature of eligibility criteria, the choice between flexibility and uniformity in assessment for eligibility, the emphasis on preventive care or maintenance, and the choice between concentrating large amounts of care on a small group having unmet needs or a small amount on a large, more diversified group. Israel has made a unique set of choices, as it has included a component of entitlement within the home-care system and, for the first time, includes entitlement to a service benefit within the social security system.

The dual system that has been created may be seen as only a step in the direction of developing a full entitlement system, or as a desirable compromise between conflicting concerns. It is clear that not only have the levels of support changed dramatically as a result of the adoption of CLTCI, but also that the dynamics of the system have been radically altered. There is no doubt that there also are difficult issues of co-ordination within this dual system that will need to be addressed if the present compromise is to be fully and effectively implemented.

NOTES

[1] The rate of poverty is defined as the proportion of persons belonging to families with an adjustable, disposable income below half the median for all families.
[2] For a single elderly person the basic pension is equal to 25 per cent of the national average wage.
[3] Income taken into consideration is that of the elderly person and spouse. For a couple, the income test is 2.25 times the average wage.

ACKNOWLEDGEMENTS

We thank Jack Habib for his contribution to the formulation of this chapter and his valuable comments, Miriam Cohen and Shmuel Be'er who provided research assistance, and Bilha Allon for her efforts in typing.

REFERENCES

Achdut, L. and Tamir, I. (1986). *Retirement and well-being among the elderly*. The National Insurance Institute, Discussion paper 34. NII, Jerusalem.

Beer, S. and Factor, H. (1989). Long term care institutions and sheltered housing: situation in 1989 and changes over time. The Brookdale Institute of Gerontology, Jerusalem.

Brodsky, J., Habib, J., Goldsher, E. and Naon, D. (1988*a*). Evaluation of a program to provide coordinated care to the elderly in the community: methodological issues. In *The evaluation of political and organizational structures and planned interventions that affect the wellbeing of the elderly* (ed. J. Munnichs). Deutsches Zentrum fur Altersfragen, Berlin.

Brodsky, I., Cohen, M., Habib, J. and Haron, T. (1988*b*). The organization of long-term care services in Israel: an evaluation. *Social Security* (Special English edn., June), 167–98.

Carmeli, M. and Morginstin, B. (1988). *Providing extensive home care services for severely dependent elderly*. National Insurance Institute, Jerusalem (in Hebrew).

Central Bureau of Statistics (1971, 1988). *Statistical abstract of Israel.*

Central Bureau of Statistics, Population and Housing Census (1983). (In Hebrew).

Cohen, S. (1988). The long-term care insurance law: background principles and organization towards implementation. *Social Security* (Special English edn., June), 4–22.

Dolev, T., Naon, D., and Factor, H. (1987). Characteristics of elderly receiving personal-care services. *Gerontology* (Israel Gerontological Society) **38–39,** 13–30 (in Hebrew).

Factor, H., Habib, J., and Shmueli, A. (1984). The role of demographic data in identifying high risk groups and projecting needs. Brookdale Institute of Gerontology, Jerusalem.

Factor, H., Habib, J., Naon, D., Bronsky, J., and Dolev, T. (1987). Relative costs of institutional and community care. Unpublished paper presented at the Ageing Well Conference, September 15–18, University of Sussex, Brighton.

Factor, H., Habib, J., and Be'er, S. (1988). Evaluating the need for long-term care services and their cost. *Social Security* (Special English edn., June), 134–54.

Habib, J. and Factor, H. (1988). Approaches to long-term care insurance law and their cost implications. *Social Security* (Special English edn., June), 69–83.

Habib, J. and Naon, D. (1987). Translating disability into service needs. Unpublished paper presented at the Ageing Well Conference, September 15–19, University of Sussex, Brighton.

Habib, J., Factor, H., Naon, D., Brodsky, J., and Dolev, T. (1986). *Disabled elderly in the community: developing adequate community-based services and their implications for the need for institutional placement*, Discussion Paper D-133-86. Brookdale Institute of Gerontology, Jerusalem (Hebrew with English summary).

Habib, J., Factor, H., Naon, D., D., Brodsky, J., and Dolev, T. (1988). *Disabled elderly in the community. Developing adequate community-based services and their implications for the need for institutional placement. Stage two: evaluation by multidisciplinary Teams*, Discussion Paper D-160-88. Brookdale Institute of Gerontology, Jerusalem.

Korazim, M. and Margulec, Y. (1986). *Organization and patterns of care in geriatric in-patient services in Israel. Day census of geriatric services*, JDC-Brookdale Cooperative Program Series, RR-1-86. Brookdale Institute of Gerontology, Jerusalem (Hebrew with English summary).

Morginstin, B. (1984). Response of formal support systems to social changes and patterns of caring for the elderly. *Social Security*, (Special English edn, June), 103–26.

Morginstin, B. (1988). *Issues related to the implementation of long-term care insurance in Israel*, National Insurance Institute, Discussion Paper 1 (Series B). NII, Jerusalem.

Morginstin, B. and Shamai, N. (1988). Issues in planning long-term care insurance in Israel's social security system. *Social Security* (Special English edn., June), 31–48.

Morginstin, B., Baich-Moray, S., and Zipkin, A. (1989). *Implementation of long term care insurance: April 1988–March 1989*. The National Insurance Institute, Jerusalem.

Shavit, N. and Levinson, R. (1988). *Home nursing visits in the districts of Kupat-Holim, 1981–1987*. Kupat-Holim Head Office, Research and Medical Economics Department, Tel Aviv.

Shuval, A. and Factor, H. (1988). *Agencies providing home-care services for the elderly in Israel, 1988*. JDC-Brookdale Cooperative Program Series RR-7-88, Brookdale Institute of Gerontology, Jerusalem (Hebrew with English summary).

Zilberstein, Y. *et al.* (1981). *Survey of medical and social needs of disabled elderly in Bnei-Brak*—needed services and their cost. The National Insurance Intitute, Jerusalem (in Hebrew).

8
Home-care services in Italy (with special reference to Genoa)

Carla Costanzi

1. Italy
2. Genoa
   2.1. The development of home care
   2.2. The aims of home care—formal policies
   2.3. The organization and staffing of home care
   2.4. The service in practice
   2.5. The achievements of home care
   2.6. New developments
   2.7. Key issues
Notes
References

1. ITALY

The first home-care services in Italy were set up in 1972 in some local authorities in the north, and towards the end of the decade in the centre and south of the country. In the north, local authorities often organized this service without any regional direction. In the south it was developed as a result of regional legislation surrounding the setting up of local health authorities, which followed the institution of the National Health Service under National Law No. 833 of 1978. Almost all the regional legislation directed the service specifically towards the elderly. However, a few local authorities[1] extended the service to children, the disabled, families, the handicapped, and the needy. In fact, most services are still aimed at the elderly, although there are variations in some regions, such as Trentino, Campagna, and Sardinia, where services to whole family units form a significant proportion of the total (see survey data in Appendix 10, Table 1[2]).

The main criteria of eligibility are:

- Residence—the first condition for all local authorities is that the claimant should be resident in the area where the service is offered.
- Age—local authorities imposing this condition define a minimum age of anything from 55 to 70 years.
- Income—in the majority of cases, clients are only considered for

home-care services if their income does not exceed the minimum pension offered by the National Institute of Social Security.

- State of physical and/or mental health—all local authorities will give consideration to elderly people with poor physical or mental health, including disability or invalidity.
- Absence of or a particular shortage of help from the family.

According to the survey,[2] chief among the range of needs put forward by clients are medical and nursing assistance, followed by home help, psychological, social, and financial support. Only 8 of the 88 authorities who took part in the survey ask their clients for any financial contribution. Contributions vary according to income.

Clients' active participation in the actual running of the service is very rare. It occasionally happens where a representative of the client group sits on the organizing committee.

Although the survey[2] used as a basis for this chapter is not comprehensive (regions such as Tuscany and Piemonte are not included, where there has been a fair amount of development in the home-care service over the past few years), the range of services covered is extremely wide. Bearing in mind the relative needs expressed by clients, there is a worrying shortfall in provision of many medical and also rehabilitational services. It should also be pointed out that only eight authorities can ensure that their clients receive a night-cover service should this become necessary (see Appendix 10, Table 2).

National provision is, above all, uneven in distribution. The service itself is not yet available in every part of the country. Where service is provided, the number of clients receiving it is so small that it cannot be considered a likely source of help, even for those who qualify. The home-care service is administered by widely differing organizational systems leading to very different levels of co-ordination and integration among the services, such that the resulting provision is itself very uneven.

The differences become even greater when average unit costs per client are taken into account; in fact it is impossible to make a comparison on this basis, given the huge disparity in services offered. It is also impossible to offer an explanation for the variety of services offered by different local authorities in terms of different perceptions of underlying need. According to the ministerial survey,[2] only 23 per cent of the authorities have undertaken an enquiry to determine the extent of need of possible candidates for home-care provision. Furthermore, this overall unevenness of provision (apart from the common negative characteristic of a lack of integration with other services) can be blamed on the slowness with which we have, in this country, accepted the notion of offering care in order to keep 'the needy' in their own homes for as long as possible.

It follows that among the many consequences of a lack of cultural awareness of the need for domiciliary care, there has been little legislation in this area. The home-care services suffer from the lack of a legal definition of key professional figures within them. A professional profile has only been defined quite recently (1984), as have the necessary qualifications for a 'home help and care services worker', by a national Commission for the study of the caring professions.[3] These provisions are still waiting to become legally binding.

2. GENOA

The remainder of this chapter is devoted to a study of home care in the city of Genoa.

2.1. The development of home care

Generally speaking, a historical perspective of the way in which a service was started up can help our understanding of how it has evolved, and this is particularly so for home care. This perspective gives a broad account of the positive elements in its development and emphasizes some of the current problems.

The home-care service in Genoa was set up half-way through the 1970s. To be precise, in 1984 the first experimental home-care centre was opened on the outskirts of the city. In 1974 the service, which had by then defined its aims more clearly, was extended to a further seven areas. By 1978 there were 15 centres (out of the 25 areas into which the city is divided). In 1979 its governing regulations were approved. At the present time each urban area has at least one centre. Although each of these hardly ever offers complete cover, in some locations, such as in the historic city centre, there are two offices in one area because of demand.

The 1970s was a time of great social upheaval in Italy as far as the question of public involvement in matters of health and social welfare was concerned, as well as in the identification of existing local bodies that were potential providers of institutional social services. The increased amount of legislation came about as a result of social pressures and cultural changes taking place in the late 1960s, and which began to take concrete shape after 1970.[4] Conference followed conference, papers were published, and new journals were floated. Intense debates opened up amongst workers, the services, and training centres, which challenged the existing structure of welfare provision and, more generally existing social relationships. Behind the grand projects to restructure the health and welfare system lay the hope of changing fundamentally the whole social structure. All this leads some writers today to describe that period as a 'movement'; for example, Manoukian (1988, p. 26) states:

> It is not by chance that the various laws were put forward not so much by the left-wing parties [the Italian Communist Party and the Italian Socialist Party] but were supported across party lines, by organizations outside the traditional party channels. I am thinking in particular of the feminist movement, which I believe has had a central role in setting up advice centres, and of the Democratic Psychiatry movement for Law No. 180 [ruling on the closure of asylums]; but also of the workers' and students' movements that worked at a local level to empty orphanages, institutes for the handicapped and special schools, and to bring about the setting up of the first integrated services.

During this period of cultural and political flux, in some local administrations there was, at times, positive co-operation between workers and certain politicians who took key roles in the administration of the service. These were often charismatic figures to whom the workers turned for support and advice when faced with problems posed by passive resistance, inertia, and downright bureaucratic obstinacy on the part of officialdom. Again, one may quote Manoukian (1988, pp. 32–3):

> It seems that the organization's bureaucracy, which is still directly or indirectly the backbone of all its activities . . . can be taken over by a new organizational order centred on teams of workers; all together, all equal, united under their powerful leader.

These people are advocates of political aims that go beyond party politics, informing the system and political institutions of the emerging demands of society at large.

The setting up of the home-care service in Genoa came about in such a context. The representative for social services for the Genoa council from 1976 to 1985 (i.e., for the duration of the left-wing administration) was a charismatic leader who made a great impression on the workers, not least because he himself was a social worker. With hindsight, this way of setting up the service was to prove something of a handicap; a radical change in political climate later led to a general loss of the impetus that was vital to the whole nature of the service in the early stages of the movement, and to a more local effect, the loss of a charismatic leader. The hypothesis on which this chapter is based is that the present crisis in the public services is not so much rooted in the paucity of and contradictions in the legislation, rather it is a feature of a transitional phase between the initial critical and innovative thrust of the emerging services, and their institutionalization through the legal system. This transition has had the effect of dampening forward planning. It has created a state of 'organizational stagnation', which, in the future, could lead either to further decline and disintegration or to new organizational and cultural developments. In my opinion this notion provides a fundamental way of tackling any analysis of the service that seeks to understand its peculiarities and its present problems.

2.2. The aims of home care—formal policies

In following the ideas and guidelines that underlay the culture of service provision at the time when home care was first being tried out and regulated, the service started out with the ambitious policy of de-institutionalization, both by reducing numbers and delaying admissions, thus providing a real alternative to residential care.

The stated regulations of Article 1 in 'The aims of the home-care service' are:

1. To enable clients to be as responsible and autonomous as possible.
2. To keep people in their own environment, giving them the necessary support.
3. To avoid the marginalization of the weakest members of the nuclear family and the breakdown, even temporarily, of the family.
4. To further the community involvement of conscientious objectors and of volunteers.
5. To avoid residential or hospital admissions unless strictly necessary.

The service aims to meet the basic needs of elderly and handicapped people. To this end the regulations set out the following priorities concerning client groups.

1. *For elderly people:*
   (a) those who have requested admission to residential care and to whom the conditions for home care apply;
   (b) requests for home care from those who are otherwise likely to need admission to residential care;
   (c) those in residential care or hospital who are fit to be discharged;
   (d) those who are healthy but who live alone;
   (e) those who live with their family, but who cannot be taken care of because relatives are away for long periods during the day, either because of work or illness.
2. *For handicapped people*:
   (a) those who do not receive any form of help;
   (b) temporary cases, to avoid admission to children's homes.
   (c) temporary and urgent cases to avoid admission into care, where the family is unable to help the person for serious reasons of work or health.

In each of the above, in selecting cases, priority will be given to those in straitened financial circumstances.

The information the management committee needs to evaluate individual cases is contained in two files, one drawn up by the doctor and one by the social worker. The social worker usually makes a report after a home visit to the elderly person who has asked for help. Most of the information on the family and social situation of the elderly person is contained in a 'descriptive' part of the file (the actual 'report'), the presentation of which can be varied (in breadth, amount of detail, accuracy, etc.)

Unlike the procedures for admission to residential care,[5] the regulations do not require central supervision of the appropriateness of the decisions for action, nor do they define the weight to be given to each criterion in assigning priorities.

The actual home-help services offered are completely free to those who qualify for them; only some social activities and summer holidays require a financial contribution from some income groups.

The workers in the field and centrally complain of the total lack of direction on objectives, strategic chores, priorities, and new initiatives. The only form of planning is the annual budget. However, even in this context an annual review is too narrow to develop significant action plans for social-work intervention. This is in contrast to the previous administration (from the inception of the service up to 1985): at that time there was an ongoing cycle of meetings between the administration and the management committees to discuss how the service was going and any new problems that arose. In this way the administration developed ideas for formulating the social policy of the service. At present the management committees meet to discuss all the most significant problems of the service (daily running and directional trends) and draw up proposals to present to the councillors. What follows from this, though, can be described in terms of negotiations between two 'opposing factions' rather than as an occasion for consultation and participation in policy decisions.

2.3. The organization and staffing of home care

2.3a. Organization

Home care is run by the local authorities. Subject to Regional Law No. 1/1974, the local authorities present annual budget requests for the home-care services as well as a report on the running of the service itself; the region draws up an annual division of finance between the local authorities. Genoa council coped with the request for financial contributions until funds were used up for annual expenditure and fixed costs. The whole issue is about to undergo radical change, following the recent law for the Ligure region No. 21 of 6 June, 1988, 'Restructuring and programming of social services in the Ligure region'.

A historical perspective of the period in which the service was set up is also helpful in understanding the importance given in the overall organization to the role of the team. The service is run at two levels (central and decentralized), each of which is divided into working groups.

The central level is made up of four teams covering the following tasks: (1) formulation of advice and proposals on social policy; (2) technical unit, co-ordinating intervention; (3) and (4) checking the accuracy of administrative processes (although the advice of the team in (1) is binding) both as regards admissions into care and the ongoing payments of financial benefits.

At the decentralized level (that is, in each of the 25 areas into which the city is divided) are the home-care centres, the actual providers of home-help services; each home-care centre is made up of: a team of workers, and a management committee. This committee is peculiar to the service in Genoa and deserves a rather more detailed description. It is made up of (a) representatives of residents in the area; (b) client representatives; (c) representatives from the work team. The task of this committee is to run the service at the local level, that is to decide to which people to offer help within the limits set by the regulations; to maintain links between the agency and the field; to give advice, opinions, and proposals on all aspects of the service. Thus it is a body of genuine social management, with responsibilities that go far beyond the formal involvement expected from other bodies. This committee carries a significant work-load and meets weekly.

In spite of this, and unlike the deep and widespread unwillingness to involve oneself in public life which has increased over the past 10 years, this management structure has amazing vitality, which suggests that, when people are asked to make decisions about concrete situations that are relevant to them, they do not hold back. Furthermore, it seems that this direct involvement has raised awareness, at least in some parts of the population (the more politically active), of the nature of the problems faced by elderly people.

The home-care service is a public service. But the private and voluntary sectors are playing an increasing role. It is mainly the laundry and transport services that need to fall back on the private sector. For some time there has been talk of offering contracts to service co-operatives for all the tasks that can be described as 'domestic help' (house cleaning, meal preparation, etc.). Special mention must be given to the voluntary sector, which over the past few years has increased its service, especially to elderly people, and is very active in some areas of the city.

Looked at in this light, the regulations seem quite out of date, having failed to foresee in any way the involvement of such a resource actually working in the field. Neither did they allow for the tasks undertaken by volunteers, which are often very valuable in broadening the service offered but which require a constant effort of co-ordination on the part of the public-service workers. In emergencies, for example, the way in which the voluntary sector is set up allows for a much more flexible, and therefore more effective, response than from the public sector. The movement towards a much greater use of the private sector by the public service, as well as the use of volunteers and other local resources, raises the question of urgently 'retraining' the public-service workers in this area.

In fact, whoever organizes the provision of assistance needs management skills (an up-to-date knowledge of resources available in the area; the ability to support and extend informal networks; and an ability to integrate different types of assistance). He or she also needs to draw upon and supervise the help offered from outside the public service (encouraging a professional attitude; checking on the type of assistance). Although within the social workers' scope many of these skills need specific training.

There is provision for institutional links with local authority lodgings, rest homes, and social centres. In fact, the service has links (though these are often beset by problems, as discussed later) with general practitioners, the hospital service, the mental health service, and the elderly and handicapped peoples' health service of the local health authority.

2.3b. Staffing

Altogether there are 200 workers in the service, divided into the 26 teams working in the field. Each team, according to regulations, is made up of social workers, home helpers, and nurses. Regulations do not set a limit on the numbers in each team. However, it has come to be regarded as standard that each team has: 1 social worker, 6 home helps, 2 nurses. While some teams are weighted in order to cope with a higher demand in a particular area, where team size is below average it is usually because of particular policy or administrative difficulties (such as an actual freeze on hiring staff).

The present distribution of professionals is: 29 social workers; 141 home helps; 42 nurses. Apart from the workers in these professions, the service also employs 9 administrative assistants, each one responsible for an area covered by two or three centres. A reorganization is being considered at the area level, which would provide for co-ordinating social workers with technical and administrative responsibilities.

The three professions of workers attached to the home-help service have different requirements for qualifications, as follows.

1. *Professional nurses* have for some time been subject to official regulation, both in terms of their functions (DPR [Presidential decree] 14/3/1974 No. 25) and in terms of the training curriculum (L [Law] 867 of 1975). Italian legislation is in line with the directions of the Strasbourg Agreement of 1967. Courses last for three years, and access to courses is limited to people with 10 years of schooling.

2. *Social workers* have only received official recognition of their profession very recently (DPR 15/1/1987 No. 14) as well as a definition of training requirements (DM ['Ministerial decree'] 30/4/1987). Training consists of a 3-year course following on from the upper secondary-school diploma. It is mainly carried out in field-work placements.

3. For *domestic assistants* and *home helps* there is still a great lack of regulation. In Genoa, training courses have been held for the past three years in agreement with the regional representative concerned. The total number of hours of training is about 700; training is usually carried out in the home-care centres.

Although admission to the training course (and thus to apply for posts) only requires completion of eight years' schooling, nearly half of the home helps now working in home-care centres hold a secondary-school diploma, and some of them even have a degree. Perhaps this fact can be seen not only as indicative of the difficulty nowadays of finding a job corresponding to one's educational abilities, but also as demonstrating the strong interest shown by young people in community work.

None of the professions represented in the service has ever had any training in specific tasks before starting work, despite the diverse institutional backgrounds and the different levels of professionalism among the workers with which the service was begun.

2.4. The service in practice

2.4a. Services available

Home-care services, according to regulations, include: (a) home making; (b) nursing care; (c) help with rehabilitation; (d) laundry; (e) transport; (f) provision of heating; (g) shopping; (h) checking suitability of facilities, advice on repairs, and house repairs that are the responsibility of the tenant; (i) ongoing financial support; (j) socialization and help with administrative tasks; (k) any other help that seems appropriate (chiropody service, meals-on-wheels, care of clothes, etc.)

2.4b. Services requested and provided

Sources of information used in this section are (i) the findings of our own study of elderly clients, which although very detailed only covers three areas of the city;[6] (ii) information given by some of the workers; and (iii) the data contained in Genoa Council's report on the home-care service for 1986 (this is the most recent document the administration has drawn up on the activities of service).

The Council's report contains, among other things, data relating to: (a) requests made to the home-help centres in 1986; (b) characteristics of the clients; (c) services offered.

Requests for home care. During 1986, 9017 people applied to the home-care centres in Genoa, in the categories shown in Table 8.1. Overall, the inappropriate referral to the service of significant numbers of people suffering hardship shows the low levels of awareness of existing public services

Table 8.1. Categories of applicants to home-care centres, 1986

	N	%
Over 70s	7281	81
Handicapped (18 to 59 years)	630	7
Others[1]	868	9
Unclassified[2]	238	3
TOTAL	9017	100

[1] The category 'others' (which had increased by 6.5 per cent over the previous year) is indicative of the economic crisis and urban change in Genoa; many people who are not elderly come to the home-help centres for help with problems of employment or housing.
[2] 'Unclassified' are those whose age was not given.

and of the help they offer. This is both because of the short time such services have been available, and the lack of public information.

The age ranges of the elderly people applying to home-care centres in 1986 are shown in Table 8.2. The types of help requested are listed in Table 8.3. There is an overall increase on the previous year (Table 8.4).

Table 8.2. Ages of the elderly people applying to the home-care centres

Age (years)	*N*	%
60–64	919	13
65–69	1117	15
70–74	1415	19
75–79	1574	22
80–84	1241	17
85 and over	1015	14
TOTAL	7281	100

Table 8.3. Types of help requested from the centres (all age groups)

Request	%
Administrative matters, including appeals, negotiation, information	30
Ongoing financial help	15
Long-term residential care	14
Occasional financial help	10
Home help	7
Help with housing	6
Recreational and social activities	5
Nursing help	3
Escort for reasons other than socialization	1
Radio-taxi service	1
Short-term residential care	1
Changes in the type of care	1
Work for the elderly	1
Work for other than elderly	1
Other types of application	4

Table 8.4. Changes in the requests for help 1985–86

Request	1985	1986	% change
Help with housing	381	544	+42.78
Escort for reasons other than socialization	70	97	+39
Work for elderly	116	130	+12
Administrative help	2927	3043	+4
Occasional financial help	984	1015	+3

The clients. Seven hundred and forty-three clients were accepted in 1986 (79 per cent of them women). This shows that only slightly over one-tenth of those applying to the service for help are accepted. This represents 0.5 per cent of the over-75-year-olds in the city. The average age of clients was 76 years, most of them living alone (Table 8.5); 83 per cent of those living alone were women.

The service did not gather information as to the degree of functional ability of the clients.

Services provided. The average number of services per month offered by home-care centres is shown in Table 8.6. As far as the frequency of service is concerned, most cases require weekly (39 per cent) or twice weekly (19 per cent) input, although quite a few (16 per cent) require daily attention.

Table 8.5. Categories of clients receiving home care

	N	%
Alone	542	73
Two-person households	125	17
Three or more people	15	2
Sheltered housing	22	3
Not known	39	5
TOTAL	743	100

Table 8.6. Monthly average number of services offered by home-care centres

	N	%
Shopping	1475	24
Cleaning	1120	18
Escort	167	3
Laundry	131	2
Meals-on-wheels	668	11
Surveillance/companionship	429	7
Administrative matters	292	5
Nursing help	1830	30
TOTAL	6112	100

The functions of the centres can be divided into two distinct areas:

1. Centres dealing with the elderly person as an individual, in which the main activity focuses on home care in the strictest sense. Here there is a fairly small number of clients, while the number of services offered tends to be higher. The clients are 'very elderly' and have been the responsibility of the home-care centre for many years.

2. Centres mainly for the elderly as a social group: the work of these tends to focus on old peoples' free time. Consequently the number of elderly people they deal with is greater, while the number of services offered tends to be lower. Also a considerable amount of time is spent on organizational and administrative work connected with implementing social activities.

2.4c. Variations within Genoa

The most relevant data from the Genoa research, such as from interviews with officials co-ordinating the activities at central level, show a wide disparity in the services offered between one centre and another. This is not only because of the different types of clients but, according to these officials, because of the wide discretion allowed in decision making. So, for example, even the instruction to select referrals for help on the basis of financial hardship is so vague as to be open to different interpretations. Only where a cash hand-out is requested is the actual income threshold clearly stated.

A study[7] of three areas in Genoa illustrates the variation in types of services provided (Table 8.7). According to these data, some centres seem to concentrate their help on particular problems, offering services in a

Table 8.7. Type of help received by a sample of clients from three home-help centres (Corn., Molo, and V. Stur)

	Corn.	Molo	V. Stur	Total	%
Socialization	22	5	24	51	68.9
Financial help	1	12	7	20	27
Social support and administration	4	8	7	19	25.6
Domestic help	9	4	4	17	22.9
Help with housing	–	7	–	7	9.4
Other help	3	2	4	9	12.1
Transport	1	2	4	7	9.4
Nursing care	2	2	2	6	8.1
Delivery of supplies	1	2	1	4	5.4
Other	3	–	2	5	6.7

specific area and, apparently, overlooking others. One can check on this by examining the type of problems that have *not* been dealt with by the service, which have been reported by nearly a quarter of the home-care centre clients in the sample (Table 8.8).[8]

Workers from the centres interviewed during the research project confirmed this view of an agency that offers services on the basis of an internal work programme ('whatever service could be offered at the time') rather than according to need. Where this way of working proves less than effective, the service tries to provide informal improvements, such as 'inventing services that have not been catered for', or offering a more generalized response (such as social activities in large groups).

To illustrate the mistakes that can arise from such strategies, workers cited the case of a couple who had referred themselves for help with shopping. On the first home visit, workers were struck by the 'very worrying' state of cleanliness of the old people and their homes. They therefore decided to increase their involvement and respond to this need as well. The

Table 8.8. Problems (absolute numbers) not dealt with by the services in three centres (see Table 8.7)

	Corn.	Molo	V. Stur	Total
Social service	3	1	2	6
Nursing care	1	6	2	9
Socialization	–	–	1	1
Help with housing	–	1	–	1
Other help	3	2	1	6

case was later reviewed, as both the elderly couple and the workers 'were dissatisfied': the clients did not want help with cleaning; they were asking for something else; meanwhile the workers realized that there are different ideas of what makes a house 'habitable'.

Clients are usually described by workers as very serious cases, likely to become worse; however, even where there is an improvement it is hardly ever possible to reduce the input of services. Cases are rarely short term. Poor living conditions are usually exacerbated by loneliness, which is often the key element in deciding to call on the service.

2.4d. Unmet needs

Groups who have suffered exclusion from the service are handicapped and elderly people who have problems in being self-sufficient. There is probably also another group of potential clients who are currently excluded from the service: all those who are so much on the fringes of society that they have no access to information that would tell them that the service exists. Indirect confirmation of this hypothesis can be found in the part of the report measuring the amount of information over-75-year-olds have about the service; among this group less than a third knew of the existence of a service providing help with housework and personal care.

Chief among the unfulfilled needs reported by workers are the range of circumstances and problems caused by senile dementia. Although accurate data are not available, it is known that the problem is consistently large[9] and that a high level of help is needed in these cases. Another group not adequately provided for at this time are those who, for various reasons, need continuous care. In fact, the working hours of the service are inadequate, as night time and weekends are completely without cover. There is a further shortfall in rehabilitation provision: when the service was set up teams also contained a physiotherapist, but since then a specific physiotherapy service has been created. This seems to have caused referral problems, leaving most clients without access to physiotherapy.

To complete the picture it should be said that our research found that many general practitioners are unaware of the existence of a rehabilitation service. Furthermore, these organizational failures and the lack of information are found in a system of public services where there is an obvious shortage (in reality an almost total lack) of intermediate provision that would ease the transition between hospital and home.

It seems unlikely that services over and above the actual needs of the client could be offered. However, it is possible, in theory, that the same family unit could receive financial help from two sources at the same time if, as well as the elderly person, there was a child in the family getting support from the mother and child welfare service. Like the elderly person, the child could receive not only ongoing financial support but also a 'bonus' because these two sorts of help are offered by two different offices that have no way of cross-checking. Given the usual financial circumstances of the client though, it is not likely that even such a duplication would give them more than they need.

2.4e. Decision-making and delivery

In practice the decision-making process described in the previous section implies, in my opinion, a series of problems that can be summarized as follows.

1. In the first place the method used allows important differences in the type of information on which a decision is based: not only can reports differ widely among themselves in the sort of information gathered (in the 'descriptive' section the writer can decide which details are relevant and which to overlook), but also within each particular file the sections on health and social factors are not comparable as different methods of evaluation are used.
2. As there are no criteria for clarifying the facts there is room for further distortion; in other words, individual, decentralized committees can interpret the regulations differently.

To sum up, it could be said that the practical and regulatory constraints attached to the means of evaluation (the file), and the lack of professional expertise necessary to make a complex assessment, allow too much discretion in the decision-making process. Thus it is possible for elderly people in similar conditions with similar needs to receive differing degrees of help according to where they live in the city.

2.4f. Contacts with other services

The service has closest links with communal housing and social centres, with both using the services of the personnel of the home-help centre in their area. Social centres are often 'offshoots' of the service, or at least in close contact with it.

There is close contact with residential homes (both independent homes and those run by the local authority), as the service acts as the point of referral to them; however, there are no other formal contacts between them. In the past few years a new use has been made of residential homes where rehabilitation schemes are offered. Here 'short-term admissions' are being tried out; in other words, the residential home is being used as a stepping stone between hospital and home.

Some of the greatest difficulties experienced in establishing links with other services are with the mental health service. These relate to conflicts of rcsponsibility, which can cause considerable hardship to the clients who can be 'off-loaded' from one agency to the other while clarification is made of their actual needs.

Even greater difficulties are experienced in contacts with hospitals, and are mostly related to the timing of discharges, and how they are undertaken. The basis of the problem is the tremendous shortage of long-stay beds on the one hand and the bureaucratic delay in providing home-help services on the other.

For many elderly people, given the absence of any intermediate facilities while their condition improves and/or home-help assistance begins, chronic illness inevitably means admission to institutional care. Neither doctors collaborating with the home-care service nor general practitioners have any say in this decision.

As the demand for home-nursing assistance is very high, given the level of resources available to the service, it has been decided to overcome this shortfall in many cases by offering financial help so that the elderly person can turn to the private sector. In 1988 about 160 people received this kind of help. This type of solution seems likely to develop at a steady rate, although obviously it will be limited by the budgetary constraints imposed in recent years. In 1988 this item of expenditure was twice that in 1987.

Other Italian regions have overcome the problem of increased demand for home care by passing the responsibility over to the National Health Service, or rather by dissociating this type of help from the services they offer. Even though this solution seems to get round the economic problem (the Health Service has a much more reliable financial budget than local authority social services) it has to be offset against other problems, first and foremost the difficulty of co-ordinating services offered by two separate administrative bodies.

2.5. The achievements of home care

Workers are convinced that admissions to institutional care should be avoided, and that independence should be maintained for as long as possible, and they quote in ongoing scheme in support of this. It is a monitoring exercise devised internally and based on the teams covering areas containing communal housing.[10] On comparing new admissions to community housing and those to residential care, it has been noticed that while the mental and physical state of institutionalized clients deteriorates very quickly, the turnover of housing tenants (bearing in mind that they are only accepted if they are self-sufficient) is very slow, or rather their physical and mental deterioration is very slow. It has therefore been suggested that a more lively social setting, for which the tenants are directly responsible, helps to maintain not only physical self-sufficiency but also mental agility, particularly memory.

Although official data show that from 1979 onwards there has been a levelling off of new demands for admission to residential care, this does not seem to be attributable to an expansion in the home-care service.[11] In fact the number of home-care clients has stayed more or less constant since the service began functioning in Genoa. Thus one could attribute the levelling off partly to a changed awareness of institutionalization in the population, and partly to the administration's policy which, by redefining the financial criteria regulating cash hand-outs, aims to tailor them to the actual needs of clients in order to give them independence. For example, clients needing constant nursing care (several hours every day) have, with financial support, been able to pay for nursing care from the private sector.

As regards the importance attached to the above mentioned aim to establish an 'alternative to admission', a recent paper (Dellacasagrande 1989) underlines the limitations of the initial approach, which by emphasizing the domiciliary nature of the service rather than the idea of community care, has meant that the service:

> provides standardized home services of a temporary nature relating to primary health or personal care needs of a clientele whose conditions would soon require an admission into care; thus its only objective is to put off for as long as possible an otherwise inevitable admission.
>
> This has meant an actual loss in practical terms, of a large part of the potential clientele and a part of the network of relationships of actual clients, resulting in a piecemeal approach to the problem and the non-utilization of potential existing resources. In short, we have run the risk of institutionalizing the home, suffocating at birth the community-based character of the service.[12]

In other words, 'bringing the services into the home' does not necessarily imply effecting a change on the combination of factors that lead to an admission to institutional care. This development has occurred over the years, leading the service to widen and fulfil its role and its expertise. It began from a recognition of the intrinsic relationship between primary and secondary needs, which widened the practical applications of the service nationwide in its various contexts:

to free the individual from the weight of mere subsistence we must act together, worker and client, to rediscover interpersonal relationships, cultural interests, educational activities, participation, to learn to describe our interests and the needs that arise from them, and to put forward appropriate answers (Dellacasagrande 1989).

With reference specifically to its clients, the service is defined nowadays by those in charge of it as at least an alternative to inappropriate admission to care (old people with financial problems, or who are isolated, but who are physically self-sufficient).

However, the re-evaluation of objectives could perhaps be even more consistent. An analysis of decision-making processes at home-care centres undertaken in an experimental project on the evaluation of the needs of the elderly[13] showed how frequently extreme solutions were resorted to, such as leaving home (and then being taken into care), even in cases not regarded by workers as 'extreme'.

It was suggested that the adoption of very strict criteria reflects the tendency to use the resources that are 'easiest' for the administration (rather than the most appropriate for the elderly person) because of insufficient personnel is allocated to the service, which results in a need to redirect referrals to other departments. Also, in considering which elements make up 'a case', workers fail to take into account resources (such as informal support) that already exist or can be easily brought into play to ease the situation of the old person, who is seen by the service outside his/her social context of relationships, friendships, and lifestyle.

This contradiction can be blamed on the gap between the formal aims put forward by the service and the more pragmatic action practised by workers in real situations. It is further made possible by the absence of an analysis of the client that draws together the problems presented. The service only systematically records the services offered.

Very few handicapped people are in receipt of home-help services. However, according to regulations they are entitled, along with the elderly, to receive these services. In 1986 they formed 6 per cent of the total client groups. In 10 out of 26 centres there were no handicapped clients on record. The only service available to them consists of vouchers for radio-taxi transport.

As mentioned above, over the years the range of services has been increased, after pressure from workers who pointed out the dangers of producing social isolation. In fact, the regulations ignore the whole problem surrounding the socialization of the elderly, although actual casework management can have a dramatic effect on it. Thus the service has instigated a series of initiatives such as holidays, social centres,[14] and good neighbour schemes.[15] These activities are mainly aimed at completely self-sufficient people.

2.6. New developments

The most consistent new development shown by workers in the service and by data in the report is the importance given to initiatives aimed at socialization. In fact, these initiatives have been extremely successful, and not only in terms of numbers of clients involved. The various activities in this category are so popular that they are breaking down the field-work boundaries of the services. To get to the social centres and take part in the activities held by them, elderly people will travel from their homes, often with considerable inconvenience, in a city that was certainly not designed with the needs of the elderly in mind; not just because of the steep hills, but also the shortcomings of the public transport system. This is proof of the widespread need for social activities, which has long been underestimated in planning services. Consequently there has been an expansion in this area at the expense of the home-care service itself: for example, during the summer, staff of home-care centres are called in to accompany groups of elderly people on holidays organized by the social centres.

There are also interesting developments in ways of using the service; the home-care centres are being used more and more as area advice centres for all types of information, and more generally as a social advice service to help people, not only the elderly, to deal with an increasingly complex social set-up. This is worth bearing in mind when assessing needs, and as far as reorganization of the service is concerned.

It seems unlikely that the planning aspect of the service will change, however much this is needed. Workers have bemoaned the lack of planning for years. However, the service is very much affected by 'external' decision-making processes due to the influence of pressure groups in the health-care professions from related fields. There is widespread awareness of the defeat suffered in the struggle against the growing 'medicalization' of all aspects of the problems of the elderly.

In this respect the service has only resisted total paralysis because some room for manoeuvre is allowed by the independent decision making won by home-care centres. This speaks in favour of allowing the service to adapt to the different needs of clients, but this would require some flexibility in decentralized co-ordination and planning. This is really the crux of the matter.

In fact, the service is based on two different organizational models: the model in the field can be defined as an 'open system' having close links with the environment in which it functions while the organizational units that make up the system are fairly independent. Centrally the model is different, being formal and bureaucratic, based on authoritarian control and carrying out instructions, so forming a hierarchical system of services and municipal offices. This uneasy mix of two contrasting organizational methods leads to a series of inconsistencies at various levels of the structure.

2.7. Key issues

This description of the home-care service in Genoa has emphasized the cultural and political climate of its early years, not because it was unusual at that time, but because it is a point that is often overlooked by other studies. Despite the difficulties of pioneering a service for which no one had professional preparation, to be part of the changes being tried out gave the workers the energy and motivation to approach those first years with vigour, setting up the basis of the service itself and establishing working methods. In fact, the whole structure of the service is designed so as to draw together the working groups (the field-work teams and the various committees at central level) and share the work between them.

When the first signs of impending crisis were seen, both workers and management approached it by studying ways of organizational restructuring. The point to be made here is that these studies have not only failed to produce any changes in the structure and working of the service, they have also neglected some important factors. Indeed, it appears that a change in organization would not be enough to deal with present problems and difficulties. The historical background of the service shows that input needs to go to the workers, to support them in working through the extremely demanding and complex evolutionary process they are having to undergo. In the absence of official interest (there has been no high-level political impetus for years), under constant threat from external pressure groups (the health service), faced with complex financial problems (increasing cuts in public expenditure), it would seem that a broadly based, long-term training programme giving workers concrete support in their development would help them to cope with frustrations and acquire a more mature professional attitude.

Another important factor that is often overlooked in forward planning is professional training of administrative officers. In Italy one very rarely comes across professionals who have made a career in administration (and it is not unusual to be transferred from one sector in the administration to another totally unrelated one). Such transfers are, for example, 'normal' when a council changes its political complexion, either because the outgoing councillor takes his 'trusted' officials with him, or because the incoming councillor removes officials in key positions who do not have enough political reliability. This causes many problems in the social services department, as in this area it is not enough to understand the administrative machinery and to have organizational and management experience. Evidence of this shortcoming can be seen in the 'wastage' in failing to make use of the wealth of experience, and mistakes, that 15 years of life have given the service. The central problem remaining is the lack of technical training of officials in the public administration, most of whom know nothing of the particular profession that they are administering or of the principles underlying the social policy of the sector.

In discussing the main problems besetting the service, some mention must be made of how the whole network of public services is run. As we have seen in this chapter, many difficulties are caused by the lack of integration of the services, as well as shortcomings in their initial planning: in particular, the lack of intermediate structures forces the existing structures to be used inappropriately. Some of these problems could be solved by setting up district health centres, which would offer all non-specialist social and health services together in one place.

Finally there is a series of problems that can be bracketed under the general heading of 'cultural' shortcomings. Public awareness in areas connected with services for the elderly is still very underdeveloped. This shortcoming is reflected in the almost total lack of authoritative representatives for the rights of the elderly and of organizations for the protection of clients of the services.

2.7a. A service for whom?

To conclude these observations on the home-care service one must ask what effects the many changes now in the air will have on demand for the service.

National legislative output (above all the long delay in producing a law reforming social-work services), together with policy decisions at the local level, have allowed an increasing medicalization of the problems of the elderly, which has led to a greatly decreased budget for the social services. As cuts in quantity inevitably lead to a lowering of quality, there is a risk of less opportunity for professional growth for workers and a growing loss of responsibility on the part of the local authority, who will find a useful alibi in the growth of the voluntary sector and private agencies offering care services.

The move towards privatization of the services, which is gathering momentum in Italy at the moment in all areas from education to health, is a further problem. As the public sector has not developed adequate methods of evaluation and standards of care, they are ill equipped to undertake a realistic quality control of the private services. Thus the citizen is completely at the mercy of a market which no one controls except in superficial ways (such as keeping within health regulations, and within administrative and accounting procedures).

The dynamic activity in the private sector will presumably have two (interconnected) possible results, that is offering services to the middle and upper classes, and making an arrangement with the public services to help with clients in the disadvantaged classes, leaving those in the middle with no alternative to residential care because they would neither be entitled to services nor able to afford the expense of private help.

If other factors are not brought into play, the service will be further stigmatized as a resource for people in financial difficulties. The shortage of financial resources means that selection is heavily based on income, and within this social group as many cases as possible are diverted towards the hospitals or residential homes.

NOTES

[1] The implementation of the service is left to each individual authority; that is to say the agency that administers it and has the power to adjust regional guidelines to specific local situations.

[2] These data, like other details of the national situation used in this part of the report, were drawn from a survey undertaken between 1981 and 1983 by the Ministry of Internal Affairs (1984*a*) in collaboration with several regions and with 88 local authorities already actively involved with the home-care sector (a total of 249 services).

[3] See Ministry of Internal Affairs (1984*b*).

[4] A concise chronological summary may help in understanding the changes that the sector has undergone:

1970
- The regions were set up, and were given a primary role in welfare and health policy, allowing a transfer of function, responsibility and property from the national welfare authorities to the local authorities.
- Divorce law.

1971
- Local authority crèches set up.
- Legislation on free availability of contraceptive advice.

1975
- Womens' health clinics opened.
- Reform of family law legislation.

1978
- Asylums closed.
- Legislation on legalizing abortion.
- Legislation setting up National Health Service.

[5] The decision-making process for admissions to residential care is centralized, and clients referred are classified into priority categories. There are six categories of priority, as follows:

Category 1: not self-sufficient, alone.
Category 2: not self-sufficient, being an excessive burden on family or living with people not obliged to support them financially.
Category 3: partly self-sufficient, alone.
Category 4: not self-sufficient, living with relatives for whom they are not an excessive burden, *or* partly self-sufficient but being an excessive burden, *or* partly self-sufficient but living with people not obliged to support them financially.
Category 5: partly self-sufficient, living with relatives.
Category 6: self-sufficient.

The process whereby each client is classified into one of these categories involves a number of stages, which are shown in the following model:

Decision-making model for residential care admissions

A ⟶ MC ⟶ AC ⟶ Classification into one of six priority categories

---

A: *Assessment* by a social worker and a doctor, each of whom draws up a report.

MC: *Management Committees* at local level. Each of these committees deals with clients in a particular locality and puts forward opinions dependent on the acceptance of the request. They follow a set of rules which are established by the authority.

AC: *Admissions Committee*. This is a committee operating at a central level, which processes applications from all the local management committees in the authority. It administers a general queueing system and placements in residential institutions. This committee does not look into the merits of decisions made by the management committee, but merely checks on the accuracy of the administrative process.

[6] The areas concerned have varying problems but each has a high proportion of complex cases and is thus not representative of the whole city as far as the client group is concerned. As well as data from a questionnaire to the elderly, the report also gives information drawn from interviews with groups of home-care centre workers, as well as from discussions with a sample group of doctors working in the three areas covered by the report.

[7] The sample of home-care centre clients was made up of exactly 100 subjects (of whom 90 were referred by the services themselves). There were 16 replies missing to this particular question.

[8] The subjects interviewed reported their main problem.

[9] According to World Health Organization data (of 1981), 5 to 10 per cent of over-65-year-olds will suffer from some form of dementia, with a higher incidence among the older age groups. This suggests that in a city the size of Genoa there are presently between 7000 and 14 000 people suffering from dementia.

[10] These are dwellings for a maximum of 8 to 10 people, meant for elderly people living alone with family support, and/or for socially deprived people who have severe housing problems and who are clearly suited to community life. The group is completely self-managed. As well as the dwelling and furnishings, the service offers financial help (towards food and other uses), social services (support and co-ordination in running the household and relationships between tenants), as well as other services normally offered by the home-help centre. In the city area there are now seven of these.

[11] Admissions into institutional care (Table 8.10). It can be seen that in absolute terms the number of admissions to residential care is fairly constant, despite the fact that the population of over-70-year-olds has increased from 23.4 per cent in

Table 8.10. Numbers of admissions to institutional care by year

1979	474	1984	568
1980	570	1985	603
1981	596	1986	558
1982	577	1987	551
1983	465		

1981 to 26.4 per cent in 1987. Therefore there has been a slight overall decrease in admissions.

[12] The critical study quoted here is from a paper given by C. Dellacasagrande (1989) at a workshop organized by the Italian Communist Party. A proposal was put forward at that forum to reorganize provision for old people unable to look after themselves (at present placed in institutions, usually very large ones) by introducing locally based sheltered housing (with 60–70 beds each) so that ultimately each area of the city would have one or two units (a total of 43 for the 25 districts) and the largest institutions could be done away with altogether.

[13] This experiment aimed to develop an evaluation tool with input from the CNR (The National Research Council) strategic project 'Expert Systems in Medicine'. For further information on the aspects referred to in the text, see Puliafito and Costanzi (1989).

[14] This is an institutionally 'hybrid' scheme as it uses public facilities but is staffed by volunteers and conscientious objectors. Its objective is to encourage socialization in the area through cultural activities, recreation and sport, etc. The running of the service is mostly undertaken by its users.

[15] These are volunteers who offer to keep an eye on neighbours, to keep them company, do odd jobs, etc., in exchange for which the council pays them a nominal fee. In fact, they have not been very successful so far, despite the importance given to strengthening informal networks shown by the relevant published record and by experience. The present number of people involved in these schemes with the service is about 80. These are mostly women (89 per cent); the average age is about 64 years (with a maximum age of 78 and a minimum of 51).

REFERENCES

Dellacasagrande, C. (1989). Relazione alla giornata di studio: Dall'albergo dei poveri alle residenze di quartiere per anziani (From the workhouse to local authority old peoples' home). Paper to a workshop organized by the Italian Communist Party, 28 January. Unpublished.

Manoukian, F. O. (1988). *Stato dei servizi. Un'analisi psicosociologica dei servizi sociosanitari*. Il Mulino, Bologna.

Ministry of Internal Affairs (Ministero Dell'Interno) (1984*a*). *I servize di assistenza domiciliare*. Direzione Generale dei Servizi Civili. (General Civil Service Department), Rome. (The home-care services).

Ministry of Internal Affairs (Ministerio Dell'Interno) (1984*b*). *Gli operatori sociali: urgenza di una normativa* Direzione Generale dei Servize Civili. (General Civil Service Department), Rome. (Workers in the caring professions, the need for legislation).

Puliafito, P. P. and Costanzi, C. (1989). Un approccio alla valutazione delle condizionidegli anziani tramite tecniche di intelligenza artificiale. In *Nuove tecnologie negli interventi per la terza età* (ed. M. Niero). Emme e Erre libri, Padova.

9
Home-care services in the Netherlands

Wim van den Heuvel and Hans Gerritsen

1. Introduction
2. The development of home-help services
3. Present provision of home-help services
   3.1. Staffing and extent
   3.2. Assessment criteria
4. The home-help service and the care of the elderly
   4.1. Home nursing and its relation to home help
   4.2. Relation between institutional and community services
5. The home-help service in practice
   5.1. Policy goals
   5.2. Service use and functional ability
   5.3. Service use and income
   5.4. The relationship between informal care and the home-help service
6. The effects of policy
   6.1. Substitution
   6.2. Co-operation
   6.3. Effects of co-payment
7. Concluding remarks

References

1. INTRODUCTION

In the Netherlands, the home-help service is largely subsidized by the government. Up to 1989 the money was allocated from general tax revenue to private organizations by the Ministry of Health, Welfare and Culture. Since January 1989, services have been funded through the Exceptional Medical Expenses Scheme (AWBZ). The AWBZ is a law which originally applied to long-term care (nursing homes; care longer than one year in general or psychiatric hospitals), but which now, under the reconstruction of the Dutch health insurance system, is gradually being extended to cover a large part of the costs of all health and social-care services (Commissie Structuur en Financiering 1987).

The home-help service is officially defined as: help of a domestic and caring nature, occasionally supplemented by help of a personal and supporting nature, offered to all inhabitants of the Netherlands who need at least help of a domestic nature related to illness, recovery, old age, handicap, death, psycho-social, and personal problems that threaten the maintenance of the household. Its objectives are to support families and individuals in need and enable them to live as independently as possible.

In this chapter a short history of the home-help services in the Netherlands is presented, followed by a description of its work and staff (numbers of organizations, intake procedures, workers, and client characteristics). Over the last five years, the home-help services have made several innovations in organization and content. Several of these innovations have been evaluated by social scientists, and the results are described in the third part of this chapter.

2. THE DEVELOPMENT OF THE HOME-HELP SERVICES

From around 1900, two 'movements' could be seen as the bases for the home-help service as it exists today. The first was related to district nursing. With the rise of district nursing as a professional and organized task it became evident that households needed (additional) care as regards housekeeping. Nurses were not qualified to do this work, so other helpers were appointed. The second movement was related to the organization of 'work for the poor'. This was traditionally part of the work of churches and charitable organizations; they distributed money, food, clothes, etc. The work was organized and 'controlled' on a voluntary basis by women from the upper classes. The 'controlling' function led to home visits, which showed the need for support with housework. This type of work could not be done by the 'upper class', so a 'helper' (unskilled) was organized to do the housework. These 'helpers' had two interrelated tasks: to improve the functioning of the household by both 'doing' and 'teaching'. This kind of help was given for a short time (maximum 6 weeks) during the day from Monday to Friday (08.00–18.00 hours), supervised by the charitable organization. Money came from private organizations and churches.

After World War II in 1947 the first government money was made available in recognition of the home-help service, followed by financial arrangements between national government and local governments (state and municipality). About half of the salary of home helpers was paid by each authority; only private organizations and churches could use these arrangements. Until the mid-1950s the emphasis of (and the motivation for financing) the home-help service was on supporting the family and the industrial process. Later, increasing emphasis was given to the care of older, handicapped, and chronically ill people. In 1955, differentiation in type of work and workers began (trained and untrained helpers; long-term service) and the financial arrangements changed as a consequence (direct funding of management tasks, training, and educational requirements, etc.). After several financial 'adaptations' (increases in salaries, etc.), a major change followed in 1967: qualitative requirements were formulated for organizations (organizational arrangements, numbers of employees, quality of staff, etc), and they received higher subsidies when they fulfilled these qualitative standards (A-institution). In 1971, the financing of the home-help service was taken over by the state (national level), which subsidized 90 per cent of the salaries of the managerial workers, 85 per cent of the salaries of the other workers, and gave an annual amount for 'organization and management'. The clients had to pay a small contribution depending on their income. Subsequently several technical adjustments were made to the financial arrangements but basically the system remains the same. Recent developments included an increase in the client contribution and plans to finance the service as part of a 'general health insurance'.

During the last 15 years (1975–1989), there have been more changes and innovations in the nature and operation of the service. Several of these innovations have now been implemented and are described in Section 3, together with the present provision of home-help services. Besides the change in client characteristics, the developments in costs were the major reasons for the innovations. During the last decade, financial restrictions have been constantly imposed on the home-help service (Maessen 1989), despite the important task it was said to have in 'controlling' the increasing demands on the health-care system due to the ageing of the population.

In 1980 the government subsidy was about fl. (guilder, *gulden*) 1.1 billion; in 1988 it was fl.1.4 billion. The client contribution increased from 98 million in 1980 to 125 million in 1986. These figures (Table 9.1), however, should be compared with the GNP, health care expenditure, and the retail price index. They show the fluctuations in the budget for home-help services due to annual cuts and changes in the regulations. The first column shows the amount of subsidy planned in the government's annual budget. In practice there is considerable deviation between planned and actual expenditure (column 2). Actual expenditure is known after two years, and often turns out to be higher. Despite the average increases in total spending, *per capita* spending on these services decreased by 11.5 per cent from 1980 to 1988 (see Table 9.2). In the same period the number of clients served increased by a quarter, but the average number of hours of home help per client increased by almost 30 per cent. The change from helping families to helping chronically ill and elderly people has been mentioned above. The help to families has decreased in the last few decades, as is shown in Table 9.3.

Table 9.1. Development of expenditure on home-help services, and other costs developments in billions of guilders. (Source: Centrale Raad voor de Gezinsverzorging 1988.)

	Subsidy to home-help services					
	Planned expenditure	Actual expenditure	Client contribution	GNP	Health-care expenditure	Price index
1980	1.141	1.287	0.098	336.12	27.680	100
1981	1.137	1.291	0.107	351.89	29.606	106.7
1982	1.224	1.350	0.118	368.48	31.693	113.0
1983	1.292	1.353	0.129	381.58	33.159	116.0
1984	1.210	1.307	0.131	398.07	34.060	120.0
1985	1.326	1.357	0.127	416.20	34.795	122.7
1986	1.251	1.336	0.125	423.95	35.933	123.0
1987	1.409	1.413	–	427.15	36.488	125.0

Table 9.2. *Per capita* spending on the home-help service in guilders (fl.), 1980–1988. (Source: Centrale Raad voor de Gezinsverzorging, 1989.)

1980	1981	1982	1983	1984	1985	1986	1987	1988
122	117	116	115	114	114	110	110	108

Table 9.3. Service hours to families, elderly and chronically ill people, in percentages, from 1980 to 1985. (Source: Centrale Raad voor de Gezinsverzorging 1988.)

	Families	Elderly	Chronically ill
1980	28	51	20
1981	27	54	20
1982	26	56	18
1983	26	57	17
1984	26	58	16
1985	25	59	16

It is evident that because of the ageing of the population the clients and the tasks of the home-help services have changed over the last few decades. The role of the service has grown, especially during the 1980s. This growth is related to the process of deinstitutionalization in the care of elderly people. On comparing the age of persons in households receiving the service with that of all households, the differences are remarkable (Table 9.4). Out of

Table 9.4. Percentage of different age groups (in years) receiving home help, 1987. (Source: Centrale Raad voor de Gezinsverzorging 1988.)

15–34	0.4	55–64	1.8
35–44	0.7	65–74	6.2
45–54	1.0	75 and over	15.3

all households in the Dutch population of 75 years and over, more than 15 per cent receive care from the home-help service, whereas this percentage is far smaller in younger age groups. The data show the relevance of the home-help service for the elderly.

3. PRESENT PROVISION OF HOME-HELP SERVICES

3.1. Staffing and extent

Home-help services in the Netherlands are offered by private organizations (foundations), which have a 'regional' function. There are 233 such organizations. About 120 000 persons work within the home-help services, two-thirds of them part time. The majority of the workers (about 114 000) directly deliver home help. The 'indirect' workers (6000) are in management and administration (2200 persons) or are home-help organizers/supervisors (3800). The organizations serve 265 000 clients annually, most of them elderly people (63 per cent are 65 years and over). The total amount of money involved is fl.1.6 billion; 90 per cent of the budget is provided by the Ministry, 10 per cent is client contributions. In general, the home helpers are employees, paid and supervised by one of the home-help organizations. The help is organized full or part time, normally as half days. The kind of help can be described as either long term or short term. Of the 265 000 clients, 22 per cent receive short-term help. Traditionally the clients are differentiated as 'families', 'elderly', and 'chronically ill'.

From 1984 to 1989 the financial arrangements were as follows. Each home-help organization received a budget from the Ministry of Health, Welfare and Culture, including direct and indirect costs. Additional budgetary sources were client contributions (income dependent), social security payments to employees (in case of illness), interest, and gifts. The Ministry subsidized about fl.1.4 billion a year; the client contribution was about fl.0.13 billion; receipts from sickness benefits were about fl.0.07 billion. From 1989 the budget has been financed by the AWBZ. The costs of the home-help service differ between regions because of distances, type of clients, organization, and investments. The cost per hour of home help is fl.31.17. About a quarter of this are indirect costs.

During the last 25 years the functions and tasks of the home-help service have become specified and professionalized. Historically, the home help began as a stand-in for the 'housewife' when she was not able to run the household, thus enabling the man in the family to continue going to work. Later, more and more old people made use of the home-help service. A special section for elderly people was later established, doing more or less the same tasks. The employees can therefore be distinguished with respect to the age group they are working for and the level of education. There are formal courses and training programmes for all types of employees. For families (Dutch, *gezin*) there are *gezinsverzorgsters* (home carers) and *gezinshelpsters* (home helpers). For elderly people, there are *bejaardenverzorgsters* (home carers for the aged) and *bejaardenhelpsters* (home helpers for the aged). Carers have more formal training than the helpers.

In addition, new types of care have been developed from these 'core disciplines'. 'Alpha care' was established as a way of providing cheaper help. This is achieved by allowing people to work as home helpers for a maximum of 16 hours a week, which is the limit below which they do not have to pay social security contributions. In 1986, Alpha care contributed 13 per cent of the total home-help hours compared with 5 per cent in 1980. The Alpha carer has the same tasks as the home help but the employer is the client. Alpha care is formally organized outside the home-help organization. However, most home-service organizations operate as an intermediary between carer and client. In addition there is the *wijkbejaardenverzorging* (community/district care for the aged), which provides service (less than 3 hours) in the evening, night, and early morning. The allocation of workers depends on the care needed and on the age group.

Thus there is a large variety of workers. This professional and organizational differentiation had started by the end of the 1970s as part of the process of deinstitutionalization. Much emphasis is now placed on adapting services to individual needs. This is called *zorg op maat* (tailor-made care). This innovation is also called '7 × 24-hour help', indicating that home help is available at all hours, seven days a week. This may include help for a very short time (for example, 15 minutes), or for longer (for example, 3 hours) at specific times, depending on the client's need. Moreover, more helpers are available for the client and the client can always reach the home-help service by phone to ask for help. *Zorg op maat* was developed to prevent (older) people from being institutionalized (especially in nursing homes and homes for the aged), to enlarge the possibilities of early hospital discharge, and to enable people to die at home. As indicated before, the innovations were partly caused by the financial restrictions ordered by the national government and partly by changing concepts of care.

Table 9.5. Staff of the home-help services by category, 1985. (Source: CBS 1986.)

	Full time	Part time	Total
Senior staff (management, home-help organizers)	1873	2695	4568
Clerical personnel	655	724	1379
Trainees			3278
Carers	4153	7157	11310
Helpers	2489	62598	65087

The numbers and types of employees of the home-help services are shown in Table 9.5. The majority of the workers are part-time helpers. In addition, there are relatively full-time carers. There is a hierarchy, depending on the level of training, from helpers to carers to senior staff.

Table 9.6 shows the distribution of hours among various client groups. The majority of elderly people are receiving 2.5 to 7.5 hours per week, while families when they are in care often receive more than 10 hours per week. The pattern of the Alpha-care group is similar to that of elderly people because the clients of Alpha care are mainly elderly. The number of hours provided to those chronically ill varies more than in the other client groups.

3.2. Assessment criteria

Another way to describe the tasks of the home-help service is to look at its intake criteria. The service has a formal and standardized intake system for

Table 9.6. Number of hours of the home-help service per week, by client group in percentages, 1980. (Source: CBS 1981.)

Hours	Elderly	Chronically ill (<65 years	Families	Alpha care
0.0–2.5	2	1	2	3
2.6–5.0	34	15	8	45
5.1–7.5	36	23	9	34
7.6–10.0	16	21	13	10
10.1–20.0	9	22	26	7
20.0	2	17	42	–
Actual number of clients	101041	21536	17871	11477

clients, called *Landelijk Indicatie en Registratiesysteem* (LIER; National intake and documentary system). This system is used by the home-help organizers to assess and allocate the quality and quantity of care. In the background of the registration system are common values about equity in the allocation of care, information for policy purposes, and a careful assessment of need. There are no research findings available on the validity and reliability of the system. Findings on a comparable system, homes for the aged, however, provide reason enough for serious doubts.

The LIER system includes four clusters of information, as follows.

- Assessment of the capacities of the client: physical capacity and capacity to handle one's own affairs and to arrange things. This also includes the possibilities for informal care.
- The nature of care to be provided: home-making tasks, personal care, or socio-emotional support.
- The quality of the worker: a home help, home carer, or Alpha carer.
- The extent and duration of care; division of tasks.

In Appendix 11 there is a translated version of a form from the LIER system. After assessment by the home-help organizer the care is allocated by matching weekly total (new) demand and available capacity. Therefore the most desirable amount of care cannot always be provided. Reassessment is made at least twice a year.

4. THE HOME-HELP SERVICE AND THE CARE OF THE ELDERLY

4.1. Home nursing and its relation to home help

Because of the change in work patterns and the emphasis on *zorg op maat*, co-operation with other professionals in the primary-care system becomes more important. In particular the tasks of district nursing are related to those of the home-help services for severely handicapped or terminally ill clients. District nursing is provided through private organizations. The costs are covered by the AWBZ. The tasks of the district nurses are: nursing as necessary; care and monitoring at home related to illness, handicap, and dying; care for mothers and babies/children; provision of facilities; and preventive visits and health promotion. Of the total client population, 72.2 per cent are elderly people. Most of this care is being provided by nurses, who have a formal education in community work. In addition there are district carers (*wijkziekenverzorgenden*) who have less training. In all regions a 7 × 24-hour service has been introduced (Leemeijer 1986).

Table 9.7. Tasks of the home-help services and district nursing. (Source: Boom and Suurmeijer 1989.)

Personal care	Who delivers in principle	Who delivers in practice	
		District nurse (%)	Home-help service (%)
Bathing (totally)	District nurse	48	2
Bathing (partially)	District nurse	20	7
Feeding	District nurse/home help	1	9
Dressing	District nurse	28	11
Mobility (in and out of bed)	District nurse	8	4
		(n=599)	(n=463)

Locally and regionally there is growing co-operation between district nursing and home help, although they are still independent organizations. However, each still have their own intake systems. Home-making tasks are often only done by the home-help service and nursing is the specific function of the district nurses, but there is overlap in the area of personal care because increasingly the home-help service is undertaking this. These differences in function are made clear in Table 9.7, which shows that while, in principle, most tasks are covered by district nursing, bathing (partly) and dressing are now also undertaken by the home-help service. Feeding is done by the home-help service, while bathing (totally) and, to a lesser degree, helping people in and out of bed are major tasks of the district nurse.

4.2. Relation between institutional and community services

The home-help service operates in relation to many other services in the care of elderly people. The Netherlands have a unique structure of the care: in particular the large capacity of the institutional facilities is remarkable compared to that of other countries. Table 9.8 provides an insight into the housing conditions of older people and the proportions using institutional or community-care facilities.

The majority of people live in the community, most of them at home, some in sheltered housing. A third of those living at home or in sheltered housing receive care from either the home-help service, the district nurse, or both. Some 1.5 per cent of all elderly people receive care from both the home-help service and the district-nursing service. Almost half the total population of elderly people lives entirely independently. Thirteen per cent of elderly people live in an institution. For those in general hospitals and non-psychiatric nursing homes, their stay is not permanent. These

Table 9.8. Housing conditions and care for those aged 65+ years in the Netherlands, 1982. (Sources: CBS 1984; Van den Heuvel 1989.)

Living independently with no formal care %	At home with formal care (%)			Living in sheltered housing (%)		Living in institutions (%)		
	Home help	Both	District nurse	Care	No care	Homes for aged	Nursing homes	Hospital
57.5	10.5	1.5	2.5	8	7	9	3	1

percentages are a cross-section. The proportion of those ever experiencing a stay in an old people's home or a nursing home is substantially higher, ± 35 per cent.

Table 9.9 shows the balance of expenditure on costs of care for the elderly between institutional and community services. In the calculation of these costs a correction was made for the proportion of users younger than 65 years. Spending is unequally distributed between community and institutional care. Large budgets are spent on institutional facilities. These are almost four times higher than the total budget spent on community care. The ratio of community care:institutional care did not change be-

Table 9.9. Expenditure on community and institutional care for the elderly in millions of guilders (fl.), 1975 and 1985. (Sources: Ministerie van WVC 1987; CBS, pers. commun.)

	1975		1985	
	N	%	*N*	%
Community care				
Home-help service	841	6.6	1 544	6.0
District nursing	288	2.3	748	2.9
Community mental-health care	182	1.4	642	2.5
General practitioners	889	7.0	1 470	5.7
Subtotal	2 200	17.3	4 404	17.2
Institutional care				
General hospital	5 584	44.0	11 108	43.5
Mental hospital	1 082	8.5	2 014	7.8
Nursing home	1 627	12.8	3 556	13.9
Old people's home	2 197	17.3	4 416	17.3
Subtotal	10 490	82.7	21 094	82.8
TOTAL	12 690	100	25 498	100

tween 1975 and 1985. Within community care, district nursing and community mental-health care (including a special section for elderly people) have received relatively larger budgets, while there has been a decrease in expenditure for general practitioners. Within institutional care there has been a relative increase in the nursing-home budget (psycho-geriatric nursing homes), while less is now spent on mental hospitals. The proportion spent on other services, including home help, has remained unchanged.

The relatively high spending on institutional care operates as an incentive for policy makers to stimulate and explore possibilities of substitution. Table 9.10 shows the supply of service relative to the number of older people in 1975 and 1985. In the Netherlands, as we have said, institutional services have a relatively large capacity. In addition, many hospital facilities are available for all age groups. If we compare institutional services over a period of 10 years, a decrease in capacity (expressed as standardized data) is visible, with the exception of psycho-geriatric nursing homes. This

Table 9.10. Developments in the availability in institutional and community care for the elderly in the Netherlands, 1975 to 1985. (Sources: NZI 1986; CBS 1988; NIVEL 1988; NK 1988; NVAGG 1988.)

	Institutional care			Community care	
	1975	1985		1975	1985
Old people's homes (places/100 of 65+ years)	9.44	8.05	Community mental-health care for the elderly (per 1000 65+ years)		0.17
Psycho-geriatric nursing homes (beds/100 of 65+ years)	0.80	1.27			
General (non-psychiatric) nursing homes (beds/100 of 65+ years)	1.78	1.61	District nursing (per/1000 of 65+ years)	2.69	3.65
			Home-help service (per/1000 of 65+ years)	21.35	20.72
General hospitals (beds/total population)	4.47	3.79	General practitioners (*n*/1000 of 65+ years)	3.11	3.46
Mental hospitals (beds/total population)	1.76.	1.68			

finding is in step with government policy, which aims to reduce institutional capacity in general and to achieve a more equal distribution across the country. For instance, places in old people's homes in areas with large capacity are being reduced, whereas some increase for old people's homes and psycho-geriatric nursing homes is allowed in areas considered to be underprovided with these facilities. In some general and mental hospitals there are units for the assessment of psycho-geriatric clients. Mental hospitals also have some long-stay facilities. Over the 10 years between 1975 and 1985 there has hardly been any increase in the supply of community services relative to the number of older people. Indeed, there has been a slight decrease in the supply of home help, although the number of district nurses has increased and some community mental-health centres have been created.

5. THE HOME-HELP SERVICE IN PRACTICE

5.1. Policy goals

The way in which the service operates in practice is largely influenced by the allocation of budgets. This is now, however, no longer a direct involvement by the government (financing directly from department budgets) because the services are under the regime of the AWBZ (see Introduction). Therefore the way in which the national government can influence the services in this regard is restricted.

The services, however, have much discretion and many possibilities in pursuing their own policy lines, although they have a national superstructure. The superstructure is relatively powerless and does not prescribe policy to the services. There is no national policy for the home-help service, apart from the desire to increase co-operation with primary health care and especially with district nursing. More important, however, is the historical fact that the services all emerged as private organizations, most of them on denominational foundations. In Dutch society the organizational principle of 'pillarization' guaranteed, in the past, considerable autonomy to private (religiously affiliated) organizations. Even now, although this principle is being eroded by secularization, government at all levels allows the services to have their own policies, even if they are largely dependent on it for resources. The home-help services can therefore develop their own policies and practices within certain limits. The assessment system (LIER) can be further refined and adapted to allocate care to lower income groups and people with severe needs. Consequently there are large regional variations.

Many changes in the home-help service took place in the past. The service is now becoming more and more relevant to the present policy goals of the Dutch government (substitution, deinstitutionalization). Both are reasons to have a closer look at the service in practice and to conduct research. Research in this field has concentrated both on existing practices and on the effects of innovations (for example, the 7 × 24-hour service). Are the goals of the home-help service achieved in practice? How efficient is the service? Are the right clients being cared for? In what way do innovations contribute to the operation of the service?

5.2. Service use and functional ability

As the formal intake criteria imply, the home-help service is intended to serve clients with handicaps and problems that make independent living without professional help impossible. Which clients with what handicaps are served? In Table 9.11, some research findings on activities of daily living (ADL), and instrumental (IADL) handicaps are presented to answer this question.

The table shows that the home-help service is relatively more often used when clients have moderate or severe problems with IADL and either no or mild problems with ADL. As ADL problems increase, while there are severe IADL problems present, the elderly person is less often in the care of the home-help service (Coolen 1982). This suggests an upper boundary of care for the home-help service. It is known that there is a hierarchy of

Table 9.11. Sample of elderly people and a subsample of clients of the home-help service, IADL by ADL and mobility handicaps. (Source: Coolen 1982.)

	ADL and mobility								
	None/mild			Moderate			Severe		
	Sample (*n*)	Users		Sample (*n*)	Users		Sample (*n*)	Users	
		n	%		*n*	%		*n*	%
IADL									
None	104	2	2	–			–		
Mild	20	3	15	[1]			–		
Moderate	24	11	46	–[2]			–[3]		
Severe	17	9	53	19	4	21	20	5	25
TOTALS	165	25		20	4		20	5	

[1–3] The respondents in these cells are included in the cells to the left[1] and below[2,3] in order to compute the percentage of users of the home-help service; *n* of sample [1] = 1, *n* of sample [2] = 6, *n* of sample [3] = 2.

IADL and ADL. ADL problems emerge after IADL are present. Clients who have ADL problems almost always have problems in IADL whereas the reverse is not true (Kempen and Suurmeijer 1989). Clients having a great need with respect to ADL are no longer in the care of the home-help service. They are likely to be either in institutions or served by district nurses and informal carers. Coolen concludes that the goals of the home-help service are being only partly attained; Kempen and Suurmeijer found the same pattern in their later study.

While there is no correspondence between need and use of the home-help service, the relation between those variables is different *within* the client population. Kempen and Suurmeijer (1989) found a correlation between need and the capacity of care allocated *within* the client population of the service.

5.3. Service use and income

Other findings by Coolen (1982) show that clients are for a large part in lower income groups. This was especially true for those with greater needs (clients with less need were, however, from higher income groups). This is confirmed by Kempen and Suurmeijer (1989). For persons in larger households, the average income was fl.1675 (net) per month, while clients living alone had a net income of fl.1300. An explanation might be that co-payment drives out middle and higher income groups (Kwekkeboom 1985). There may also be cultural factors whereby the use of social services is seen as 'improper behaviour' by higher income groups, and may induce such people to hire private help.

5.4. The relationship between informal care and the home-help service

The relationships between the home-help service and the availability of informal carers are complex. Two different models are possible. Complementarity exists when a high level of formal care coincides with a high level of informal care. Substitution is the case where formal care replaces informal care or vice versa.

Coolen (1982) found complementarity for handicapped people living alone. When there was relatively less informal care the elderly people were less often in the care of the home-help service, while extended informal care corresponded with care provision by the home-help service (see Table 9.12). For handicapped people living in larger households the relationship changed into substitution: more informal care kept out the home-help service. A possible conclusion is that the allocation of care by the home-help service has no relation with the availability of informal care (Coolen 1982). However, the finding of substitution is biased by the fact that a

Table 9.12. Use of the home-help service by those living alone and those with more persons in a household as related to the availability of informal care. (Source: Coolen 1982.)

	Potential informal care relations	
	Few	Many
Handicapped, living alone		
Users	24	50
Non-users	76	50
Handicapped in larger household		
Users	44	24
Non-users	56	76

'baseline' of informal care was already present in larger households. Therefore the Coolen's findings are more in favour of complementarity.

Kempen *et al.* (1986), who studied comparable client groups, argued that the relationship between informal and formal care might depend on the nature of the tasks. Therefore three broad categories of tasks were distinguished: ADL (personal care), IADL (home making), and supervision (socialization, etc.). Table 9.13 shows an overview of the Pearson correlations between the number of activities jointly carried out by the informal care provider and the 'total' home-help service.

Although the correlations are not particularly high, they point out a relationship of complementarity. Less personal care–ADL by the client is associated with more personal care–ADL by *both* the informal carer and the home-help service. An equal relationship is present for supervision,

Table 9.13. Pearson correlations between the number of activities carried out by the elderly person, informal care provider and 'total' home-help service. (Source: Kempen *et al.* 1986.)

	Elderly person–informal care provider	Elderly person–total home-help service
ADL	−0.39*	−0.43*
IADL	−0.12	−0.15
Supervision	−0.47*	−0.34*
TOTAL	−0.44*	−0.31*

* $p<0.05$

while for home-making tasks–IADL, neither substitution nor complementarity could be found. This might be due to the existence of a number of other people and/or organizations such as private help and meals-on-wheels, who cater specifically for this type of activity. Moreover, the number of IADL carried out by the elderly people themselves is low, which also influences the correlations.

The correlations with respect to ADL–personal care between the elderly person and home help have been analysed by distinguishing between the 7 × 24-hour service and the traditional home-help service. It appears that the correlations with regard to the 7 × 24-hour service are higher (−0.40, $p < 0.05$) than those of the 'ordinary' home help (−0.25, $p < 0.05$). As for the remaining two activities (IADL and supervision), this is not, or is to a much smaller extent, the case. In this sense it can be said that the 7 × 24-hour service clearly performs a separate function, i.e., providing more personal care.

A general conclusion from these studies is that there is more evidence in support of complementarity between formal and informal care, even when a distinction is made by different tasks.

Van den Heuvel (1985) and Kempen *et al.* (1986) studied the division of tasks of the elderly, their informal carers, and the home-help service according to the answers given by the elderly people or their care provider. The results are based on interviews with elderly people who received the 7 × 24-hour service. In the research period, 67 period received this service. Of these 67, 34 were interviewed (the rest were either too ill, died, or refused). Interviews were also held with the informal carers. For the 33 elderly people not interviewed, information was collected through 16 interviews with care providers living in the household, and through 17 interviews with care providers living outside it. Some characteristics of the 67 clients were: 53 were women and 14 were men; the average age was 78 years; and 37 clients lived alone. Elderly people and 'informal care providers' were asked which activities had been carried out and by whom. The answers were listed in Table 9.14.

The elderly people generally carried out the ADL themselves (1 to 7 in Table 9.14), and to a lesser extent the supervision activities (16 to 20). It appeared that the IADL were often not carried out by elderly people (9 to 15). Here the patterns shown in Table 9.11 are reflected, indicating the needs of elderly clients with respect to IADL, while those with ADL problems can manage (almost) independently. Home-making tasks were therefore a major area for support by the informal carer and the home-help service. Assistance in personal care and supervision was, in particular, provided by the informal carer (living with the client) and the 7 × 24-hour service. The informal carer provided many personal-care, home-making and supervision items, and was thereby an important support for the

Table 9.14. Percentages of situations in which activities were (co-) performed by clients, persons from their social network, the 7×24-hour service and the 'normal' home-help service. (Source: Kempen *et al.* 1986.)

Activities	Client	Informal carer		7×24-hour service	Normal home help
		Living in	External		
ADL					
1. Getting in/out of bed	46	50	13	48	22
2. Moving around the house	54	33	3	40	15
3. Dressing/undressing	25	50	5	52	22
4. Sitting/up lying down	60	46	3	30	11
5. Visiting the WC	52	54	5	40	15
6. Eating/drinking	67	17	5	25	7
7. Washing the elderly person	36	25	8	27	15
Subtotal	49	39	6	38	15
IADL					
8. Preparing meals	6	71	28	61	44
9. Making up beds	4	29	10	61	67
10. Washing (clothes)	4	42	23	36	70
11. Ironing	4	21	15	37	67
12. Sewing	15	29	21	21	37
13. Light cleaning chores (dusting)	7	25	13	46	81
14. Heavy cleaning chores	1	8	15	34	74
15. Shopping	10	83	54	36	44
Subtotal	7	38	22	42	61
Supervision					
16. Supervision: carrying out of medical advice	33	75	8	31	15
17. Receiving visitors	1	79	8	18	7
18. Accompanying elderly person on hospital/GP visits	7	50	28	37	15
19. Financial/administrative business	3	79	41	6	7
20. Warning other authorities	4	67	33	12	11
Subtotal	33	70	24	21	11
N (number of situations)	67	24	39	67	27
TOTAL (average %)	28	47	17	35	32

elderly person, covering all tasks. Where the care provider lives in, many more activities will be carried out than when the provider visits from outside (average 11.2 against 6.6).

The home-help service mostly provided home-making activities, and to a lesser extent personal-care activities, and hardly any supervision. Personal care is more often the province of the client, the informal carer, and the 7 × 24-hour service, but is also provided by services like district nursing. The home-help service concentrates on home-making tasks. The 7 × 24-hour service, however, clearly included more personal-care activities than the 'normal' home-help service, and scored higher for all activities. Except for some supervision, the pattern of care tasks of the 7 × 24-hour service was similar to that of the informal carers living with the client. Personal care therefore exists as a separate function of the 7 × 24-hour service, but normal tasks are also surprisingly often carried out by this special arm of the home-help service.

6. THE EFFECTS OF POLICY

So far the functioning of the home-help service has been analysed in terms of client characteristics. The functioning can, however, also be analysed in terms of policy objectives (does it contribute to substitution? do primary care organizations co-operate? etc.), and in terms of the consequences of new regulations (for example, the effect of client contribution on patterns of use). Some findings will now be presented that deal with 'the effects of policy' in relation to the functioning of home-help services.

6.1. Substitution

In the studies of Van Sonderen *et al.* (1985), Goewie (1987), and Kempen *et al.* (1989), attention was paid to the potential for substitution by the home-help service. Substitution is here defined as 'replacement of one service by another which has the same function and effect'. Van Sonderen *et al.* evaluated the effects of the introduction of the 7 × 24-hour service on the home-help service. To what extent the 7 × 24-hour service contributes to a substitution from institutional care to out-patient care/independent living can be examined in various ways. One method, as used by Van Sonderen *et al.*, is to make use of the judgement of experts. Another method is to ask the opinion of the elderly people themselves; their care providers can also be asked. Such data are presented in Table 9.15.

Elderly people and informal care providers largely share the opinion that through the 7 × 24-hour service early discharge from hospital is possible. As to the possibility of substitution for residential or nursing-home care, it

Table 9.15. Substitution perceived by elderly person and informal carer—living in/external. (Source: Van Sonderen *et al.* 1985.)

		Informal carer	
	Elderly person (%)	Living in (%)	External (%)
Substitution by early dismissal from hospital	64	50	71
Substitution by (no or later) admission to residential home	15	42	47
N	34	24	51

is particularly the elderly people who are not convinced. It may thus be concluded that substitution through the 7 × 24-hour service is certainly a possibility. It has been suggested, however, that instead of substitution between institutional and community care, the 7 × 24-hour service might substitute for informal care. The argument is that with the coming of professional care, informal care is reduced or withdrawn. Through experience it is then thought (socially desirable) that without the 7 × 24-hour service, independent living (at home) will not be possible. However, the findings for the relationship between formal and informal care that point to complementarity (see above) seem to contradict this suggestion.

Goewie (1987) examined the relationship between the homes for the aged and the home-help service. His study included groups of elderly people who have the home-help service and/or are assessed for a place in a home for the aged. The conclusions were that the home-help service is a reasonable alternative for some 18 per cent of the elderly clients on a waiting-list for a home for the aged. If the possibilities for home-help service were extended and more elderly people on the waiting-list applied for it, this proportion could be increased to 35 per cent of the waiting-list for the homes. Of the total client population of the home-help service, 14 per cent is on a waiting-list or will get an assessment when they apply for it. For a majority of these clients the home-help service is an adequate substitute. The care offered by that service is mostly restricted to heavy, home-making tasks. For substitution, extension of capacity is considered necessary. A comparison of the costs of the home-help service and the homes for the aged shows that the home is less expensive when more than 10 hours of home-help service per week have to be provided (NEI 1984; Goewie 1987).

Kempen *et al.* (1989) asked clients and professionals whether they thought earlier discharge from a hospital or delay or prevention of admission was associated with home-help availability. Approximately one-third of the clients thought that home-help provision made earlier discharge possible. Fewer clients (13 per cent) thought that admission to institutional care was prevented or delayed. Kempen *et al.* asked home-help organizers, home helpers, and district nurses whether they thought that the introduction of 7 × 24-hour services had had any effect on substitution. According to 59 per cent of all professionals there was sometimes delay or prevention of admission (8 per cent replied 'often'), and 47 per cent thought that discharge from a hospital was possible earlier (5 per cent replied 'often').

6.2. Co-operation

As mentioned before, co-operation between professionals in the care system, and especially between district nursing and the home-help service is a policy objective. Kempen *et al.* (1989) studied the co-operation between the home-help service and the district-nursing service. Major impediments to co-operation according to professionals from both services are: (a) differences in expectations concerning co-operation; (b) differences in the 'culture' of the services; (c) differences in status; (d) lack of clearly defined responsibilities; (e) lack of coherence in assessment; (f) differences in education; (g) differences in procedures concerning discharge from hospitals; (h) differences in financial arrangements; (i) differences in organization; (j) competition between services.

Desirable improvements, according to the professionals, include better exchange of information concerning style of operation, blockages experienced, and clients in the care of both services. More co-ordination is thought to be necessary as well. A common intake for all clients, whether they use one or the other service, is not desirable according to the professionals, except for clients in the care of both services. The effects of better co-operation could be improved efficiency and more possibilities of earlier discharge from hospital.

6.3. Effects of co-payment

Since 1976 the home-help service has a standardized, nationwide, co-payment system. Before then, services used their own standards of co-payment. The clients' contribution depends on their income. Between 1983 and 1986 a distinction was made between short-term and long-term care. When the expectation was that the care would last no longer than 12 weeks, a higher fee was charged. Long-term care had lower co-payment from the start. Short-term care therefore became substantially more expensive. In 1986, this distinction was abolished because the higher tariff was too much for many clients. In 1990, the minimum tariff was fl.3 per week; the maximum *per hour*, fl.8.25. An elderly person having a net income between fl.1325 and 1349 who is receiving 3 hours of help per week will pay, in 1990, fl.22 per week. This is 6.5 per cent of his/her monthly net income. The co-payment system is maintained under the new regime of the AWBZ, but a common co-payment for the home-help service and district nursing is to be established.

Research has shown that use of the home-help service is far more expensive than other primary care services: district nursing, social services, and general practitioners (Kwekkeboom 1985). Because co-payment is dependent on income, the financial burden is particularly high for middle- (and upper-) class clients. Therefore, many are forced to restrict the period in care. From statistics on the home-help service, 15 per cent explicitly mention financial reasons for ending the period in care or for having fewer hours of care per week. As co-payment gives rise to a more critical attitude to the home-help service, it is assumed that this percentage is actually much higher; often financial reasons for discontinuation are concealed by other explicit reasons like dissatisfaction with care provision. It can be concluded that particularly in middle-income groups, handicapped people refrain from care uptake or clients restrict care as much as possible. This shifts a higher burden to the client him/herself or to the informal carer (when available).

7. CONCLUDING REMARKS

The home-help service is an important community service, which supports a substantial number of elderly, handicapped people living at home. The service can play a significant part in reinforcing primary care in order to prevent admission. Governmental policy, however, is not consistent in this respect. Budget cuts (in spite of a policy in favour of primary care) in recent years and co-payment arrangements have impeded the effective operation of the service. Groups of clients who are most in need can often not be cared for adequately. This can largely be attributed to government policy, because the home-help service is a relatively innovative service, open to co-operation and experiments, and not hindered by a strong, self-centred, professional ideology. Until recently (January 1989) the home-help service was particularly vulnerable to budget cuts because it was directly dependent on the annual government budget. Now, however, the service is under the regime of an indirect mechanism, the AWBZ, which is far less subject to political whims. District nursing and general practitioners are financed within the same system. In the future, all care facilities from medical to social origins will be included in this law; this will facilitate co-operation. The home-help service and district nursing often co-operate already. Therefore, a more consistent approach can be expected in future home care, especially for elderly people. With this and the financial re-arrangements that will be carried out in the next two years (1990–91) the differences between organizations will decrease. They are now free to offer a variety of services and they are no longer restricted, for example, to in-patient care. In future, they will receive funding for the individual functions they perform rather than as 'institutions'.

Another political development is to stimulate the market mechanism in the care system. On the one hand, this could stimulate co-operation between services to offer a better, cheaper, and more complete product to the clients. On the other hand, each care organization may offer the same service, trying to find their place on the market. They will concentrate on low-risk groups, which would be more 'profitable'. High-risk groups could become excluded from care. The home-help service may play an important role in the restructuring of the care system. Probably the service will be the key institution, together with district nursing and the homes for the aged, that will serve independently living, chronically ill, handicapped and aged persons. The out-patient services of hospitals will increase and create an additional market for this new service.

REFERENCES

[Translations of titles are not by the authors of the respective publications.]

Boom, R. C. and Suurmeijer, T. P. B. M. (1989). *Thuiszorg in beweging* (A change in home care). Vakgroep Gezondheidswetenschappen, Groningen.

CBS (1981). *Cliëntenonderzoek gezinsverzorging 1980.* Staatsuitgeverij, 's-Gravenhage.

CBS (1984). *De leefsituatie van der Nederlanse bevolking van 65 jaar en ouder, 1982* (The living conditions of the Dutch population of 65 years and over). Staatsuitgeverij, 's-Gravenhage.

CBS (1986). *Statistiek van de gezinsverzorging en gezinshulp 1984 en 1986* (Statistics of the home help service 1984 and 1986). Staatsuitgeverij, 's-Gravenhage.

CBS (1988). *Statistiek van de gezinsverzorging 1984/1875.* Staatsuitgeverij, 's-Gravenhage.

Commissie Structuur en Financiering Gezondheidszorg (1987). *Bereidheid tot verandering* (Willingness to change). Staatsuitgeverij, 's-Gravenhage.

Coolen, J. A. I. (1982). *Bejaarden en maatschappelijke dienstverlening. Een empirische studie over bereik, inhoud en gevolgen van gezinsverzorging* (The elderly and social services. An empirical study concerning the range, contents and effects of the home-help service). TH, Twente.

Goewie, R. (1987). *Gezinsverzorging, een alternatief voor het verzorgingstehuis?* (Home-help service, an alternative to the home for the aged?). NIMAWO, 's-Gravenhage.

Kempen, G. I. J. M., van Sonderen, F. L. S., Suurmeijer, T. P. B. M., and van den

Heuvel, W. J. A. (1986). Formele en informele hulpverlening bij ouderen. Een onderzoek naar de taakverdeling tussen bejaarden, informele hulpverleners en de gezinsverzorging (Formal and informal care among the elderly. A study of the division of tasks among elderly, informal carers and the home help service). *Tijdschrift voor Gerontologie en Geriatrie*, **17**, 227–32.

Kempen, G. I. J. M. and Suurmeijer, T. P. B. M. (1989). *Thuiszorg nader bekeken* (A closer look at home care). Vakgroep Gezondheidswetenschappen, Groningen.

Kwekkeboom, R. (1985). *Op de vlucht gejaagd? Een onderzoek naar de effecten van de eigen bijdrage regeling in de gezinsverzorging* (Deterred? An inquiry into the effects of the co-payment arrangements of the home help services). NIMAWO, 's-Gravenhage.

Leemeijer, M., Suurmeijer, T. P. B. M., and van den Heuvel, W. J. A. (1986). *Thuiszorg door 7 × 24-uurs kruiszorg* (Home care by the 7 × 24-hour service of district nursing). Vakgroep Medische Sociologie, Groningen.

Maessen, P. (1989). *Bezuinigingen op de gezinsverzorging. Besluitvorming in de verzorgingstaat* (Budget cuts in the home-help service. Decision making in the Welfare State). Porefschrift, Leiden.

Ministerie van WVC (1988). *Financial Overzicht Gezondheidszorg en Maatschappelijk Welzijn 1987* (Financial review of health care and social services). Staatsuitgeverij, 's-Gravenhage.

Nederlands Economisch Instituut (NEI) (1984). *Oud en zelfstandig: een onderzoek naar de voorzieningen voor ouderen in Zeeland.* (Old and independent: a study into service-provision for the elderly in Zeeland). NEI, Rotterdam.

NZI (1986). Instellingen van intramurale gezondheidzorg. Basisgegevens 1-1-1985 (Institutions in health care. Basic data). National Ziekenhuis Instituut, Utrecht.

Van den Heuvel, W. J. A. (1985). Interaction between formal and informal care in primary care for the elderly. Unpublished paper prepared for the ESF workshop 'The elderly and their families. Patterns of mutual caring'. Jerusalem, 11–13 November.

Van den Heuvel, W. J. A. (1989). Use of care facilities of psychogeriatric patients. In *The future of psychogeriatrics* (ed. D. H. Sipsma and L. M. Punt), pp. 46–55. Psychogeriatrisch Verpleeghuis Nieuw Toutenberg, Noordbergum.

Van Sonderen F. L. P., Suurmeijer, T. P. B. M. and van den Heuvel, W. J. A. (1985). *Op maat gemeten* (Measuring the home-help service). Vakgroep Medische Sociologie, Groningen.

Part Three

Home care from a cross-national perspective

INTRODUCTION TO PART THREE

The following chapters will address issues of home-care services and policies from a cross-national perspective. Without repeating the findings and arguments presented by the contributors of each of the national chapters, I shall draw upon these and highlight some of the key points. My aims are, first, to give a descriptive overview of policies and practices across the different countries, and in doing so, to identify key similarities and differences; and secondly, to point to some of the factors that could be said to explain some of the differences in the way in which the home-care services operate and in the policy measures taken—or not taken—to promote home care.

Chapter 10 will compare home-care provision from the point of view of formally stated policy aims and of practices. It aims to highlight similarities and differences in the extent and nature of provision, client characteristics, and the processes of service allocation.

In Chapter 11, the final chapter, I discuss the achievements of home care, and consider policy trends, past and recent, in an attempt to understand the factors affecting policies and the direction of future changes.

10
Home-care provision and allocation

Anne Jamieson

1. The aims of provision—the range of possibilities
2. The formal policy aims of home care
   2.1. Policies or services: which came first?
   2.2. Home care as an alternative to health or social institutions?
   2.3. The role of informal care
   2.4. Target population
   2.5. Conclusions about formal policy aims
3. Home care in practice: patterns of provision and use of services
   3.1. Quantity of provision
   3.2. Nature and organization of home care
   3.3. Who receives home help?
   3.4. What kind of help do people receive?
4. The process of service allocation
   4.1. Who is involved in the decision-making process?
   4.2. Allocation criteria—needs or standard solutions?
   4.3. Factors affecting service allocation
   4.4. Conclusions
References

1. THE AIMS OF PROVISION—THE RANGE OF POSSIBILITIES

Policies for older people in most countries emphasize the need to enable them to remain at home for as long as possible, and this is stressed as an important aim in relation to home-care services. However, there is considerable cross-national variation and a great deal of ambiguity on questions concerning the role of the state, the relation between home care and various forms of institutional care, and the expected cost implications. By reviewing espoused policy aims across several countries, it is possible to identify a range of possibilities, which are first itemized.

1. *Impact on the use of hospitals.* In all systems the concept of 'bed blocking' is a familiar one. It refers to what is seen as inappropriate use of hospital beds, partly by people who have completed treatment but are too frail to be discharged home, partly by people who are admitted to hospital

for non-medical reasons. Home-care provision is seen as one of the ways of freeing beds.

2. *Impact on the use of residential/nursing homes.* In policy statements everywhere, home care is seen as an alternative to long-term institutional care. The philosophy of the 'deinstitutionalization movement' is well known in all countries and, of course, is not confined to the care of older people but includes those mentally or physically ill, and handicapped people. The philosophy is that many of those who have in the past been confined to institutions, isolated from the rest of the community, are able to live normal lives, provided that there is adequate support for them in the community.

3. *Impact on informal carers.* Informal carers, in particular families, are mentioned in policy statements in most countries, but in different ways that express some very important differences regarding the expected role of the family in providing care. It is possible to distinguish between at least three different 'ideal types' of arguments. One is that the state must *replace* the family, which can no longer be expected to look after older relatives. This differs from the second approach, according to which the family is seen to carry the main responsibility for care, with the state fulfilling a kind of *residual* function, filling in gaps where there are no families available to provide care. Finally, there is the argument that the role of the state is to *encourage and support* families, by providing services which both complement and support them so that that their burden does not become so enormous that they totally relinquish their role. This argument does not necessarily exclude one of the two others, but it does represent a different emphasis with possible implications for practice.

4. *Impact on older people.* One should not, of course, forget the possibility that the aim of home-care provision could be to improve the quality of life for older people. This may seem an obvious point; indeed one of the reasons for the popularity of home care is precisely that it is seen to provide what most older people want. Yet, as argued below, the needs of older people are not all the same, and some may lose out at the cost of others in attempts to achieve other aims. Furthermore, the needs and wishes of older people are certainly not always the prime consideration of policy makers.

5. *Impact on costs.* Finally, it is possible that the aim of home care is to reduce spending on services. If admissions to hospitals and residential homes decrease as a result of increased home care, the argument goes, not only will this improve the quality of life for people but it will save money.

I have set out these four sets of expected effects of home-care provision as a framework for an analysis of policies and practices. It does not claim to describe what actually happens. Indeed, as the analysis will attempt to show, priorities vary between countries, and these apparently simple and expected effects or objectives are, in fact, far from straightforward. They often conflict, and the relationship between them is unclear and open to interpretation and argument. In the following I will consider these policy aims as they are expressed through *formal policies* on home care, as manifest in explicit statements about aims, or implicit through legislation and regulation about service provision and the target clientele.

2. THE FORMAL POLICY AIMS OF HOME CARE

2.1. Policies or services: which came first?

The formulation of national policies—the setting of objectives, the passing of legislation, and the making of regulations—is often a response to changes that have been taking place over a long period of time, a response to existing practices rather than a break with these. This is certainly true of home care for older people. In many countries, home-care services existed long before any policies for elderly people had been formulated. Thus, in Belgium, Denmark, Germany, the Netherlands, and the UK, home-help services developed in the immediate post-war period, primarily as a *family service* aimed at maintaining the labour force intact by relieving 'housewives' in times of sickness and childbirth. However, the pattern of demand and use of this service changed through a combination of factors, such as the increased number of women participating in the labour force, the changes in household structures and living arrangements, and the growing number of older people in the population. Thus, by the end of the 1960s, the vast majority of home-help consumers were older people, most of whom needed the service longer term than had been the case for 'housewife substitutes'.

In most countries, a great deal of this care had been provided by voluntary organizations, and although this continued in many cases, the state began to take on an increasing role through the provision of finance and through regulation. Thus public statements began to appear more frequently in the 1970s, emphasizing the need to enable older people to remain in their own homes for as long as possible. Demographic trends were one factor that accounted for this development. But equally important was the increasing realization that expenditure on services, in particular health services, could not go on increasing indefinitely. Policies for older people developed in conjunction with the introduction of planning and cash limits in the health and welfare sectors in general. Thus, during the 1980s, one of the intentions behind maintaining older people at home became more clearly spelled out: to contain the rising costs of care by reducing admissions to institutions or minimizing the need for further provision of institutions. In the final chapter, I shall return to the question of policy formulation and implementation and consider more closely whether and in what ways policy measures were actually taken to develop home care for older people. In this chapter the focus is upon current aims and practices in home-care provision.

2.2. Home care as an alternative to health or social institutions?

In most of the previous chapters there are references to the debate about the containment of *health-care* costs and the inappropriate use of acute hospital facilities by older people in need of care rather than treatment. But there is very little clarity about the extent of such 'inappropriate use', or about the relationship between home care and hospital use. In most countries the provision of home *nursing care* has developed within the health-care sector, almost separate from the wider consideration of home care for older people. The *separate* organization, funding, and, in many cases, philosophy of the health-care sector from that of the *social*-care sector has meant that nearly everywhere there has been, and still is, a division between home health care—which includes professional nursing—and other forms of home care, a separation which is clearly manifest in the actual provision and operation of the service.

But this division, it seems to me, has also had the consequence of making general policy statements about the care of older people extremely vague, inconsistent, and difficult to implement. The relief of the burden on hospitals is only one of the espoused policy aims. Another aim is to reduce or prevent an expansion of the number of people entering various forms of residential-care institutions. Implied in the policies is a *continuum of care*, from home care to residential care to hospital care. In other words, it is assumed that the freeing of places in nursing homes through the provision of home care will in turn free beds in hospitals by enabling them to discharge some of the old people to nursing homes. Although this may be true to some extent, it is, in my view, questionable whether this model continuum always applies. The relationship between home care, residential care, and hospital use is a complex one. So much depends on the nature of the home care available. For example, crisis intervention service provided to people in their own homes may prevent some acute, emergency admissions to hospital, but not admissions to long-term care of the permanently frail. A less intensive service provided routinely may prevent admissions to residential care, but may result in greater use of hospitals for acute crises than would have been the case if the people involved were living in an institution. The relationship between these different types of care does not appear to have been given much, if any, attention in the debate about home-care policies. I shall return to this in the final chapter, where I attempt to assess the degree to which policies have been successfully implemented.

The relative emphasis on the prevention of hospital as opposed to residential-care admissions differs between countries. In Germany, health insurance organizations are primarily concerned with care in connection with medical treatment. German policies in relation to insurance-funded care therefore emphasize the importance of relieving hospitals: the provision of home care is conditional upon the need for medical treatment, the aim being to treat people of any age at home as far as possible. The health insurance organizations provide funding for home nursing care for those in need of medical treatment, and it is only recently that a new law was passed enabling frail people in need of care rather than treatment to receive financial support for this. The German contributors point to the absence of a coherent set of policies specifically for older people. Frail people in need of help with daily activities have to pay for their own care, whether in their own home or in a nursing home, unless they are entitled to social welfare, in which case the state will provide some limited care. There has been home-care provision in Germany for a long time, but it is still primarily aimed at families with young children in the same way as it used to be in countries like Denmark and the UK 20 years ago. This is not to say that there are no atempts to reduce the use of residential care; but the point is that such efforts are not linked to the provision of home care as an alternative. Policies aimed at reducing the number of beds in residential homes have been practised separately from any home-care strategy.

In France, the concept of *maintien à domicile* (see Chapter 5) developed in the 1960s. It implied an emphasis on maintaining people at home as opposed to any kind of institution, whether hospital or residential home. However, since the 1970s, the measures taken reflect a concern, above all, to unblock hospital beds. Thus in addition to the provision of (some limited) funds for home care, efforts have been equally, if not more, focused on the improvement of the residential care, most notably by enabling institutions to add on medical facilities to avoid hospitalization of their residents.

Whereas France and Germany tend to stress the importance of freeing hospital beds, other countries put greater emphasis on the need to reduce the proportion of older people in residential homes. In this connection it is, of course, important to bear in mind that the degree of institutionalization of older people varies between countries. As Table 10.1. shows, the cross-national variations are considerable. This is an important factor in affecting policy aims concerning residential care, although the quality of provision can be equally important, as the example from France demonstrates. In

Table 10.1. Proportion of population aged 65+ years currently in residential care[1]

	%	Relative category
Netherlands	12	'High'
Denmark, Belgium, UK, France, Germany	Between 5 and 7	'Medium'
Israel	4	'Low'
Italy	1.5	

[1] Excluding hospitals and sheltered housing.

countries with very low provision of institutions, like Italy and Israel, home care can be seen as a way of compensating for lack of residential facilities rather than as an attempt to reduce the use of institutions. The Netherlands is at the other extreme, with an unusually high proportion of older people living in institutions. Policy aims here are explicitly directed at reducing this number. In between these two extremes are countries with a 'moderate' proportion of elderly people (5 to 6 per cent) living in institutions. Here policy aims are directed at limiting the growth, and possibly reducing the proportion, although it is not at all clear what is perceived as the ideal target or norm in these countries.

2.3. The role of informal care

The question of what may be regarded as ideal targets of provision, whether institutional or home care, depends, among other things, on the attitude or ideology regarding the responsibilities of the families themselves for care. In other words, whether formal services are expected to replace, support, or complement family care. Here, countries are divided, although the principles behind stated policies are not always clear. In Denmark the role of the family is hardly debated. It is assumed that offspring will not and should not take on any major role in providing care for their elderly parents. State provision is seen as a right for all. The role of spouses is different, however. Policy objectives for home help specify that priority should be given to those living alone. In Germany the responsibility of the family, including children of older people, is stated very explicitly in the principle of subsidiarity guiding social welfare. Families are obliged to provide either care or financial assistance towards care for their frail relatives. Social services perform a residual function as a safety net for those too poor and without families to care for them. Only health care is provided as a right as part of the general insurance system. In none of the other countries reviewed do policy statements seem to stress so unambiguously the responsibility of the family. In Italy and Israel, services are still so scarce that the reliance upon families is almost taken for granted, whilst at the same time accepting that there is a need for formal provision. However, in most countries the importance of building upon existing patterns of informal care is stressed, and it is often emphasized that the provision of formal care should not drive out informal care. This is the case in Belgium, France, the Netherlands, and the UK. In these countries an increasing amount of research has focused on the relationship between formal and informal care, and espoused policies have begun to stress the importance of services focusing not merely on the needs of the older people but on those of their carers.

Very broadly speaking, it is possible to see the following *continuum of aims*:

replace informal — care	support/encourage — informal care	provide a safety net for those with no informal networks.

As far as policy aims are concerned, the countries reviewed would place themselves on this continuum in the following way. Denmark is closest to the left-hand side, services seemingly aimed to replace informal care; in the middle are the UK, the Netherlands, Belgium, France, and Israel; and towards the right-hand side of the continuum are Germany and Italy, where home-care services aim to fulfil a residual function.

2.4. Target population

Statements regarding the role and responsibilities of informal carers do, to some extent, define the target population, but there are other dimensions and formal criteria of eligibility that help to define this, and that display some striking similarities as well as differences between countries.

2.4a. Income criteria

The distinction between health-related and other forms of care is crucial for an understanding of the problems that have been encountered in the development of home-care services. The distinction is important in two ways: in terms of organization and of criteria of eligibility. The very fact of their separation is one of the factors affecting the implementation of policies. The separation of health and social services is also manifest in the criteria of eligibility which apply. In all the countries reviewed, basic health care is accessible to all as a right, and it is strongly perceived as such in their populations. This applies irrespective of whether the countries have a national health service funded out of general taxation—such as Denmark, the UK, and Italy—or whether they have some kind of insurance-based system. In both types of system the population is entitled to some health-care treatment. The quality of the treatment and the speed with which people receive it does, of course, vary but this does not affect the basic principle. Nursing care in the narrow sense of this word is included in this, and in all countries people have a right to such care whether in a hospital or in their own homes. The rationing of this does not take place through the formulation of specific criteria of eligibility other than medical/health criteria. In so far as people do not receive adequate health, including nursing, care, this is a function of lack of supply. The social services sector is very different from this. Here, a number of explicit criteria of eligibility affect the perceptions of right, and so ration demand.

There exists an important distinction between countries where a principle of universality applies to the public provision of home help, and those where home help is provided only to 'the poor', i.e., in conjunction with social welfare. Thus, in Genoa, home care is provided free of charge, but only to those on basic social welfare. This is similar to what happens in Germany, unless home care is needed in conjunction with nursing care, which itself can only be provided for people undergoing medical treatment. In France, personal care is delivered by the home-nursing services and is not conditional upon income. But for home-help services there is a 'two-tier' system: the public sector pays for home help for those eligible for social welfare, and the private insurance funds for pensioners provide services for people above this level of income, and with a great deal of variation between the various funds. In contrast to Germany, the right to insurance-funded home help in France is not conditional upon people undergoing medical treatment. In these three countries, home help, that is, help with activities of daily living (ADL) for frail elderly people, only has a residual function as far as any state commitment is concerned. In all other countries, home-help services are not exclusively for those in the poorest income group, but in most some form of co-payment exists, which is mostly graded according to means. Denmark is now an exception to this, as after July 1989 all those in need of permanent home help have been entitled to receive it free of charge.

2.4b. Criteria of health and functional ability

As regards help with personal care and home-making, i.e., that which we broadly refer to as home help, most countries, in their general policy statements, stress that this is for people who are unable to manage without help, who are frail and infirm. In other words, the general national criteria are extremely broad and widely open to interpretation by local decision makers. But even at local levels, the studies show that there is very little in the way of formal policy guidelines for those who actually carry out the day-to-day decisions about service allocation.

Some exceptions should, however, be mentioned. First, the regulations in Germany, as already pointed out, whereby strictly medical criteria determine the eligibility for home care funded by the health insurance organizations. For those eligible to help under the social welfare provision, however, there do not appear to be any specific criteria of health or functional ability. The second exception is Israel, where criteria of eligibility under the new Community Long-Term Care Insurance law are very clear. Home care is aimed at those who are most frail, and this is specified in terms of a clearly defined ADL scoring system which has to be followed in allocating services, and which forms the basis of entitlement. Finally, the Netherlands has a national system of ADL assessment, which all providers are expected to follow. However, this does not in itself specify the levels of disability at which care can or cannot be provided.

2.5. Conclusions about formal policy aims

The main points to emerge from a consideration of formal policy aims are, first, that home-care policies cannot be understood in isolation from the existing supply of other services, in particular the extent of institutionalization, which varies widely between countries. Some countries, like, for example, France, may still see a need to expand and/or improve the supply of residential homes, whereas others, most notably the Netherlands, appear to have a more urgent wish actually to reduce the number of institutions. Such different aims are likely to affect policies and practices of home care. The second and most important difference between the countries reviewed relates to the role of the state and its relation to the role of the family. Thus, in countries with a strong family ideology and where the state has historically played a residual role in social welfare, one can expect policies and service provision to be very different from that in countries with a more universalist welfare state. Finally, apart from these major and important differences, what most countries appear to have in common is a general lack of explicity defined aims and policies for home-care services. Israel and Germany, through their specification of entitlement criteria, are exceptions to this general pattern. In most cases, when it comes to *practices*, there is ample scope for interpretation and variation, both between and within countries.

3. HOME-CARE IN PRACTICE: PATTERNS OF PROVISION AND USE OF SERVICES

3.1. Quantity of provision

It is often claimed that in cross-national research one must compare like with like. The units of comparison must be the same. Whilst this would, of course, be desirable, in practice this is not always possible, for the very simple reason that often there are some very fundamental and important differences between countries that cannot and should not be reduced to the same entity. This is certainly the case when it comes to comparing home-care provision. First, there are some 'technical' problems in that national statistics are not available in equal amounts in the different countries. But more importantly, because of the differences in the units of comparison, i.e., the nature of the services in the different countries, it is impossible to compare like with like. But this should not keep us from attempting to make comparisons, indeed it does not generally seem to deter researchers or practitioners from doing so. The point to bear in mind is that many statistical comparisons have to be interpreted with caution; often the best we can get are approximations or broad trends. An attempt to put together a 'simple' table (Table 10.2) showing the proportion of those aged 65 years

Table 10.2. Proportion of population aged 65+ years currently receiving home help/nursing

<table>
<tr><th></th><th>Home help (%)</th><th>Home nursing (%)[1]</th></tr>
<tr><td>Denmark</td><td>17</td><td>12[2]</td></tr>
<tr><td>Netherlands</td><td>12</td><td>4</td></tr>
<tr><td>UK</td><td>9</td><td>5</td></tr>
<tr><td>France</td><td>7</td><td>0.6</td></tr>
<tr><td>Belgium (Antwerp)</td><td>6[3]</td><td>–</td></tr>
<tr><td>Israel</td><td>6</td><td>3</td></tr>
<tr><td>Germany</td><td>max. 3[1]</td><td>max. 10[1]</td></tr>
<tr><td>Italy (Genoa)</td><td colspan="2">0.5</td></tr>
</table>

[1] Included in these figures are people receiving home help as well as home nursing. It is not possible, therefore, to add up the two columns.
[2] In any one year—this means that the number of people currently receiving home nursing is considerably smaller.
[3] Percentage of population aged 60+ years.

and over receiving home care in each country exemplifies the problems well. Yet, because there are some significant differences, these show up, despite the lack of perfectly comparable data.

There are no national figures for Belgium, Germany, or Italy (Table 10.2). This is partly due to the regional variations in service provision within each of these countries, and partly due to lack of adequate information systems for collecting such data. The figure for Belgium is based on calculations from Antwerp and refers to people over the age of 60. It would presumably be higher if the cut-off point was 65 years as it is for the other figures. The figures for Germany are based on research data from Berlin, which we know is relatively well provided with home care. So even these figures are probably an overestimate for Germany as a whole. Only a very small proportion receive home help only. Because of the criteria of eligibility, whereby the need for nursing is a requirement for insurance cover for other forms of home-care services, most people receiving home care would do so in conjunction with nursing. In the survey conducted by Garms-Homolová (Chapter 6.2), no distinction could be made between nursing and home help because the clients themselves just did not know the difference. The figures are not directly comparable to those of the other countries, as they refer to people receiving these services during a year and not to people currently receiving the services, which would be a far smaller number. In Genoa, home care is integrated in such a way that statistics do not distinguish between home help and home nursing. Thus the figure here refers to any kind of home care. But despite such problems of definition, the trend is clear: both Genoa and Berlin have extremely low levels of provision compared with the other countries; and at the other end, Denmark and the Netherlands have the highest proportion of older people receiving home help.

The proportion of elderly people receiving home care/home help does not, of course, tell the whole story. One needs to know how much help is received, and how it is distributed. Table 10.3 gives an indication of the quantity of home help provided. The pattern suggested by the figures on overall service receipt is further emphasized and points to Denmark and the Netherlands as the two countries with the most provision—not only covering the largest proportion of the elderly population but also providing more to the recipients. Israel is interesting in that although the overall number of older people receiving home help is relatively small, the amount they receive, in hours, is very high. Services in Israel are much more concentrated and heavily targeted, as one would expect in the light of the clearly stated eligibility criteria.

The overall picture for the quantity of home-care provision (whether or

Table 10.3. Home-help hours received per week (in percentages) by country and age groups (in years)

Hours per week	Denmark		UK		France	Netherlands	Israel
	67–79	85+	65+	75+	65+	65+	65+
1–6	84	67	94	93	97	72 (1–7 h)	71 (10 h or less)
7+	16	33	5	6	3	27 (> 8 h)	29 (15 h)
TOTAL	100	100	99	99	100	100	100

not home nursing is included) is as follows: (1) 'High provision' countries—Denmark and the Netherlands; (2) 'medium provision' countries—at the top end of this group the UK, followed by France, Belgium, and Israel; (3) 'low provision' countries—Germany and Italy.

3.2. The nature and organization of home care

From the clients' perspective, home care in all countries suffers from varying degrees of *fragmentation*. In other words, from their point of view there is no such service as a 'home-care service'. Rather, there are a number of different services, catering for different needs and delivering different kinds of care. However, the degree of fragmentation varies between countries.

First, there is, in most countries, a barrier between health-related care and social care, which in home care is manifested in the separation of nursing care from other forms of home care. In countries like Belgium, Germany, Israel, and, until recently, the Netherlands, home nursing is provided from sickness insurance funds, operating their own specific criteria of eligibility, separate from any other home-care needs. Similarly in France, where home nursing and home help are subject to the same form of regulation but their day-to-day operations are separate.

The separate funding of services in most countries is reflected in the separate organization of the *providers*. In systems with a taxation-funded national health service, such as Denmark, Italy, and the UK, health and social services are also separately funded and organized. In Denmark and in Genoa, however, home nurses are part of the social-service organization. The problem in Genoa is dominated by a general scarcity of services. But even in Denmark, where nurses and home helpers are funded from the same source (the municipalities), the lack of co-ordination between the two has been a long-standing problem. Efforts are increasingly directed at improving this, and more and more local authorities are beginning to organize home care in multi-disciplinary teams, comprising nurses, home helpers, and other relevant home-care providers. In Denmark, this is a relatively easy task, facilitated by the funding and organizational context. But in other systems there are similar efforts to provide integrated services through local teams. Thus in Israel, for example, despite the separate funding and organization of nursing and other forms of care, there has been a great deal of local, inter-agency collaboration. This is being formalized through the national implementation of neighbourhood teams. Thus it would appear that the problems arising from the separate funding and organization of services can, at least to some extent, be overcome if there is a commitment to do so on the part of policy makers as well as the professionals themselves.

Germany is another example of an attempt to overcome the barriers between nursing care and home-help care. Here home nurses are part of the 'social stations', and therefore the social-service sector. Yet the services are not very well integrated in practice because the separate funding of nursing care dominates day-to-day activities. As already mentioned, nursing care as part of medical treatment is funded by the health insurance organizations via complex rules and regulations for health criteria, whereas home care for frail elderly people is funded by the municipalities via a means test. Bureaucratic processes of assessment, form filling, and funding applications overshadow any attempts to provide integrated care packages.

The need to co-ordinate, if not integrate, nursing and social care is obvious. Older people often present a complex of health and social problems. But more importantly, the boundaries between the different professional domains are unclear. The consequences are 'borderline disputes', duplication of efforts, and the risk of leaving gaps in provision. One of the origins of the separation is the primacy given to medical and medically related treatment compared with social care, which in many systems has been relegated to the status of support for the poor and is separate from health care (or rather, from medical treatment). Yet this is only one factor. Even in systems like the Danish one, where the social-services sector performs far more than a residual function, it is still separate from the health-care sector; and even though home nurses are an exception and part of the same organization as other home carers, the division still exists. In other words, the 'separateness' of nurses, which characterizes all the countries, is more than a funding or organizational issue. It has to do with *professional specialization and division of labour.* And this is not confined to a division *between* health and social care, but applies equally *within* each of these sectors. Furthermore, it is not some historically inherited legacy which the system is trying to abolish. On the contrary, the trend toward specialization and therefore an increased risk of further fragmentation is continuing, and there is plenty of evidence of this from several of the countries reviewed in this book.

Most countries have for a long time worked with a division between qualified nurses and nursing auxiliaries, the auxiliaries doing the non-technical tasks related to personal care. Home help developed originally as a non-technical, non-professional job concerned with helping with general household duties. It gradually took on a wider range of tasks, especially personal care and general social support for older people, and it developed from being voluntary to paid work. In nearly all countries, home help has been and still is performed by relatively unskilled people, mainly women, and there are very few national standards or requirements for qualifications and training. In practice, most countries offer some kind of training for home helpers, mainly in the form of a short induction course. However, this is increasingly seen as inadequate for people who are not only carrying out a clearly defined set of tasks, like cleaning, making beds, or washing older people, but also have to be skilled in social relationships, and in assessing and dealing with a range of social, psychological, and emotional problems. But at the same time there is also increasing demand for home care, arising from the increasing number of the very old people (people over the age of 80), which is occurring at the same time as the pressure to economize and use resources most efficiently.

The result of these different pressures—the need to professionalize home help on the one hand, and the need to be cost effective on the other—can be seen in some countries in the form of yet more specialization and subdivision of the home-help tasks. This is most clearly manifest in the separation of personal care from home-making/cleaning tasks, as in Belgium, the Netherlands, and Israel. Financial considerations, certainly in Belgium and the Netherlands, seem to have been the main impetus behind the change. Thus in Belgium, the long waiting-lists for home help were reduced at a stroke by the introduction of the cleaning service. This service is cheap for the providers because it is staffed mainly by long-term unemployed people. The waiting-lists now are longer for the cleaning service than for home help. In the Netherlands the introduction of the so-called Alpha help has again been a way of providing help as cheaply as possible. The employment status of Alpha helpers is such that they do not have to pay national insurance contributions (self-employed and working part-time). They are used to provide cleaning services. At the same time, more 'caring type' services, like 24-hour care, have been introduced for people needing round-the-clock personal care. In Israel, personal-care services have long been distinct, and indeed separately funded, from home-making services, one being under the auspices of the Ministry of Health, the other under the Ministry of Labour and Social Affairs. The recent new community-care law is complementary to the existing arrangements, but provides for personal care as well as home-making services. Yet, the distinction is maintained, and policies have been directed mainly at the provision of personal care for the most disabled groups of elderly people.

The separation between different types of home help, like the distinction between personal care and home-making/cleaning services, is linked to the question of target population. It could be argued that the existence of a home-making service alongside a personal-care service is an acknowledgement of the different types of clientele, an acknowledgement of the right of people to receive some home help, even if they are not terribly frail and in need of help with personal care. In other words, it could be a sign that the aim of home-care provision is to spread certain services thinly over a larger proportion of the population, and concentrate other more intensive and specialized services on those with a higher level of need.

In Britain, the question of targeting of services is very high on the agenda. The change in the home-help service is towards a higher degree of professionalization. Many local authorities have renamed the service 'home care', emphasizing personal care more than mere home-making. The trend is going in the direction of concentrating services on those with the highest levels of functional disabilities, i.e., those seen to be most at risk of institutionalization, *instead of* rather than *as well as* providing a little help to the many more 'lighter cases'. Therefore, there has not yet been any serious debate about splitting up the home-help service.

In Denmark, like the UK, home help is one service only, providing help with a range of tasks from cleaning to personal care and even 'socializing' (see below). The wish as well as the financial ability is (still) there to keep the service integrated, yet providing differing levels of help. Holstein (Chapter 3) concludes that the best solution is for the service to be aware of the different needs in the population, many of which are, for example, emotional and general rather than specific and task oriented, and to match the different qualities of the staff employed in the home-help service to these needs. This, he suggests, is preferable to any kind of specialization whereby the flexibility of the service as a whole might be jeopardized.

Although it is possible to understand the reasons for the increased specialization and division of Labour in the home-care services, it is equally possible to see the problems this trend can present in providing continuity and flexibility of care. The more specialized and divided the services, the more important becomes the process of needs' assessment and care planning. Before looking at this process, let us first turn to the question of who actually receives home care.

3.3. Who receives home help?

3.3a. Age and functional ability

This section focuses on the distribution of home help rather than of any wider range of home-care services. This does not mean that the distributiobn of services like home nursing is not important. But as in most countries nursing services are offered on the basis of more clearly defined and often short-term nursing needs, less attention has been paid to issues of distribution, in research as well as in discussion of home-care policies.

In asking who receives home help, one of the aims is to see whether the services reach those for whom it was intended, and whether those who need the services most are those who actually receive them. The concept of need is, of course, complex and can be defined in terms of many different combinations of variables like: inability to perform any number of activities of daily living (ADL or instrumental (I)ADL); self-reported ill health; living alone; living in an isolated area. As already pointed out, explicit policies regarding the needs towards which home-help services should be directed are, in most countries, formulated in very general terms. But most policy aims imply that services should be for people with functional disabilities, and that priority should be given to those living alone. How far are services in practice distributed to those most 'in need', and what concepts of need are implied in the way the services are distributed in the different countries?

As discussed above, overall provision of home-help services varies considerably between countries, which means that the total proportion of beneficiaries is much larger in, for example, Denmark than in France or Israel. The potential for needs' coverage, therefore, is far better in some countries than in others. Given these differences, how are the individual countries distributing the resources available? Comparable data are not widely available, but a number of research studies do point to certain trends. On looking at the distribution of home-help services in different *age* groups, one can see that in all countries service use increases with age. But on comparing those countries for which comparable data exist (Table 10.4), it is clear that the differences between age groups are not the same. In the UK, for example, services are more heavily concentrated upon the oldest elderly people than in Denmark and France. Denmark is so well provided that all age groups seem able to share in the services, and it is particularly remarkable that, compared with the UK, three times as many young elderly people receive home help in Denmark. In France the service is rather thinly spread over all age groups, and because of the overall low levels of provision this means that the very old people receive relatively little home help.

Table 10.4. Proportion (per cent) in each group receiving home help

Age group (years)	Denmark	UK	France	Netherlands
65–79	6	2	3	
				6 (Age 65–74)
70–74	11	6	4	
75–79	22	11	8	
				15 (Age 75+)
80–84	34	22	12	
85+	38	34	14	
ALL 65+	17	9	7	12

The increased use of home help with age is hardly surprising. Functional disability and the likelihood of living alone increase with age, and however vague and general the policy statements, they all emphasize those two factors. Looking at the distribution of home help by *functional ability*, the general trend is clear in all the countries from which information is available. In broad statistical terms, service use increases with increasing functional disability, however this is measured. But the degree of correspondence between service use and functional disability is not the same for all countries. Looking first at the population of *recipients*, the question is: to what extent can they said to be 'in need' of home help, where 'need' is defined in terms of some measure of functional disability?

Very broadly speaking it seems possible to distinguish between countries where nearly all the clients of the home-help services have problems in performing ADL, and those where a considerable proportion of clients do not appear to have any impairments. Among the former countries are Israel and Germany (Berlin). In contrast to these countries, studies from France, the Netherlands, the UK, and Denmark all indicate that many users have no or few functional disabilities. France appears to have the largest proportion of such users. Henrard (Chapter 5) quotes a study of home-help beneficiaries showing that more than half of them have little or no disability, and only 6 per cent are very 'bad cases'. In the other three countries mentioned, there are also a number of users with no apparent disabilities, although detailed comparable data are not available. As the chapter (4) on the UK shows very clearly, much depends on the definition of 'disability'. Three different definitions are used here to calculate the number of users without 'need', and the proportion of clients in need ranges between 36 and 67 per cent depending on the definition. Ability to perform daily activities is, as already stressed, only one possible definition of 'need' and perhaps the most one can say about the clients with few problems is that they appear to need the home-help service 'less badly' than certain others. It would be wrong to conclude from this that such clients do not benefit from the service.

3.3b. Unmet needs

The question of service distribution cannot, of course, be answered merely by looking at the characteristics of the client population. It is also a matter of the extent to which people with need do not receive any services. For the countries where most recipients have disabilities, the vast proportion of older people do not receive any home help. The basic problem in these countries is shortage of services and not inadequate targeting. In Israel the scarcity of home-care provision is managed relatively successfully in the sense that recipients meet the very explicit criteria of functional disability; but research indicates that nearly a third of those eligible do not receive care. In Berlin, services are also scarce, and although recipients are generally needy, the criteria for funding mean that many, although in need of care, are not eligible. Many of those excluded from the service are not necessarily less disabled, rather their problems are different in the sense that they do not require medical attention. The data from Genoa do not tell us anything about the functional ability of the clients but they do indicate very clearly the enormous gap in provision. Only 10 per cent of those referred to the home-care centres were successful in obtaining any help; furthermore, demand would be much higher, according to Costanzi (Chapter 8), if people actually knew about the existence of the services. Less than a third of those over 75 years included in the study knew about the home-care service.

In those countries where a certain proportion of the client population was thought to be in little need, there is also, with the possible exception of Denmark, a significant proportion of elderly people with high levels of disability whom services do not reach. The French, Dutch, and British studies all show evidence of this. The most comprehensive data are those from the UK, where information based on the General Household Survey indicates that only a third of those who are 'disabled and lacking in support' receive home help. In Denmark, the home-help service reaches between 80 and 90 per cent of those with functional disabilities and living alone.

3.3c. Need/demand

The British and the Danish contributors introduce a note of caution about the use of functional ability as a measure of demand or potential demand for services. People's perceptions of their own health and abilities as well as their attitudes to receiving services play an important part. Holstein (Chapter 3) claims that only 1 to 3 per cent of those in poor self-assessed health do not receive services, and among his population of elderly people only about 3 per cent of those not receiving home help expressed an unmet need. Whether 'objective' measures such as functional ability or subjective measures such as self-assessed health or expressed demand for services are the better indicators of need is a delicate question. Attitudes towards services are a function of the nature of the services themselves and the prevailing culture and norms. The more services are associated with stigma and charity the more this will suppress demand and keep unmet needs at bay. In countries like France, Germany, and Italy this clearly is the case. The reluctance on the part of the German insurance organizations to accept funding responsibility for home care other than that associated with medical treatment is based on a fear that if this was accepted as an insurance-based *right*, people's attitudes towards the services would change and result in an enormous increase in demand. Interestingly, this is what has happened in Israel, where home help was earlier excluded from health-care insurance. The new community-care law has created new rights, which in principle are legally enforceable, and has changed people's perceptions. This is seen as part of the reason for the increased demand for home-care services. In Denmark, on the other hand, home-help services are so widely used and known that any reluctance to accept them is more likely to express a person's ability to cope than any antipathy towards receiving help from the public sector.

3.3d. The role of informal care

The attitudes of potential clients as well as the providers towards service use are inextricably linked to the whole question of the role of informal carers. So far, I have concentrated on the association between functional disability and use of home help. But the availability of support from informal sources is another important factor which influences demand as well as supply of home help. Everywhere there is an expectation that for at least some older people a certain amount of help will be forthcoming from their own informal networks. Thus in all countries there is a clear preponderance of people living alone among the clients of home help. Precise, comparable figures do not exist, but the trend is the same everywhere. In Denmark, for example, 36 per cent of elderly people (between 70 and 95 years old) living alone receive home help, and 'only' 17 per cent of those living with others. In England and Wales the equivalent figures for people over 65 are 19 and 4 per cent, respectively.

The general importance of the family and other informal networks in providing support and care is now widely acknowleged; this whole question is dealt with in more detail elsewhere (Jamieson 1990). Broadly speaking, the overall levels of provision and the household structures are the most important factors in predicting the extent of tasks performed by the informal networks. Thus, for example, in Italy and Greece the family carries most of the burden of care. However, one of the questions that have for some time occupied the minds of policy makers and researchers alike is how far the provision of formal services 'drives out' informal care, and what the optimal balance between the two is and should be. The evidence provided by the Danish, Dutch and to some extent the French contributors in this book is that formal services *complement rather than substitute* for informal care. In other words, those people who receive home help also tend to receive help from informal sources. This, at least, is the case for people living alone. Indeed it could be argued that the provision of some formal services helps to encourage not only the family but also friends and neighbours to contribute some help because it gives them some reassurance that they will not have to take on the total responsibility for the old person.

A great deal of evidence suggests that the informal network living outside the household performs *different tasks and with less regularity* than the formal services. The Dutch contributors (Chapter 9) quote a study which shows that carers outside the household help with shopping, transportation, and administrative matters, whereas formal services tend to provide personal care and cleaning, bed making, washing, and ironing. This trend is confirmed in a survey of older people in Denmark (Holstein 1988), which shows that they have much contact with their children, although no longer living with them, and that they provide a great deal of social support and help with occasional tasks. The more regular daily activities, however, whether home-making or personal care, are done by the old people themselves or by the home-help service.

The situation for those not living alone is different. The Dutch as well as the Danish data suggest that spouses are expected to care for each other and that the patterns of care which have prevailed throughout the lives of married couples will continue if they become disabled. Thus the Danish data suggest that the traditional gender roles are continued into old age: more women living with a spouse and more men living alone receive home help. In other words, women look after their spouses as well as themselves to a larger extent than do men. The question which Holstein (Chapter 9) does not answer is whether this distribution of the service is a function of discrimination on the part of providers or whether it reflects differential demand originating in traditional gender norms and attitudes.

3.4. What kind of help do people receive?

In discussion of the role of informal care, I touched upon the possible division of tasks between formal and informal services. What do we know about the kind of help that people receive, and the extent to which this is actually what they need? First, most help is provided regularly, and most home help is long term, although in some countries a distincion is made between temporary and permanent help. Some evidence suggests that too often home help is provided as a permanent service, despite changes in the situation of the clients. Lawson and Davies (Chapter 4) point to the lack of reassessment as one of the reasons why so many people with seemingly low levels of need continue to receive help. Home nursing, on the other hand, is usually provided as short-term help with very specific tasks, mostly related to illness and medical treatment. In countries like the UK, where nurses perform some personal tasks like bathing people, the help tends to be more long term.

The nature of help provided by the home-help services is very similar in most countries, although there are some interesting deviations. First, the balance between help with personal care and other tasks is very similar everywhere, with the exception of Israel and France. Personal care constitutes a very small proportion of the tasks of the home-care services in all countries except Israel, where home care is targeted towards those needing personal care. More than 4 per cent of those over 65 years receive personal care (or personal care combined with home-making), whereas just under 2 per cent receive help with home-making. The opposite is the case in France, where the home-help service is only supposed to deliver help with household tasks and not personal care, which is still the domain of the home nurses. The figures from the UK and Denmark suggest that less than 10 per cent of the help received from the home-help service is personal care. By far the most important activity of the home-help service is housework, especially cleaning. Shopping is the second most important activity. In this context it is worth remembering that the home-care service in Israel is a relatively recent innovation, developed specifically for frail elderly people, whereas in the other countries mentioned it developed as a home-making service, which 'drifted' into becoming a key service for older people.

The proportion of time devoted to personal care, although still relatively small, has actually increased as a consequence of the needs of the 'new' clientele. Personal care was originally undertaken by the home nurses in conjunction with their professional nursing tasks. Whereas this continues to be the case in France, in most other countries the home-help service has gradually taken on more and more personal-care tasks. In several countries there is now a great deal of ambiguity in the division of tasks between nurses and home helpers. However, the increased importance of personal care delivered by the home-help service is widely acknowledged, but at the same time it is clear that most of the help delivered is, in fact, cleaning.

This tension within the service around the question of its core function has had different consequences in the various countries. In the UK there is increasing pressure to develop the home-help service into a more skilled, more 'targeted', personal-care service for those with clear problems in ADL. As already mentioned, several local authorities have renamed the service 'home care' and are trying to provide better training for the providers in an attempt to make it less of a cleaning service and more of a personal-care service. This strategy is not without its critics, who point to the danger that cleaning will be pushed out of the domain of the public service (Morton 1989). In Belgium and the Netherlands, on the other hand, the same tension has been approached by splitting the service into personal care and cleaning.

The data from Denmark on the activities of the home helpers include the category 'conversation', an interesting item that does not figure in any of the material from other countries. These data come from a study of a sample of home helpers, who were asked how they spent their time. They said that 13 per cent of their time was spent on conversation, the second largest category of 'activities' after cleaning, on which they reported spending 37 per cent of their time. The data suggest that in Denmark social support is accepted by service providers as an important function. The relatively large proportion of people receiving home help supports this interpretation that services are targeted not only to those who have physical disabilities and who might be at risk of entering an institution, but also to those who feel isolated and for whom the home-help service 'merely' contributes to improving their quality of life. It is, of course, important to bear in mind that the data quoted from other countries are based on questions to clients, and the exclusion of the category 'conversation' reflects either the clients' perceptions or possibly the researchers', depending on the method used. In either case, it does not necessarily mean that home helpers in other countries do not spend time on conversation with the clients, but it does raise the question of whether this is a function that is underestimated, or perhaps not accepted as part of the tasks of the home helpers. Henrard (Chapter 5) mentions that in France there is a great deal of ambiguity around the role of the home helpers. According to him the service provides a great deal of psychological support, but the official criteria explicitly state that physical needs should be the main criterion for service allocation.

Whether the intention is to provide personal care for a relatively small group of highly disabled people or to provide a wider range of services including cleaning help to a larger group of people, it is evident that, at present, most home-help services provide a wide range of help. But the question is whether people actually receive the kind of help they want and need. One way of throwing more light on needs' coverage is to go beyond the very broad, statistical indicators and consider in more detail how decisions are made about care allocation. In the next section, I will discuss some of the findings from the decision-making studies that are part of the ACRE project.

4. THE PROCESS OF SERVICE ALLOCATION

One of the aims of the decision-making analyses was to see if and in what ways the service responded flexibly to the individual needs of potential clients, and whether clear criteria were being applied in determining the amount and type of care to be provided. In this book, some of the results from these studies are reported from Belgium, Berlin, Denmark, and Genoa. The chapter (4) on the UK refers to some material, and to supplement this I will also refer to the study conducted in Scotland, which, although not included in this book, forms part of the ACRE project (Hunter *et al.* 1988).

4.1. Who is involved in the decision-making process?

The decision-making process starts at the point of referral. In most of the systems studied, it is rarely the old people themselves who make the referral. Someone makes the referral on their behalf. The exclusion of the elderly people from the whole decision-making process is characteristic of most of the countries studied, although in the Scottish system there was some considerable negotiation between them and the home-help manager during the assessment. In Denmark, the lack of involvement of the old people themselves is described as one of the major faults of the system. Here, as elsewhere, relatives play a part in referring and deciding on services, sometimes against the wishes of the elderly people.

The role of the informal carers in the decision-making process was discussed at some length in Jamieson and Illsley (1990). Studies from Scotland and England show that informal carers often have an active role as advocates and in mobilizing services. The data now presented suggest similar trends in Denmark and Belgium, where the decision-making process was studied in some detail. But, as Twigg (1990) argues, carers can also be seen as clients of the services themselves, although providers are reluctant to take their needs into account. The debate in the UK has long centred on the need to provide adequate support for carers, not just for clients. The studies in this book from Denmark, Belgium, and Genoa suggest that formal service providers pay little attention to the needs of informal carers, although there is not enough material to indicate the feelings of the relatives. An interesting aspect of the Danish and Belgian studies is the reluctance of older people to give permission for the researchers to interview their relatives. The reasons given by the Danish respondents were that they were not relevant. Similarly, many of the Belgian respondents did not want their relatives 'to be bothered'. One cannot conclude from this that the relatives do not play a part in the whole 'care process', but it does seem to indicate that the older people themselves may wish for some independence of their relatives and are using formal services in an attempt to achieve this.

The most typical sources of referrals in most countries are the general practitioners and the hospitals. The part played by the general practitioner varies between countries. In Scotland they accounted for the largest number of referrals, and although in some cases the contact between them and the home-help service was made by a receptionist's phone call, in most cases there was a great deal of discussion between the home-help organizers and the doctor about the needs of the client. General practitioners here seem to have better contacts with the home-help service than in most other countries. In the Danish case studies the practitioners do not receive much attention: although their role as the patient's advocate is mentioned, they do not actually make many referrals themselves. There are considerable barriers between the general practitioners and the local authority social services, more so, it appears, than in the UK, where the problem also exists. In general the findings from the Danish case studies show that the decisions are dominated by the professionals—the home-help organizers with or without the hospital social workers. This trend was also evident in Belgium, where in case of discrepancy between the views of the clients/carers and the social workers, the views of the latter prevailed.

In Berlin, the doctors' interest in and knowledge of social problems and social services is very low, irrespective of whether they are hospital doctors or general practitioners. Yet, because of the formal service criteria whereby medical prescriptions are needed for the insurance organization to pay for care, the doctors play a crucial role in the decisions. People often end up in hospitals because of lack of home care, and sometimes the doctors have the role of 'relabelling' them so that they are entitled to care. The hospital social workers form the link with the community centres. They make the referrals, but backed by the doctors' prescriptions. General practitioners are often reluctant to get involved with the problems of older people, and the staff in the 'social stations' spend much time searching for co-operative general practitioners. In their view, most general practitioners know very little of the world of social services. In this system the key decision makers are partly the doctors and partly the 'social station' staff, but they in turn are so constrained by the rules of the system that their decisions are based not on professional but on bureaucratic criteria. The result from the clients' point of view is that they receive inadequate or inappropriate services, which are often interrupted or discontinued, leading to further deterioration of their condition.

All the studies suggest very strongly that the older people themselves have the least influence in the decision-making process. Their relatives have, at times, some influence, although this is variable and seems less so in Denmark. Everywhere decisions are dominated by the professionals in the system: in some systems the general practitioners have a great deal of say, whereas in others social workers or home-help organizers figure more prominently. In the light of this, the question one might then ask is: what criteria do these professionals apply? to what extent are decisions made on the basis of an assessment of the needs of the older persons?

4.2. Allocation criteria—needs or standard solutions?

Lawson and Davies (Chapter 4) point out that nearly all those referred to the home-help service are allocated help and that the response is usually quick. This is confirmed by the *Scottish* data (see above), which are based on the most detailed investigation of the decision-making processes. Not only did the investigators in Scotland interview the parties involved, but in one area they used participant observation of the process. In both England and Scotland the home-help organizers make a visit to assess the needs of a person referred to the service. One of the important findings from the Scottish study was that the assessment process was not so much a matter of deciding *whether* a person needed home help, but of deciding *how much* help to allocate. The process itself was characterized by a great deal of informal negotiation with the client and sometimes the carers. There were no clear policy guidelines, and the investigators stressed that it was difficult to see what the allocation criteria were, except that in terms of the speed of the decision, priority was given to people living alone and to people who had just been discharged from hospital. The people were assessed within a few days. The fact that the providers did not like to turn anybody down meant that the service was rather thinly spread over a large number of people. The clients themselves expressed satisfaction and gratitude, and from this perspective the service clearly did meet the expressed needs of the older people themselves. The service managers interviewed expressed a wish to target services more on particular groups of clients, but this was resisted by the home-help organizers themselves, who believed that even a single session with a client was a point of contact which would be greatly missed if it was taken away. It is quite clear from this study that because of the absence of strict policy guidelines those who actually shaped 'policies' were the practitioners themselves, i.e., the home-help organizers. The point about these 'policies', however, was that the principles underlying them were not very clear, and in practice there was a great deal of variation in service allocation and a thin spread of the service.

The 'reactive' decision-making process manifested in the absence of refusals to provide help to people referred is not confined to the British system, but also seems to occur in *Denmark* (Chapter 3). The Danish case studies included only those who were allocated at least four hours weekly home help, and this limits the extent to which one can draw any conclusions about the way in which the service is distributed. According to the Danish contributors, however, very few referrals are refused. This they see as a positive aspect of the service, and the possibility that people without needs receive home help is not considered. Whilst it is true that Denmark is extremely well provided with home help compared with all other countries, it is also true that provision varies between geographical areas by as much as 100 per cent. Some older people are clearly better provided for than others. Similarly, the allocation criteria vary between local authorities, some using a rigid ADL scoring system, others more flexible *ad hoc* criteria. Assessment for home help is undertaken by the home-help organizer, as in Britain. The case studies showed that this process was far from satisfactory; follow-up studies of clients showed that the home helpers did not always provide the kind of help they needed. Standard solutions seemed to be applied, irrespective of need. Some of these problems stemmed from deficiencies in the assessment process, but others had to do with the limitations of the service. Thus the most obvious gap in provision was rehabilitation, and the reason for this was that the local authorities are not formally obliged to provide rehabilitation, which is seen as a matter for the health service. Yet, despite these problems, the general conclusion drawn from the Danish case studies is that the great majority of the clients in the sample (i.e., those receiving four hours or more of help) had a large number of physical and social problems, and, according to Holstein, without home help they would have had to move into an institution.

The *Belgian* case studies (Chapter 2) did not include refusals. However, among the cases selected were people who were put on a waiting-list. The assessment is made by a social worker, and the process involves two questions: does the client need home help or cleaning help? is the need acute, or can the client be put on a waiting-list? The existence of a waiting-list means that services are insufficient in meeting the demand, but it may also be a result of what appears to be a rather rigid way in which services are 'packaged' into standard quantities. The cleaning service was created in order to alleviate the pressure on the home-help service, and the result is that waiting-lists for home help have been reduced, whereas there are now long waiting-lists for cleaning help. Both home help and cleaning help tend to be offered as standard packages. Home help is offered as an 8-hour service, cleaning help as a weekly 4-hour service (or even a fortnightly 8-hour service to reduce transport costs). Providers work within fixed budgets, and excess of demand over supply therefore means that, instead of spreading the service more thinly, waiting-lists are created. No strict ADL criteria are stipulated as a guide, but in practice these are used. But equally important is the availability of informal care, which often determines whether a person is put on a waiting-list or not. Many providers were found to operate a queuing system, whereby a certain number of people already on the waiting-list will receive help irrespective of the urgency of the need, but, at the same time, some people referred for the first time and deemed to be in acute need will be placed on waiting-list. As regards the choice between home help and cleaning help, there is remarkable correspondence between what the clients want and what the professionals judge to be the need. The Belgian contributors point out that the professionals tend to perceive demand as needs. In short, the decision-making process appears reactive and rigid, and there is little evidence of flexible response to varying needs.

Service- rather than needs-determined criteria also influenced decision making in *Genoa* (Chapter 8). The pattern of provision in the different areas studied varied, and this was due to differences in services available rather than to differences in the pattern of need. Care providers were aware of the problems of inadequate services and attempted to solve these as flexibly as possible. They had some scope for discretion, for example in relation to the income assessment, which was so complex that it allowed for interpretation. There was a tendency to respond to the general lack of services by spreading them thinly in order to reach as many as possible. Thus much of the help provided by the centres was to do with group social activities rather than help to people in their homes.

Decision-making processes in *Berlin* are almost totally dominated by financial criteria and bureaucratic procedures. The needs of the elderly people are subordinate to the regulations of the system; thus the assessment process is concentrated upon the person's financial situation and upon negotiating 'prescriptions' with the doctors. The providers at the 'social stations' do not even always make a visit to assess the needs of the clients referred. If they are prescribed home care in conjunction with treatment, and the funders are satisfied that the medical criteria are met, providers have to deliver the service, even if they find that the clients do not need the care. What comes across very strongly in the Berlin case studies is that, although the professionals take the decisions, the criteria they use are becoming increasingly bureaucratic rather than professional.

4.3. Factors affecting service allocation

On the basis of the cross-national comparison I will attempt to highlight some of the most important factors that affect the ways in which decisions are made about the allocation of home care.

4.3a. Budgetary versus entitlement criteria

There is an important difference in those countries where the supply of services is determined by the amount of money allocated in the *budget*, whether this is set locally or nationally. In this case, decisions focus on the 'fairest' distribution of existing resources, and a great deal of discretion is left to the providers to determine needs and allocate services accordingly. This is what happens in countries like Belgium, Denmark, Italy, the Netherlands, and the UK. In contrast, the principle of *entitlement* operates for part of the services in Israel and Germany. In Israel the new community care law gives people some insurance-based rights. If the services are not available, people have a right to cash so that they can buy in their own help. Although the service is supposed to be funded from earmarked contributions, the state guarantees to make up for any shortfall. On this background it is hardly surprising that the criteria and process of assessment have been specified very rigidly. There is no evaluation yet of this system, and of whether it is perceived to result in a fair distribution of services. It is clear though that the stringent ADL criteria do exclude those with minor problems, who in other systems get their share of the cake. Many of these people were expected to obtain some care from existing services. The new entitlement-based system was aimed to be complementary to the existing system of budget-limited services, and one of the unintended effects has been a reduction in the supply of these services. On the other hand, the uptake of the new services has been very high because of the principle of entitlement.

In Germany, those home-care services funded by the insurance organizations are similarly characterized by insurance-based rights. But the criteria of entitlement are medical and the amount of services to which people are entitled is specified in complex regulations. In this system the providers themselves make the decisions, and the control is exercised through the regulations. The consequence of this is that the task of the providers is extremely bureaucratic; their activities are dominated by the need to raise money for the clients in order to avoid the risk that the providers themselves will end up having to pay for the care. A great deal of time, therefore, is spent on assessing the precise rights of the clients, and a great deal of effort is put into ways of 'playing the system', i.e., upon ways of defining the clients' needs that will entitle them to services. Providers depend on doctors to co-operate in this process, the medicalization of people's problems becomes inevitable, and those who cannot be defined as 'ill', however frail, tend to lose out.

4.3b. Separation of funding and provision

Providers, whether motivated by profit, professional considerations, or by charity will tend to do what they can to preserve or expand service provision. This applies irrespective of who funds the service, but in systems where the funding is separate from the provision, regulation of the providers is perceived as more urgently needed. In Israel and Germany such regulation is implemented through entitlement criteria, as described earlier. Belgium offers an example of a system where funding and provision are separate, and where service allocation is through insurance-based entitlements. Providers are 'controlled' in two ways: first, through a fixed budget, and secondly, through regulations which stipulate the maximum hours of home help and cleaning help a person can get, and which stipulate that a social inquiry into the needs of the clients must be conducted by a social worker. In practice the maximum hours stipulated by the funders (central government) are used as the *norms*. By and large, people get either eight hours a week of home help or four hours a week of cleaning help, or nothing at all. Furthermore, because the funding only takes into account the hours delivered, providers try to save money on transport by concentrating these hours on one day a week or even one day a fortnight. The interpretation of 'maximum' as 'norm', when combined with budget ceilings, results in waiting-lists, and a person's place on the list sometimes takes precedence over the current needs. The existence of waiting-lists is widely known, and it encourages clients to refer themselves at an early stage so that they can get on the list. At the same time, it discourages hospitals from discharging old people back to their homes because they tend to believe that help cannot be provided instantly, although, as the case studies show, this is not entirely true. The situation in Belgium is not only a function of the separation of funding and provision, but also is equally due to the way in which the control is exercised. It does, however, point to the strong possibility that the survival of the provider organizations takes precedence over professional judgement.

In countries like Denmark and the UK, where the local authorities are funders as well as providers, there are few guidelines for service providers and the control is exercised from within. In the UK, the need for better quality control and for more efficient use of resources is widely discussed, and the way in which the Conservative government intends to improve efficiency is to separate funding from provision by making local authorities contract out more services, leaving them to concentrate more on the managerial and regulatory functions. Whether this will result in more efficient use of resources is debatable. The experience of other countries like Belgium or Germany indicates that the separation of funding and provision should not necessarily be seen as a panacea for more efficient service allocation. Much will depend on how much and what form of control over the process of assessment and care planning is retained by the local authorities, as well as the kind of criteria set for service allocation and quality.

4.3c. Service characteristics and professional attitudes

In the absence of entitlement criteria and regulatory norms, service allocation is very much at the discretion of the providers 'at the grass roots'. The case studies from Denmark and the UK show that the service tends to be reactive rather than responsive. In both countries the service was judged to be producing standard solutions rather than solutions geared to individual needs. In other words, the assessment process is less one of clarifying a person's *needs*, and more one of assessing *suitability for a service* as defined by professionals. Allocation of care is to a large extent service led rather than needs led, and it is therefore important to consider the service characteristics that affect decisions.

First of all, the *range of services* available is, of course, important in determining what people get. In most countries the lack of an adequate, 24-hour service is mentioned as a serious gap in provision. Rehabilitation is another gap which the home-help services have not sufficiently taken on board. In Denmark, for example, rehabilitation is a health-care responsibility, which therefore many local authorities do not provide, despite a need for this among many older people living at home. This is linked to the fact that the extent and nature of the fragmentation of the different aspects of care play a part. From the point of view of home help, it is partly a question of the range of care for which the service is responsible and is able to offer. But although the degree of specialization and division of tasks vary between countries, there is everywhere some division of labour and organizational separation between different relevant parts of the system.

What matters as much is the nature of the *relationships between the parts* and not merely the fact that they are in some way separate. For example, in all countries the health-care system is separate from the home-help service. Hospitals are separately funded and organized, and general practitioners are independent of hospitals and home-help services. Home nurses, with the exception of Denmark, Genoa, and Berlin, are usually part of the health-care system. But decision-making practices do not depend on the existence of such organizational barriers alone. *Professional perceptions and interests* are as important. The Danish case studies show a very high degree of co-ordination and planning of services for people discharged from hospital, better than for those referred from their own home. The possible explanation is that hospitals have a strong interest in relieving their beds and therefore have an interest in co-operating with community workers in making arrangements for home care. But their interest in quick discharge is not the only factor that accounts for their co-operation. Professional norms, expectations, and knowledge of alternative services play a part. Thus, in the Flanders case studies, hospital social workers did not refer people to home help/cleaning services because they had poor expectations and inadequate knowledge of how the service operates. Instead, people discharged from hospital were destined for institutions or, if they went back home, only the home-nursing service tended to be involved.

The role of the general practitioner is another example which shows that formal, organizational arrangements only tell part of the story. In the Scottish case studies, the practitioners were very important as referring agents and as a party to the home-care planning. Although the home-help organizers did not, to the same extent, contact the general practitioners, the practitioners themselves seemed highly aware of the existence and potential of the home-help service. This is not the case in many other countries. The general practitioners hardly make any referrals to home help in Belgium, and in Germany, although they are needed to prescribe care and thus exercise a great deal of power, their interest and knowledge about 'social type' services is very low. In the Danish case studies, the general practitioners did not figure very prominently, although they are mentioned as occasionally playing the advocate's role for the clients. They appear remote from the home-help organization, and the home-help organizers seem quite happy to exclude them.

The status and power generally of the social-service system in Denmark is relatively high. Many problems have been successfully 'demedicalized'. The tension between the medical and the 'caring professions' (nurses, social workers, and home-help organizers) seems to manifest itself in a desire on the part of each party to exclude the other. The social-services sector seems less in a position of subordination to the health-care system than in many other countries. The organization of home nurses within the domain of local authorities has further enabled the home-care services to develop team-based care allocation. This is an innovation which is only practised in certain local authorities, but it is significant that these teams include social workers, home helpers, nurses, and other paramedicals, but not general practitioners.

4.4. Conclusions

If one were to assess procedures for service allocation on the basis of a model of 'rational' decision making, whereby services were allocated according to clearly stated policies and according to the needs and wishes of the population of older people, none of the cases reviewed meets these requirements. This, however, is hardly surprising; no system could ever expect to be fully 'rational' in this sense. First of all, each individual case has its own specific set of problems, which can never be predicted and allowed for in regulations and guidelines. Flexibility is always necessary, and therefore a certain amount of discretion needs to be left to those allocating services. But it would be unrealistic to expect this discretion to be exercised to the full satisfaction of all parties involved in every single case. The needs and problems of the clients are not static; they can change from one day to the next. Nor are they always clear and unambiguous. But even if they were, there are other actors in the system with needs that often conflict with those of the older people themselves. Their relatives, for example, may have different interests and needs, which have to be weighed up against those of the old people. Service providers also have 'needs' or interests that inevitably influence the decision-making process. At a given time, for example, the balance of the existing case-load of a service may determine which client is given priority. Indeed, the Scottish study demonstrates most clearly and explicitly how the assessment process is often more to do with assessing people's suitability for services rather than their needs. As Hunter (1990, p. 887) argues, '. . .we do no service to anyone, least of all the users, by continuing the pretence of assessment being a rational, objective and value-free activity. It is not.'

This is not to say that services and service systems cannot be improved, simply that there is no one, perfect solution. This comparative review shows that some systems seem to function better than others, but it also shows that different systems choose different strategies of service rationing, and that in many respects one cannot be said to be 'better' than another. The overall extent of provision clearly makes a big difference. In Denmark the extent of home-help provision is such that deficiencies in the targeting of services matter less; they can afford quite a few 'misses'. At the other extreme, some systems, as in Genoa, have so few services that any attempt even to begin to allocate them according to rational criteria of need is almost certainly doomed to fail. In between these extremes are systems with a significant but more or less limited supply of services, where the targeting process becomes more important. The nature of the systems in which the providers operate, as we have seen, affects the ways in which this process operates. The more fragmented the organization of funders and providers, the more their conflicting interests are likely to divert attention from the clients' needs. Also, some providers work within the constraints of rigorous eligibility criteria, imposed 'from above', which allow little scope for discretion and indeed do not take the needs of many older people into consideration. Others operate within extremely loose frameworks, where policy aims appear to be either absent or confusing.

Whatever the system, it seems quite clear that the solutions to the problems of service allocation cannot be found solely through 'top down' policies. As the investigators in the Scottish study conclude (Hunter *et al.* 1988, p. 159):

> If policies are to make sense to those at street level, certain preconditions would seem to be necessary. We list three but there may be others: (a) policies need explicitly to allow for provider discretion (which will occur anyway) by being sufficiently flexible; (b) policies need to allow for difference among elderly people—they are not all the same and nor are the circumstances of those of their carers; (c) policies need to be discussed at *all* levels in the organisation so that they become accepted and 'owned' by everyone.

These, I would say, are necessary but not sufficient preconditions for home-care services to function. Other requirements must be met, not least the commitment of a certain amount of resources to their development. Resources will always be scarce and no allocation will ever be perceived as 'enough'. The resources devoted to services for older people depend not only on the economic capability of a country but also on political priorities.

Thus, although service providers 'at street level' shape policies through the decision-making process—in ways which depend on factors like professional attitudes and relationships, managerial leadership and organization—the wider context within which providers operate sets the parameters for their actions. Factors like availability of resources, funding arrangements, and the degree and nature of regulations are of overall importance. These are the factors that are, in principle, subject to national policy making. 'Top down' policies therefore are necessary, if not sufficient for services to function adequately. The final chapter will turn to a consideration of these, asking the question: what have been and what are currently the policy measures taken to enable older people to remain at home for as long as possible? and how do we explain such policies?

REFERENCES

Holstein, B. (1986). *The elderly in Denmark. Health and social situation.* Report for ACRE, University of Copenhagen.

Hunter, D., McKeganey, N., and MacPherson, I. (1988). *Care of the elderly. Policy and practice.* Aberdeen University Press.

Hunter, D. (1990). Redraw the lines. *Health Service Journal*, **100,** 5205.

Jamieson, A. (1990). Informal care in Europe. In *Contrasting European policies for the care of older people* (ed. A. Jamieson and R. Illsley). Avebury/Gower, Aldershot.

Jamieson, A. and Illsley, R. (ed.) (1990). *Contrasting European policies for the care of older people.* Avebury/Gower, Aldershot.

Morton, J. (ed.) (1989). *Achieving change in home care services.* Age Concern Institute of Gerontology, London.

Twigg, J. (1990). Carers of elderly people: models for analysis. In *Contrasting European policies for the care of older people* (ed. A. Jamieson and R. Illsley). Avebury/Gower, Aldershot.

11
Trends in home-care policies

Anne Jamieson

1. An assessment of home-care measures
   1.1. Trends in provision and distribution
   1.2. The impact of home care on institutionalization
2. Past and recent trends
   2.1. Policies—a model of aims and means
   2.2. 1960s and 1970s: growth without policies
   2.3. 1980s: policies without growth
3. Factors affecting policies and their implementation
   3.1. 'Systems' factors
   3.2. 'Non-systems' factors
4. Conclusions
References

1. AN ASSESSMENT OF HOME-CARE MEASURES

All the chapters on home-care provision in individual countries discuss problems and shortcomings in that provision. But what exactly have been the successes and failures in the different countries? There is, of course, no one way of measuring this, but I will try to summarize some of the trends discussed by the different contributors in order to get some way towards an understanding of policies and their implementation.

1.1. Trends in provision and distribution

In all countries the provision of home-help services increased considerably in absolute terms during the 1970s and until the middle of the 1980s. However, with the exception of Denmark, the increase hardly or only just kept up with the rise in the number of older people. Indeed, when measured per 1000 elderly persons, home-help provision in the UK fell during this period. The response to the growing demand for home help in most countries has been to spread the services more thinly to a larger proportion of older people. Belgium, or at least the region of Flanders, is an exception to this trend. Here the proportion as well as the absolute number of beneficiaries has declined, whereas the number of hours per client has grown. It is not clear what has brought about this development, but it could be a consequence of the tendency by many providers to allocate the maximum number of hours possible to all clients, irrespective of needs. Home-nursing provision has increased in all countries, but with the exception of Germany, home-nursing care is provided to a relatively small proportion of clients compared with home help, and an increasing number of personal-care tasks are being taken over by the home-help services.

Although age, functional ability, and the availability of a relative in the household are the most important predictors of home-help use, severe doubts are raised by several contributors about the extent to which services are matched to needs. Lack of provision for people with severe disabilities is a problem in all countries except Denmark and possibly the Netherlands. The data from the Netherlands are ambiguous. The chapters on France (5) and England (4) in particular suggest that a certain proportion of home-help clients does not appear to need or benefit from the service. Data on the allocation of home help indicate that there is insufficient regard to the clients' needs and that they do not always receive the kind of care they need. Thus, whilst overall shortage of provision is the most serious problem, inadequate assessment processes and lack of co-ordination with other services are also serious symptoms of the failure of policy implementation.

Yet the views of the clients, in so far as they are known, tend to be highly appreciative. Some would like more help, and more continuity, but there seems no doubt that in most places the home-help service is popular and staunchly defended by its clients.

1.2. The impact of home care on institutionalization

One of the espoused aims of home-help provision is to prevent institutionalization. If one considers trends in the proportion of each age group living in some form of residential care, it is difficult to discern any dramatic changes. There has been a slight decrease in the Netherlands and Denmark in the late 1980s, but elsewhere the proportion has either remained stable or has increased. As already stressed, it is important to bear in mind that not all countries have aimed to reduce their number of institutions, rather home care has been a way of making up for a shortfall of residential places, as for example in Israel, Italy, and, to some extent, France. The Netherlands has by far the largest number of institutions, and a reduction in these has been high on the policy agenda for many years. But, as in most other countries, the concept of 'deinstitutionalization' does not merely entail a simple reduction of institutional places, and its success or failure therefore cannot be measured simply by looking at figures for total provision. It is as much the structure of provision that is the object of the policy aims.

First of all, national figures for service provision conceal enormous geographical differences. We (the project group) cannot identify a single country where provision of institutional and home-care services does not vary by at least 100 per cent between localities. Policies in Denmark and the Netherlands explicitly take such variations into account. In the Netherlands there are specific measures to equalize distribution of institutional provision, and in Denmark the recent legislation that bans the setting up of new nursing homes makes exceptions for certain areas where there is relatively scarce provision. Thus, although the Dutch contributors do not provide the evidence, it is possible that the figures for total institutional provision cover some degree of equalization between geographical areas.

Whether such changes are associated with changes in the actual provision of home care is another question. Studies of different localities in the UK concluded that between 1979 and 1983 there was no correlation between the increase in the scale of the home-help service and the decrease of permanent local-authority places (Bebbington and Tong 1986). Thus there was no evidence of any clear planning process of substitution.

Another aspect that must be taken into account concerns the fact that there are different types of institutions, and policies aimed at reducing the use of one type may result in greater use of another, whether or not this is intended. This is a particularly important issue in relation to the use of *hospitals*. As mentioned in the analysis of formal policy aims (Chapter 10, Section 2.2, pp. 243–5), home care is at least in part expected to reduce the use of hospitals. Policies in most countries have the clear aim of reducing the number of older people relying on hospitals for *long-term care*, and there is some evidence that this aim is being achieved. On the use of hospitals for *acute* care, there is no clear statistical evidence of trends, and only more qualitative analyses will tell us something about possible trends.

Whatever the trends in the use of institutions (including hospitals), these are not enough to draw any conclusions about *causal links* between alternative types of provision. The question is: to what extent would people have entered an institution were it not for the provision of home care? In other words: does home care substitute for institutional care? In Britain, there has for some time been a great deal of debate and research around this question. The answers are ambiguous. The evidence discussed by Lawson and Davies (Chapter 4) suggests that the amount of home-help input makes little difference to the eventual probability of admission to an institution. Yet other commentators have put forward the view that it is a mistake to see domiciliary care as an alternative to residential care, because services have rarely been delivered in sufficient quantities to provide a realistic alternative (Sinclair and Williams 1989). Both views imply that, given the way services are at present distributed, the direct effect of home-help provision in preventing institutionalization is, for the most, not obvious.

The data from the Netherlands also seem to question the extent to which home care substitutes for residential care. Holstein *et al.* (Chapter 3), on the other hand, in their study of Danish recipients of four or more hours of home help, judge that without this help most people would have had to enter an institution. This may point to another factor that plays a part in the question of substitution—the extent to which informal carers substitute for lack of home care. Although, as discussed earlier, formal provision does not appear to 'drive out' informal care, it is possible that the resources of informal carers are stretched far further in the UK and, to a lesser extent, the Netherlands, than in Denmark, and that in these countries you can 'get away with' providing less home care than in Denmark, in the sense that lack of home care in Denmark would be more likely to manifest itself in a higher demand for residential care.

The question of the impact of home care on demand for acute hospital care is even more complex. From what we know about the nature of home-care provision it is possible, however, to deduce certain likely effects. Thus, most commentators point to the lack of 24-hour provision of home care, without which it is not possible to intervene in crises. Evidence certainly suggests that, in so far as 24-hour care is available, this tends to reduce acute hospital admissions. The problem is that this service is still only provided in limited amounts. Attempts to maintain people at home when the supply of home care is restricted may well lead to more use of hospitals for crisis relief. The most obvious example of this is the German one, where not only the lack of 24-hour care but also the restrictions upon access to home care actually encourage the use of hospitals. They in turn become reluctant to discharge people back home and prefer to find a residential solution in order to avoid further acute admissions. Indeed, there is evidence from the Berlin study (Chapter 6.2) which suggests that the original intention of avoiding the hospitalization of older people has been perverted. Instead of a reduction in admissions, a significant number of older people are admitted to hospital *in order to* obtain home care, as this route is the easiest from the point of view of the clients as well as the providers of home care.

In short, the effectiveness of home-care provision in preventing the use of residential and hospital care is not clearly visible. It is possible that in the majority of cases the key function of home help has been to improve the quality of life of older people, for example by helping to make their homes clean and tidy or by providing social stimulation; and to improve the quality of life of their relatives, by relieving the burden on them and by providing general support.

2. PAST AND RECENT TRENDS

Going back now to the original set of aims expressed in policy statements, we have seen that the extent to which these appear to have been achieved is variable. Provision of home care, in particular home help, is seen as inadequate in most countries—least so in Denmark. What does exist is not always distributed according to need; the effectiveness of the service in reducing admissions to institutions is questionable. In an attempt to understand some of the variations and the extent of success and failure, let us consider what policy measures were actually taken, and the factors that affect their implementation.

2.1. Policies—a model of aims and means

By policy measures we refer primarily to action taken by central government, as our interest is in measures that are intended to affect society as a whole. Policies are, of course, also developed at local levels, or even 'from the bottom up'. We are interested in this in so far as it is a consequence of central policies, but we are not here considering 'local experiments' *per se*. The model in Fig. 11.1 illustrates, first, that there are different policy

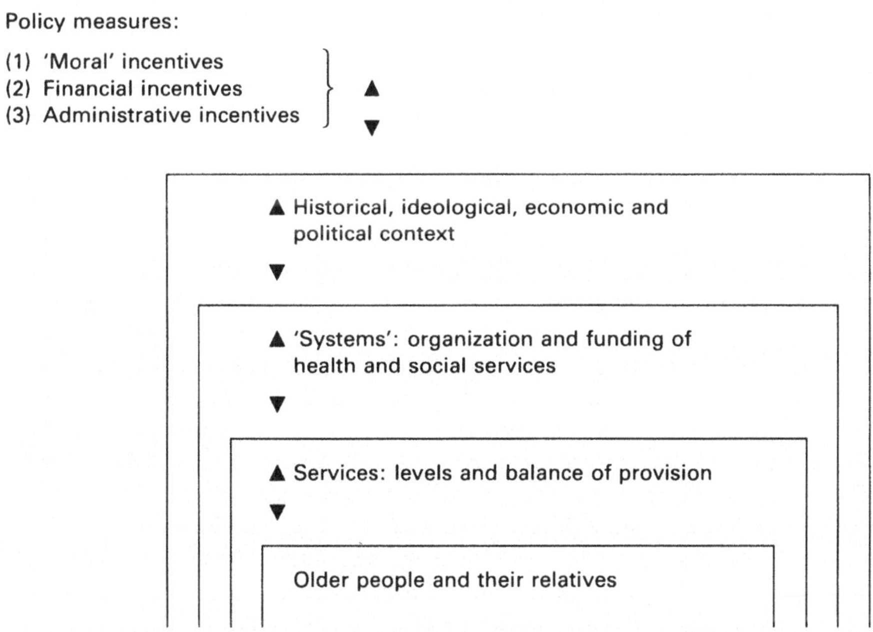

Fig. 11.1. Policy measures: targets and means.

measures (Rodwin 1984), i.e., 'moral' incentives, which aim to change the values and norms of providers and clients. Secondly, financial incentives are ways of changing behaviour through the provision of funding for particular programmes or through the structure of funding whereby providers have incentives to act in certain ways. Finally, 'administrative incentives' are legislation or regulations actually telling providers or clients to behave in certain ways.

Policy measures can be directed at the systems, attempting, for example, to change the organization of services or the balance between health and social services, or between private and public services. Measures could also be directly focused on the extent of provision, for example by allocating funds for home help, or on the pattern of provision, for example by shifting resources from institutions to the community, or from health into social services. Finally, measures could be directed at the individual older person and their family, attempting to change behaviours either through moral incentives—for example by stressing the importance of family responsibility—or by financial incentives—for example by providing a carers' allowance. However, policy measures, although directed at these different levels, are themselves affected by existing systems and the extent and pattern of provision. Existing systems and patterns of provision are the result of historical, economic, ideological, and political factors, all of which form the wider context within which policies operate. Thus, if we are to understand policies at any given time, we need to understand this wider context as well as the nature of the systems and existing provision.

2.2. 1960s and 1970s: growth without policies

On looking at policy trends in relation to home care for older people, we can distinguish between the earlier period of the 1960s and 1970s on the one hand, and, on the other, the more recent period of the 1980s. The earlier period was characterized by two important developments: the acceleration of the increase in the proportion of older people, and general economic growth, which although decreasing in the 1970s, was even then accompanied by an increase in spending on health and social welfare.

This may be called a period of 'growth without policies', because it appears that, in most of the countries, services for older people, including home-care services, developed more as a result of pressures 'from below' and a general increase in welfare provision than as a result of a coherent set of policies. True, some political interest in older people did surface as early as the 1960s, but with few practical implications. Thus, in France, the 'Laroque report' appeared in 1962, stressing the need to maintain older people at home, and a few 'pump priming' resources were allocated, with limited and temporary effect. In most other countries, government reports did not appear until the 1970s or even early 1980s. But despite these, policies during this period can at best be described as incremental, and developments as provider led rather than the result of clear planning. Some measures, however, were taken to encourage providers in certain directions.

Taking first the 'moral incentives', the stress on enabling older people to stay in their own homes for as long as possible can be seen increasingly in statements and government reports from the various countries, especially during the 1970s. In the Netherlands, for example, several reports during that decade pointed to the need to reduce the number of institutional places. This is not surprising, in view of the large proportion of older people living in institutions in that country. In many other countries the stress on home care for older people was part of a wider movement towards community care, focusing especially on mentally ill people and the move to close the large psychiatric intitutions. This can be seen in particular in Italy, but also in the UK and Germany. Thus, despite variations in emphasis and focus, there seems no doubt that by the beginning of the 1980s the general aim of maintaining people at home for as long as possible was well established and widely accepted as a basic value, by politicians, practitioners, and the populations themselves. What remained open, however, was *how* this aim should be achieved, and *how far* it should and could be achieved.

Financial and administrative measures taken during this period were mainly directed at the *overall extent* of home-care provision. By this I mean that a number of financial measures were set in motion involving the allocation of funds towards home help. This happened in several countries, most notably in the Netherlands and Denmark. In the Netherlands this funding was, however, cut many times during the 1970s in attempts to curb public spending. In Denmark, central government paid 80 per cent of local-authority expenditure on home help, a financial incentive that encouraged the expansion of home-help provision. In other countries like, for example, France and the UK, funding was more modestly allocated in the form of 'pump priming', short-term experiments. In most countries, some limited administrative measures were taken, specifying eligibility criteria, but these were generally very broad and left most of the decisions to local providers.

2.3. 1980s: policies without growth

The debate about older people and their care needs increased during the 1980s in most countries, and in some it only just began. A number of factors account for this. First, although the decline in economic growth had started in the previous decade, there was a time lag in policy responses to this. When they came, during the 1980s, issues of cost containment in health-service spending in particular and public-sector spending in general were at the top of the agenda. This period saw the introduction of *cash limits* and with this an increased emphasis upon *cost effectiveness* and upon *planning* in health and social services. Services for older people were no exception to this, and the renewed focus on their care must be understood against this background, but also perhaps in the light of the realization that the proportion of older people in institutions had not decreased during the previous decades. During the 1980s a number of policy themes developed, which make up the agenda for the most recent policies. These themes do not all recur in all countries, indeed there are some important differences, which can, in part, be traced back to the different nature of the systems, but even more importantly seem to reflect differences in the welfare principles of the different countries and differences in current political ideologies and attitudes.

2.3a. Expansion of home-care cover—the 'late developers'

Whereas in most of the countries reviewed, policies in the previous decades had been mainly concentrated on extent of provision, some did not actually begin to take any measures at all until the latter part of the 1980s. Thus Israel developed its community-care programme towards the end of that decade, mainly in response to general lack of services (including residential services) for older people. Germany, too, did not see any significant change until the 1980s, and even then it is doubtful whether the changes introduced can be called significant.

It is interesting to compare these two countries, because they both have an insurance-based health service and a means-tested, limited provision of social services. In Israel, however, the political will was there to extend and earmark a proportion of insurance contributions to cover home care. In contrast, German policies have been dominated by two factors: first, strict adherence to the health-insurance principle and the principle that the insurance organizations decide what they wish to include in this; and secondly, the principle of subsidiarity guiding social welfare, whereby the state plays a residual role and the family carries the main responsibility. There has not been any political move to break with these principles, but some limited action has been taken in response to pressure from providers. First, the government has attempted to put pressure on the insurance organizations to accept liability for some care of frail, but not necessarily ill, old people. In 1991, new regulations were implemented whereby a limited amount of care qualifies for insurance-based funding. But it is strictly limited, and not meant to cover all home care because of the fear of escalating costs and rising demand.

In the social-welfare sector in Germany, the state has provided funding for the 'social stations' to be set up, but again the funding is strictly limited.

As Dieck (Chapter 6.1) points out, the interest in services for older people is very low; the measures taken are minimal and mainly adopted in an attempt to curb demand for health and hospital care. The measures do not form part of a coherent set of health and social policies for older people, and it is doubtful whether, in the foreseeable future, there is likely to be any significant change away from what is largely family-based care combined with the back-up of a highly sophisticated and well-developed system of medical treatment.

2.3b. Better 'targeting' of services

The targeting of services to match needs has become an important item on the agenda in many countries. In other words, the focus in many places has shifted towards ways of distributing *existing resources* more effectively. This interest is reflected in the growing number of research and evaluation programmes concerned with the needs and characteristics of the population of older people in institutions compared with those living at home, and comparing home-care clients with those not receiving services at all. The body of research on these questions is particularly large in the UK and the Netherlands and, to some extent, in France and Italy, as is evident from the contributions in this book.

As discussed above, the problems of matching services to needs can broadly speaking be due to one or more of the following factors. First, the lack of variety and flexibility of the services available; secondly, inadequacies in the process of assessment due to lack of clear measures and lack of competent care managers; and thirdly, the fragmentation of the service system, either through organizational and/or financial separation between the different, relevant parts of the system. In lack of variety and flexibility there is some evidence of change, most notably, perhaps, the development in many countries of a 24-hour service. It seems that this innovation, as well as many others, came mainly 'from below' and is not the direct result of policy decisions from above. This means that, whilst it is possible to identify many innovative practices, these tend to be local and rather limited in scope. Of measures intended to improve the assessment process itself, an example is the introduction of nationally applicable standard assessment forms in the Netherlands, albeit not a very successful example according to the Dutch contributors (Chapter 9). Little attention has been paid to the need to improve the level of training of care managers such as, for example, home-help organizers, and again this is an area where change would appear to depend very much upon local initiatives.

The third problem, the fragmentation of provider systems due to organizational and financial separation, has received increasing attention in the 1980s. It has become more and more obvious that, if the notions of service substitution and of flexible responses to individual needs are to be practised in any meaningful way, then the different types of services must be not only co-ordinated but also interrelated organizationally and financially. Some national policy measures in a few countries have been directed at these problems.

First, in the Netherlands, the law on the Exceptional Medical Expenses Scheme (AWBZ) is a recent change whereby all services, medical, nursing, and social, are financed within the same scheme in order to promote co-ordination, especially between home-nursing and home-help services. Furthermore, the financial arrangements for agencies have become more flexible in order to allow provider agencies to offer a mix of residential and home care.

In the UK, problems arising from the separate funding of a large part of residential care and from the separation of health, including community health, from social services were addressed by a government-sponsored inquiry known as the Griffiths Inquiry (Griffiths 1988). The new Community Care Bill, introduced in Parliament in the Spring of 1990, proposed a number of measures. Among others these were to concentrate the funding of residential as well as community care with the local authorities, thus removing any financial incentives to refer people to institutions, until then partly funded by central government. Furthermore, local authorities are to be given the total responsibility for community-care allocation, although home nursing is to remain within the health-care sector. To overcome this continued separation the new Bill stipulates that local authorities' social services departments must plan services jointly with the health authorities. Thus the measures taken to overcome structural impediments are mainly managerial rather than a change in the structures themselves. The main criticism of this new Bill has been that no resources have been set aside by central government to develop home-care services. The main burden is to fall upon the local authorities. In the summer of 1990, however, the implementation of this new bill was postponed for political reasons: the wish on the part of central government to keep down local authority spending—and thus the level of local taxation—was stronger than any concern with older, mentally ill and mentally handicapped people, all of whom were to benefit from the new law.

In Denmark a government commission on elderly people was set up in the early 1980s, and some of its recommendations resulted in a new law implemented in 1988. Like the British Community Care Bill, this seeks to remove the incentives to rely on institutional care through the creation of financial incentives towards less institutionalized forms of care, and it went further than the British law by actually stipulating that no more nursing homes were to be created. The contents of this law and its aims are a radical break with much previous thinking, and I will consider it in some detail in a separate section below.

2.3c. Privatization and increased reliance on market mechanisms

As we have seen, independent providers—whether non-profit making or for-profit—have long been part of the home-care scene in many countries, and continued to exist with increasing public financial support. The notable exceptions have been the UK and Denmark. However, there is now in many countries a trend in the direction of further privatization and encouragement of private providers to compete on the market. This trend is part of a widespread disillusionment with public-sector planning and provision, manifest in the capitalist as well as the socialist world, and in some countries it is beginning to have an impact on policies for the care of older people.

In Europe, the Thatcher government, which has dominated politics in the UK for more than a decade from 1979, has been the most ardent proponent of privatization and reliance on the markets as the best way of distributing resources. As far as health care is concerned, the popularity of the National Health Service as a public enterprise has so far prevented the government from considering its privatization. Instead, market mechanisms are being introduced by encouraging units (especially hospitals) within the health service to 'opt out' of the control of the health authorities, whose task will be confined to the planning and 'purchasing' of services from the providers. In the area of community care, however, the new Community Care Bill directs local authorities to contract out as many services as possible to private and voluntary providers, whilst retaining and, so it is believed, improving the role of the public sector in planning and controlling the quality of provision.

No other European country has witnessed such concerted efforts in this direction as the UK, but both the Dutch and the Italian contributors here point to trends towards further privatization and reliance on market mechanisms. Whether such developments will help improve the quality of home-care distribution and provision is an open question, and many point to potential problems. As the Dutch contributors conclude: 'High risk groups could become excluded from care' (p. 234). This indeed is what is actually happening in the German system, where, as the German contributors argue (Chapter 6), private organizations are not interested in clients with complex, long-term care needs because of the risk of lack of financial coverage. The German experience indicates that a great deal depends on the ways in which providers will be funded and the ability of the funders to manage what would become a fragmented sector of providers. This is also borne out by the French experience, which shows that the extreme fragmentation of funding as well as provision of services is one of the major barriers to the functioning of home care.

2.3d. Increased emphasis on the family

The family has always played a major role in supporting and caring for older people, although the extent to which they carry this burden varies between countries. However, policy statements in most countries, Denmark excepted, are putting an increasing emphasis on their role. In the UK, 'care in the community' means 'care *by* the community', as far as the present (Conservative) government is concerned. In the Netherlands, the concept of 'the caring society' is increasingly stressed in policy statements, and in France and Belgium there are similar signs of renewed emphasis on the responsibility of the family. In Germany this has always been explicit, and in Italy it is a continuation of existing practices. In other words, rather than considering ways of extending and improving home-care provision for older people, governments are beginning to withdraw, on the basis that the growing number of very old people presents too great a burden on 'society', i.e., the tax payers. It is recognized that the state may play a part in encouraging and maintaining the ability of families to provide care, and this is manifested in attempts to target services and cash payments to carers in the form of respite care and payment of compensation. Thus carers have increasingly become the focus of policy making. Although to some extent this development is a response to some real needs, some would point to the dangers of such policies. Thus, policies directed at 'carers' tend to assume not only that families care but also that they *ought to* care, thereby attempting to shift more of the burden of care on to families.

2.3e. A new concept of 'home care'

Some of the recent policy trends in Denmark alluded to by Holstein *et al.* in Chapter 3 are important, because they represent a radical break with previous concepts of care provision. Thus, in principle, the new law on housing for older people aims to separate *care* from the *locus* of care. In other words, the principle behind the new legislation is that care should be delivered to people as they need it, irrespective of where they live. Their status and the people caring for them should not change as the old people become more frail. People should never have to move into an institutions; there should be no such things as nursing homes. It is recognized that the reason people have to move when they need a high level of care is most often that they live in dwellings unsuitable for them. Policies are therefore directed at improving existing housing stock and building new dwellings that are all independent units, but which are adapted for people with handicaps (Christiansen 1989).

Before the new law, central government in Denmark provided subsidies to local authorities' housing according to a complex set of rules, which differed depending on whether the dwellings were 'old age housing', sheltered housing, housing collectives, or 'nursing homes'. Now, subsidies are all streamlined and related to 'housing for older people', i.e., dwellings of a certain size with independent facilities and adapted for handicapped persons. Subsidies from central government are generous and encourage local authorities to improve existing housing stock and to build new dwellings. This is clearly an ambitious aim but already some local authorities have completely abolished nursing homes (Wagner 1989). All their older people are offered independent housing, but with teams of home helpers, nurses, and others providing care as necessary. If people have to move into more suitable housing, sometimes in the 'elderly centre', they continue to receive care by the same personnel. They continue to pay rent and live independently as far as they can. In such local authorities there are no more 'nursing-home residents'. Thus, although this new law is only beginning to be implemented, it is a practical step in the direction of realizing what observers in many countries are increasingly pointing out: that institutions have been used to solve problems, many of which come from poor housing conditions and an environment that is not 'people friendly', let alone 'elderly people friendly'.

3. FACTORS AFFECTING POLICIES AND THEIR IMPLEMENTATION

This brief review of some of the main policy trends points to certain similarities between countries, but also differences. Both need to be explained, and in this discussion I have already suggested a number of reasons for policies or lack of policies in the different contexts. These can be summed up under two headings, 'systems' factors and 'non-systems' factors, and in the following I will give some examples of how each of these sets of factors affects policies.

3.1. 'Systems' factors

The very factors that we have found to impede good practice, and which are therefore a focus of policy making, do themselves pose constraints upon policies and their chances of being successfully implemented. This is, perhaps, most clearly manifested in the *separation of health and social services*, not only organizationally and financially, but also in terms of different principles underlying eligibility for services. It is generally agreed that policies ought to address the problems of lack of integration and collaboration between health and social services, and that the balance of resources should be shifted in the direction of social services rather than health, and of home care rather than institutions. This is clearly very difficult to achieve in all the systems here reviewed, but mostly so in systems like the German one, where health and social services have separate funding principles, criteria of eligibility, and loci of responsibility.

This makes any co-ordinated policy of health *and* social care extremely difficult. There are similar problems in France, where a highly fragmented system with a multiplicity of actors with conflicting interests has made any far-reaching changes virtually impossible. Henrard *et al.* (Chapter 5) do not conclude on a very optimistic note as regards future policies. In the Netherlands, national policies have been constrained by the organizational principle of 'pillarization', whereby the (religiously affiliated) organizations have traditionally had a great deal of autonomy.

In systems like the UK and Denmark there are fewer actors and less fragmentation. Yet the separate organization of health and social services in these countries has also formed a barrier to fully co-ordinated policies. In the UK, policies have for some time attempted to encourage collaboration between health and social-service sectors through the provision of 'joint finance' for jointly planned services (Hunter *et al.* 1988). However, this was a limited measure and not entirely successful. The latest changes, which are yet to be implemented, seek to address this structural problem by stipulating by law that health and social services must produce joint plans and work closely together in providing services. Whether these measures go far enough in solving the problems arising from the structural barriers is highly debatable.

In Denmark, the development of home care has proceeded almost without the involvement of the health services. Compared with the UK, Denmark has the advantage that community nurses are organized within the social-services sector, and this clearly has facilitated the development of more coherent home-care policies and practices. But, as the Danish contributors indicate, the problem of hospital admissions and the relationships between hospitals and home-care services have still not been fully solved.

In all the countries reviewed, organizational, financial, and professional structures contribute to making coherent and integrated policies difficult if not impossible. Such 'systems' factors are particularly at play at operational levels, posing barriers, as we have seen, to effective allocation and planning of services. However, in national policy making, other 'non-systems' factors are at least as, if not more, important, and these are now discussed.

3.2. 'Non-systems' factors

3.2a. Welfare traditions

Whatever the structure of existing systems, these are in many ways a manifestation of historically rooted, welfare ideologies. Thus service provision and policies in all countries are formulated within the context of long-established welfare traditions which pervade attitudes and expectations and which have resulted in particular arrangements regarding the role of the state and the extent and criteria of welfare provision.

Esping-Andersen's (1990) classification of welfare-state regimes is illuminating in this respect. He argues that when comparing cross-national variations in social rights and welfare-state stratification there are qualitatively different arrangements, which are clustered by 'regime types'. He distinguishes *three* different regimes: first, the '*liberal*' welfare state, in which means-tested, modest, universal transfers predominate. The norms of the liberal work ethic predominate and the limits of welfare equal the marginal propensity to opt for welfare instead of work. Benefits are limited, and the state encourages the market, either by guaranteeing only a minimum or by subsidizing private welfare schemes. Typical examples of this type of regime are the United States, Canada, and Australia. The second type of welfare regime is the '*conservative*' or '*corporatist*'. In this the liberal obsession with market efficiency was never important. The state took on the role as welfare provider, but in a way which preserved class and status differences. Such corporatist regimes are typically shaped by the Church, and therefore strongly committed to the preservation of traditional family relationships and thus to the principle of subsidiarity. Countries like France, Germany, and Italy are examples of such welfare regimes. Thirdly, there is the '*social-democratic*' welfare regime, where principles of universalism and state dominance prevail. Rights and benefits were made available to all, irrespective of class and market position. Furthermore, the family is freed from its social obligations, individual independence rather than family dependence being the aim. This type of welfare regime is found in Scandinavia.

Esping-Andersen analyses these different welfare regimes in detail and along a number of key dimensions. His objective is to compare welfare states, to explain their origins, and to assess their effect on national economies. Our aim here is not to explain the origin of welfare regimes or indeed the origin of policies for older people, but, more modestly, to begin to understand some of the factors influencing present-day policies for the care of older people. Esping-Andersen's analysis points to the relevance of considering this question within a wider framework.

In the present analysis, which is confined to services for older people, some of the important questions to ask for each country are: does the state provide benefits universally to all citizens, or are entitlements conditional upon insurance contributions, which themselves depend on people's position on the labour market? does the state play the dominant role in providing care, or does it play a residual role, leaving the main responsibility to the family? The answers to these questions go some way towards explaining differences in policies of care for elderly people. This can be illustrated by comparing three countries, each of which represents a different type of welfare state.

Taking first *Germany* (with a 'corporatist/conservative welfare regime'), the separation of two distinct domains, with their different principles of distribution and access, is crucial in conditioning the plight of frail old people. The dominance of the insurance principle in health care, and behind this the vested interests of the labour-market partners, has had the effect of largely excluding older people needing long-term care or rehabilitation. They are left to rely on inadequate, 'residual-type' social services, which have always been very explicitly guided by the principle of subsidiarity. For the state to replace the family or in any substantial way to ease the burden upon families would be counter to well-established principles of welfare. The prospect of any erosion of these principles would only be likely to come from demands from the labour market to free women for work.

In contrast to Germany, indeed in contrast to all the countries reviewed in this book, *Denmark* has a tradition of comprehensive state intervention and institutionalized social- as well as health-care entitlements based on universal coverage and solidarity ('social-democratic welfare regime'). This has been highly conducive to the care and welfare of older people and to their families. Women are no longer expected to be full-time carers at any stage in their lives; the responsibilities of the state are well established, and this explains why, in Denmark, policies for older people have been more consistent and far reaching than in any other country in the European Community.

The *British* system has more aspects in common with the Danish than the German one. But there are differences. Both Britain and Denmark have a tax-funded national health service which is universally accessible, and which has the strong support of all classes. But in social welfare the British state has never taken on such a degree of universality and comprehensiveness as the Danish state. Whereas in Germany and Denmark the underlying principles of the welfare state have been more firmly entrenched from the very beginning, the welfare state in Britain never obtained the degree of general, in particular middle-class, support necessary to sustain the development of a comprehensive, universal regime. If one adds to this the fact that the electoral system has tended to polarize politics, it is not surprising that questions of social policies have been subject to change depending on which political side has been in government. Mostly this has been the Conservatives, and the last decade has seen Conservative rule of a radical, neo-liberalist persuasion. In Esping-Andersen's terms, the British welfare state regime is becoming increasingly 'liberal'. Yet the effort of the Thatcher administration to roll back the frontiers of the welfare state have not been entirely 'successful'. Traditions and commitments from the past cannot easily be swept aside, although given more time the radical objectives of this government may well be realized.

The present time is still characterized by a great deal of conflict between opposing forces in the UK. This can be seen, for example, in policies related to 'carers'. Whereas in Germany, carers are low on the policy agenda because they are simply expected to fulfil their obligations to care, and in Denmark they are low if not absent from the policy agenda because they are not expected to play an important role, in Britain their centrality on the policy agenda reflects to some extent the lack of a consensus about their role. There is pressure from across the political spectrum to focus policies upon carers, and nowhere are the dilemmas inherent in such focusing more obvious: to the government this represents an opportunity to shift more responsibility on to families; to those representing the interests of older people and their families the objective is to provide further support and relief for this group.

Welfare regimes, developed historically out of a constellation of economic and political factors, are embodied in the structures of health and social services and in existing power relations. Thus an understanding of this context will help us to understand policies and assess the possibilities and direction of future change. But policies are not solely 'predetermined' by such historical legacies. Within this context, policy measures can vary and welfare regimes can themselves be subject to change or modification. At any given point in time, economic and political factors are powerful in affecting policies.

3.2b. Economic factors

Whilst the concept of home care is attractive to those who have the interests of older people at heart, there is no doubt that the expectation that it is cheaper than institutional care has made it popular among decision makers, whatever their political persuasion. If in many countries, as I have argued, relatively little has happened to develop home-care services, economic considerations are certainly among the causes. Increasingly, doubts are being raised as to whether the provision of home-care services is actually the cheapest solution.

Two factors are behind this. First of all, the costs and actual expenditure on existing alternatives (i.e., institutions) affect the degree to which home care is viewed as a cost-saving measure. And these vary immensely. The Dutch contributors, for example, quote figures to the effect that for anybody needing more than 10 hours of weekly home help, living in a home for the aged would be cheaper. Such calculations are not likely to encourage politicians to devote a vast amount of resources to home-care services. The costs of institutional care in Denmark, on the other hand, are much higher; and this therefore goes some way towards explaining the high level of commitment to home care in that country. Thus some calculations show that as much as 30 hours of weekly home help is still cheaper than a place in a residential home. In other words, other things being equal, home-care provision is cheaper the higher the level of spending on institutional care. This means that in countries with little or cheap institutional care, the economic incentive to develop home-care services appears weak.

There is a second reason, however, behind the apparent decline in enthusiasm for home-care services, and this is the uncertainty about their effectiveness as a substitute for institutional care. Much of the research quoted in this book and elsewhere points out that the relationships between the use of different kinds of services are unclear. As discussed earlier, there are no unambiguous answers to questions like: in what ways do services substitute for each other? does the expansion of home help, for example, necessarily lead to a decline in the rate of institutionalization? is it possible to target home-care services to those who might otherwise have entered an institution or do they merely create new demands? if more people remain in their own homes, is it likely to lead to an increase in the use of hospitals for acute episodes, for crises, and for relief of carers? As long as doubts remain about the answers to these questions, the cheapest, though by no means the most desirable, option may well be to leave older people and their families to cope and merely to provide a safety net of institutional care for those with no families or who are too frail to live at home.

Neither the 'liberal' nor the 'conservative' welfare states have ever sought to take on tasks that traditionally have been seen as the responsibility of the family, unless of course there are strong pressures for this to happen, and these are usually economic. Just as the state developed child-care facilities where necessary to free women for paid work, the growing interests in family care in many countries reflects the realization that this is cheaper than providing services. It has become increasingly obvious that families in all countries, Denmark excepted, provide the main bulk of care and support for older people, and that any decline in the will of families to continue to care could have costly service implications. Consequently, policy debates are increasingly focusing on the provision of support—services or cash—to carers. The introduction of carers' allowances of various kinds is an attempt to ease the burden on services. This development seems most widespread in the 'liberal' welfare states and fits in with the reliance on 'market incentives'. In 'conservative' regimes, such as in Germany or Italy, where moral incentives are still more heavily stressed, measures to support carers are likely to be even more modest for fear of eroding the sense of family obligation.

3.2c. Political factors

Policies at any given time are the result of political decisions. The structure of the systems, the welfare traditions, and economic factors all impose certain constraints upon the extent to which politicians can influence events. But within these constraints, priorities and options chosen are a function of the interests and beliefs of governments. Most of the contributions in this book show evidence of the importance of political factors in influencing service provision. For example, the Community Care Law in Israel was passed despite the fact that the existing system was divided in its criteria and functions, and the new law cut across these existing divisions. Another, different, example is the Netherlands, where the system itself has been the focus of policy makers. Thus changes are gradually being introduced that aim to increase central control over providers, thereby facilitating further change through government initiatives.

Whether the direction of changes promotes home care for older people is another question and depends on prevailing political priorities and beliefs. The trend towards privatization, for example, apparent in many countries and most obvious in the UK, where it is also most clearly linked with the wish to replace public-sector planning with markets, can best be understood as a political move, guided by neo-liberalist ideas rather than by clear evidence that such changes will improve the quality and distribution of services. Indeed, as some commentators have pointed out (Hunter 1990), regardless of what is happening in health-care delivery, there is a desire to do something different precisely because it *is* different. While Eastern European countries and the UK are showing interest in market systems, the USA is looking for ways of moving towards more collective forms of provision. As Hunter says, 'We cannot be sure of the virtues of the market place, because there is no evidence'.

The extent to which governments are able to realize political objectives is itself a function of 'systems' factors, i.e., the amount of central control of health and social services' funding and provision. In the UK, the National Health Service is largely controlled by central government whereas social services are within the domain of locally elected authorities. However, these are themselves subject to central legislation and regulation, and this has increased during the last decade of Conservative rule. Thus the very strong commitment of the Thatcher administration to reducing public spending, to reducing the role of the public sector as providers, and to the introduction of market mechanisms has had considerable impact on health as well as social services. These political aims have always taken precedence over any wish to improve community care for older people. Thus, although the government appeared to be concerned with improving community care when they set up an inquiry into this (Griffiths 1988), the implementation of the recommendations of this inquiry has been modified and delayed purely for political reasons: the government wishes to limit local-authority spending in order to limit local taxation and local-authority autonomy.

The opposite trend can be seen in Denmark, where there is strong political support for local government, and where consequently municipalities have been able to develop home-care services and set up innovative experiments with the support of, but without interference from, central government. Costanzi's account of service developments in Genoa (Chapter 8) emphasized how the lack of political will has meant that there are no social-service policies for the country as a whole. Decisions are local; the planning as well as the operation of social services are almost totally dependent on the (ever changing) local political leadership, and hence subject to a great deal of discontinuity and unpredictability.

4. CONCLUSIONS

This book has focused on home care in terms of broad trends in what could be called 'mainstream provision'. It builds on the premise that home-care provision, as the contributors have defined it, remains the most important ingredient in the policy mix aimed at enabling older people to remain in their own homes for as long as possible. The key focus throughout the book has been upon '*home help*' in the sense of help with various activities of daily living, especially personal care and household tasks. The rationale behind focusing on this type of help (rather than, for example, medical or nursing help) was the view that the amount and nature of home-help provision in a country is an indicator of the extent to which the specific needs of frail older people (as opposed to the general medical needs of the population) are being recognized as a matter for the state as a public domain of policy making. In doing so it was, of course, necessary to consider the context of home help, firstly because of institutional variations between countries, and secondly because one of the aims was to examine the extent to which this kind of service could be seen to operate as part of a co-ordinated network of services and within a clear strategy of home-care policy.

The starting point for the study of 'Age Care Research Europe', of which this book is only part, was a problem that seemed to be of common concern to all countries: the blockage of pathways into and through the services (see Chapter 1). The initial hypothesis was that such 'blockages' were due partly to the inadequacy of the total volume of services, but also to two other factors: the relative over-concentration of resources upon medical and residential institutions as opposed to preventive use of support for people living in their own homes; and the widespread organizational and professional fragmentation of existing services.

Our combined examination of home-care provision points to a number of conclusions. First, there are enormous cross-national variations. What constitutes 'adequate' provision is, of course, to a large extent a matter of judgement, dependent on perceptions of needs and demands. Yet it seems safe to say that in many countries provision is inadequate if the aim is to enable older people to remain at home in a dignified way, and if espoused policies are to be implemented in practice. However, although inadequacy of provision is one of the major problems in many systems, several of the findings reported in the national chapters suggest that the distribution of existing resources is far from optimal. The studies of the decision-making processes show how 'systems' factors, such as the organization of services and funding arrangements, affect the ways in which services are allocated to individuals and result in a distribution that cannot be explained solely by reference to the needs of the population, however these are defined. Although to some extent these problems can be said to be due to 'organizational and professional fragmentation', this is not the only explanation. Lack of clear policy directions, managerial leadership, and professional competences are equally important problems, which cannot be solved purely through reorganization of service systems.

Our review suggests that one needs to be cautious in accepting the hypothesis that some of the problems stem from over-concentration of resources upon medical and institutional forms of provision. True, in all countries more resources are spent on health care and on institutional care, but this, we would argue, is not the main *reason* for lack of home care. First, from the point of view of individuals' service needs, there is no clear empirical evidence of substitutability between different types of services; the 'continuum of care' model does not operate clearly in practice. Secondly, trends in service developments show no correlation between residential and non-residential services, and indeed policies aimed at reducing institutional provision have not been clearly linked to the development of home-based care as an alternative. This, we would argue, is not merely due to the fact that the different services are separated in their organization and funding; this separation is to a very large extent a manifestation of some underlying factors. I have here examined policy trends and some of the factors affecting these. The conclusion was that the problem of home care cannot be reduced to one of organization or of shifting the balance between different budgets. We need to go behind these symptoms and consider the welfare traditions and ideologies, the political priorities and economic pressures, if we are to understand the successes and the failures of home-care policies and practices, and if we wish to assess the likelihood of change.

A wide range of ideas about the world as it *ought* to be is found in abundance in the published record and at international meetings. These ideas are often interesting and thought provoking, and a necessary part of our attempts to find new ways of looking at the world. But any serious analysis of policies must go further and inquire into the possibilities and conditions of change. This we have attempted to do, and what we have found is not totally encouraging from the point of view of the interests of frail older people. The policy agenda for this group, as for any other group, will be influenced more by economic and political factors than by any 'humanitarian concern' for older people *per se*. A great deal, therefore, will depend on the measure of political power which they and their representatives are able to wield. But it will also depend on the extent to which the interests of older people coincide with those of other groups in society, and in many respects they are, of course, not necessarily in conflict.

Two important areas seem worthy of more attention in future research and politics. The first concerns the development of *health services*. Researchers and advocates for older people alike—and this book is no exception—have tended to point to the inappropriateness of a medical approach to the problems of old age, and therefore the need to shift the balance of services from health to social care. As I have discussed, this has been difficult to achieve. At the same time we have also seen how, in all the countries reviewed, health care is perceived as a universal citizens' right—in contrast to social care. Without forgetting the limitations of a medical approach to the problems of old age, one should not underestimate the role of health-care services in providing support in various forms for older people and in making them fit to live independently. The popular, and therefore political, support in many countries for health-service systems compared with social services should perhaps be exploited more fully and the potential for older people explored more positively.

A second area relates to *environmental issues*, which are becoming increasingly important on policy agendas throughout the world. These include not only issues of chemical pollution, but increasing pressures from different groups to improve the living conditions for all human beings through changes in areas like housing, transport, roads, and public facilities, areas which all affect older people and their ability to remain independent. The relevance of such issues to older people is increasingly being recognized, and is already manifested in existing research and in projects like the World Health Organization's Healthy Cities Project.

Whilst the future for older people will much depend on the extent to which policies are formulated and implemented, it will also, of course, depend on trends in demography, health, and labour markets. In other words, the *characteristics* and *needs* of older people are not likely to remain static. One of the quetions that are increasingly occupying policy makers and observers alike is whether the proportion and number of frail older people is going to rise dramatically and present a serious strain on the economy and on systems of formal and informal care (OECD 1988; van den Heuvel *et al.* 1991). The vast majority of those aged over 65 years are active, healthy, and independent, and the image of 'old age' is changing accordingly. Those who are frail and in need of support are a small minority. But will they continue to be so? Will the rising number of very old people (80 years and over) necessarily mean that the need for care will rise, or will future octogenarians be healthier? Will their problems be different? Will families continue to be able and willing to provide present levels of care? Will labour market needs change the patterns of work and retirement and reduce the availability of informal care? These are just some of the questions that will continue to be on the research agenda of those concerned with what has so far, in the majority of European countries, been of limited interest to policy makers: the plight of frail elderly people and their families.

REFERENCES

Bebbington, A. and Tong, M. S. (1986). Trends and changes in old people's homes: provision over twenty years. In *Residential care for elderly people* (ed. K. Judge and I. Sinclair). HMSO, London.

Christiansen, S. P. (1989). Aeldreboligloven i praksis (The elderly housing act in practice). *Gerontologi og Samfund*, **5**, 47–50.

Esping-Andersen, G. (1990). *The three worlds of welfare capitalism*. Polity Press, Cambridge.

Griffiths, R. (1988). *Community care: Agenda for action*. Report to the Secretary of State for Social Services by Sir Ray Griffiths. HMSO, London.

Hunter, D. (1990). Paradox on the market. *Health Service Journal*, **100**, No. 5209.

Hunter, D, McKeganey, N., and MacPherson, I. (1988). *Care of the elderly. Policy and practice*. Aberdeen University Press.

OECD (1987). *Ageing populations: the social policy implications*. OECD, Paris.

Rodwin, V. G. (1984). *The health planning predicament. France, Quebec, England and the US*. University of California Press.

Sinclair, I. and Williams, J. (1989). *Welfare provision for the elderly: the contribution of the tatutory sector*, Report for ACRE. National Institute for Social Work, London.

Van den Heuvel, W., Illsley, R., Jamieson, A., and Knipscheer, K. (ed.) (1991). *Opportunities and challenges in an ageing society*. Elsevier, Amsterdam.

Wagner, L. (1989). A proposed model for the care of the elderly, *International Nursing Review*, **36**, 50–3.

Appendices

Appendix 1: Demographic and economic background of the study in Belgium

Table 1. Number of elderly, aged 60+, in the total population of the Flemish, the Walloon, and the Brussels regions, 1981. (Source: Dooghe and Van Den Boer 1987.)

	Total population (1)	Elderly, aged 60+ (2)	(2) as % of (1)
Flemish region	5 630 129	986 784	17.5
Walloon region	3 221 225	615 744	19.1
Brussels region	997 293	222 236	22.3

Table 2. Population of Greater-Antwerp by sex, age and marital status in 1981; absolute numbers. (Source: NIS 1981.)

Age (years)	Males				Females			
	Single	Married	Widowed	Divorced	Single	Married	Widowed	Divorced
60–64	626	9922	715	483	956	8998	3050	631
65–74	1173	17746	2842	789	2379	15035	12846	1184
75–80	320	4546	1715	160	935	3299	7745	306
80+	212	2413	2249	73	932	1415	9117	208
TOTAL 60+	2331	34627	7521	1505	5202	28747	32758	2329
TOTAL 65+	1705	24705	6806	1022	4246	19749	29708	1698
TOTAL 75+	532	6959	3964	233	1867	4714	16862	514
TOTAL 80+	212	2413	2249	73	932	1415	9117	208

Table 3. Government expenditure on health care for the elderly in Belgium in BF, 1975–1985. (Source: OECD, RIZIV, NIS.)

	Total		% spent on the elderly[1]	
	1975	1985	1975	1985
Total government budget	1 028 342	2 518 360	2.0	2.3
Government budget directly spent on health-care services	106 700	268 000	2.0	2.3

[1] Pensioner widows without profession are classified in another category and are not included in the figures.
Total government expenditure on health care in 1987 was 7.9 per cent of GDP

Appendix 2: Background data from Denmark

Table 1. Estimated expenditure on health and social services for the elderly: Denmark, 1984. (Source: *Statistiske Efterretninger, Social sikring og retsvæsen, 1987:1* and *1987:2*.)

Service	Expenditure (Millions Dkr.)
Community care	
Home help, home nursing, and other domiciliary care	3 542
General practitioner and other primary health care	1 308
Rent subsidies	1 959
Institutional care	
Hospital treatment	12 500
Nursing homes, residential institutions	10 557
Old-age pensions	32 387
TOTAL	62 253

Table 2. Expenditure on pensions, health and social services: Denmark, 1984, total population. (Source as in Table 1.)

Service	Expenditure (Millions Dkr.)
Health services	39 000
Social services	59 356
Pensions and cash benefits	98 043
TOTAL	196 399
GNP	559 874

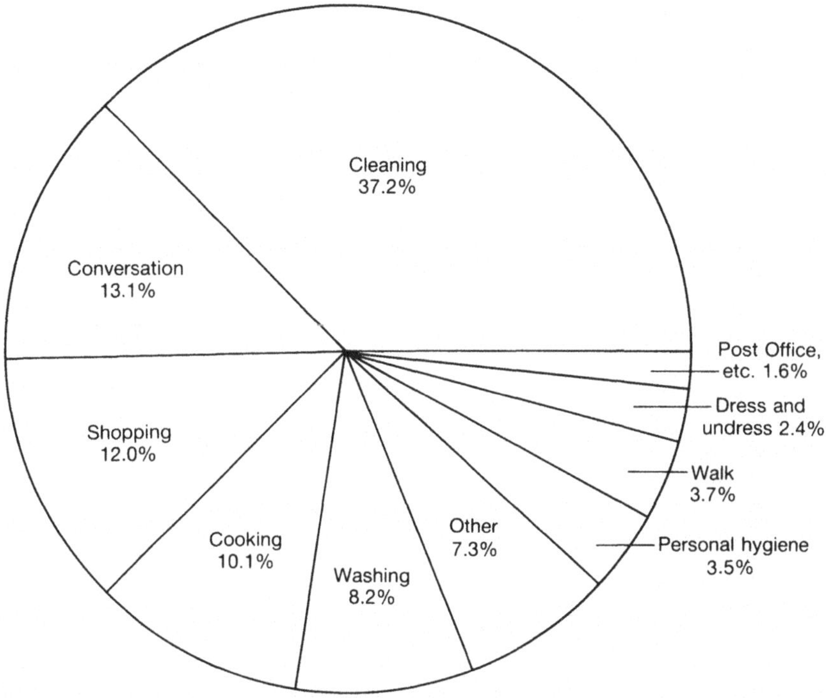

Fig. 1. Home helpers' reported use of time during one week in one commune.

Table 3. Home-helper activities during night hours (Næstved, 1 March 1982 to 28 February 1983). (Source: Hansen and Werborg 1983–84.)

Activity	Acute visits	Planned visits
Administration of medication	45	16.595
Observation	90	15.633
Dress or undress the client	122	15.422
Helping into or out of bed	142	11.758
Serve dinner	14	10.778
Personal hygiene	96	8.190
Helping to the lavatory	146	6.410
Prevention of bed sores	35	5.361
Changing colostomy bag/urine bag	26	3.169
Changing bed-clothes	33	1.265
Other activities	139	17.736
Total number of activities	888	112.317
Total number of visits	421	45.565

Tables 4 to 12 are derived from our survey of older people living at home (see Section 2.2)

Table 4. Proportion (percentages) using services during last year.

Service	Men	Women	Age (years)			Total
			70–74	75–79	80–95	
General practitioner	80	86	81	86	85	84
Hospital treatment	21	17	17	19	20	18
Ambulatory hospital treatment	13	14	12	15	15	14
Practising specialist	22	28	25	26	25	26
Dentist	30	31	39	27	20	31
Physiotherapy	7	12	11	11	9	10
Home nurse	9	13	7	11	23	12
Home help	20	29	13	26	49	26
Meals-on-wheels	6	5	2	4	14	5
None of these services[1]	29	23	27	25	21	25
Three or more of these services[1]	23	30	22	28	35	27

[1] General practitioner services not included in this index.

Table 5. Proportion (percentages) of elderly clients who think they are in need of (more) of these services.

Service	Men	Women	Age (years)			
			70–74	75–79	80–95	Total
General practitioner	6	6	7	6	7	6
Practising specialist	3	4	3	4	4	4
Dentist	5	6	5	6	6	6
Physiotherapy	3	4	3	4	4	4
Home nurse	2	2	1	1	4	2
Home help	7	9	5	9	13	8
Meals-on-wheels	2	1	1	1	2	1
Equipment	6	2	3	6	7	5
Chiropody	6	10	6	10	11	8
Other	3	3	3	3	4	3
None of these[1]	77	75	79	76	69	75
Two or more of these[1]	8	9	7	9	12	9

[1] General practitioner services not included in this index.

Table 6. Proportion (percentage) in need of (more) specific service provision among users (within the last year) and non-users of these specific services

Service	Users	Non-users
General Practitioner	7	1
Practising specialist	9	2
Dentist	7	5
Physiotherapy	21	2
Home nurse	13	1
Home help	24	3
Meals-on-wheels	13	0

[1] Differences between users and non-users are all statistically significant; $p < 0.001$.

Table 7. Percentage receiving home help by demographic characteristics in combination

Characteristic		Receiving help	
Living alone	Men, 70–79 years	35	41
	Men, 80–95 years	54	
	Women, 70–79 years	26	35
	Women, 80–95 years	48	
Living with others	Men, 70–79 years	9	12
	Men, 80–95 years	26	
	Women, 70–79 years	15	22
	Women, 80–95 years	58	

Table 8. Percentages having home help by functional capacity and household composition

Functional capacity	Leaving house	Cleaning the house	Washing and bathing
Living alone, having home help			
No impairment	25	9	27
Difficulty	61	19	68
Unable	86	85	92
TOTAL	36	36	36
Living with others, having home help			
No impairment	10	3	12
Difficulty	37	24	41
Unable	78	52	71
TOTAL	17	17	17

Table 9. Proportion (percentages) receiving home help by household composition and household income

Household income, 1985	Receiving home help	
	Living alone	Living with others
Less than 50.000 Dkr.[1]	41	24
50.000–100.000 Dkr.	31	20
More than 100.000 Dkr.	22	6
TOTAL	36	17

[1] Danish krone.

Table 10. Variables associated with (a) receiving home help and (b) having an unmet need of home help

Variable	Receiving help	Unmet need
	Largest frequency	Largest frequency
Socio-demographic		
Commune	NS	NS
Sex	Women (29%)	NS
Age	80+ years (45%)[3]	80+ years (14%)[2]
Household composition	Live alone (36%)[3]	Live alone (13%)[3]
Social class	NS	NS
Household income	Low (37%)[3]	Low (14%)[3]

Table 10. (*cont.*)

Variable	Receiving help	Unmet need
	Largest frequency	Largest frequency
Perceived health status	Poor (50%)[3]	Poor (17%)[3]
Functional capacity		
Able to:		
leave home	Not able (83%)[3]	Not able (33%)[3]
walk 15 minutes	Not able (75%)[3]	Not able (15%)[3]
climb stairs	Not able (88%)[3]	Not able (23%)[3]
move around indoors	Not able (100%)[3]	Not able (20%)[3]
get out of bed	Not able (100%)[3]	NS
wash and bathe	Not able (88%)[3]	Not able (21%)[3]
dress	Not able (100%)[3]	Not able (13%)[3]
do light domestic work	Not able (76%)[3]	NS
do heavy domestic work	Not able (76%)[3]	Not able (15%)[3]
use public transport	Not able (76%)[3]	Not able (17%)[3]
do own shopping	Not able (78%)[3]	Not able (17%)[3]
chew regular food	Not able (60%)[3]	NS
reach toilet in time	Not able (70%)[3]	Not able (32%)[3]
remember recent information	Not able (45%)[3]	NS
remember the day's programme	Not able (61%)[3]	Not able (17%)[1]
hear (converse with one person)	Not able (56%)[3]	NS
hear (converse with several persons)	Not able (40%)[3]	Not able (14%)[1]
read normal print	Not able (49%)[3]	NS
Utilization of health services		
Frequency of contact with general practitioner	Every month (35%)[3]	Every month (13%)[3]
Hospitalized in last 12 months	Yes (46%)[3]	NS
Social network		
Frequency of contact with children	NS	NS
Ability to help children	Not able (50%)[3]	Not able (19%)[3]
Children's ability to help their parents	No help (35%)[2]	No help (16%)[1]
Aggregate social network	NS	NS
Activity		
Frequency of:		
leaving home	monthly (75%)[3]	monthly (22%)[3]
receiving visits	NS	NS
paying visits	None (47%)[3]	NS
Personal resources		
Future perspective	Not future Plans (34%)[3]	NS
Feeling lonely	Often (55%)[3]	Often (23%)[3]

Table 10. (*cont.*)

Variable	Receiving help	Unmet need
	Largest frequency	Largest frequency
Feeling forgotten	Often (61%)[3]	Often (25%)[2]
Feeling superfluous	Often (58%)[3]	Often (26%)[3]
Feeling old	Often (65%)[3]	NS
Mood	Poor (72%)[3]	Poor (17%)[3]
Coping style		
Try to forget the problems	NS	NS
Escape the problems	NS	NS
Discuss problems with others	NS	NS
Try to solve problems	Not at all (48%)[2]	Not at all (23%)[2]
Quality of life		
Perceived:		
quality of housing	NS	Very dissatisfied[2]
economic situation	NS	NS
quality of life	Very dissatisfied[3]	NS
quality of social relations	NS	NS

[1] $p = 0.05$; [2] $p = 0.01$; [3] $p = 0.001$; NS = Not significant.

Table 11. Proportion (percentages) of respondents receiving home help scored against two social network characteristics

Characteristic	Score	With home help (%)
Social network index[1]	Weak, 0 points ($n = 282$)	27
	Medium, 1 points ($n = 489$)	27
	Strong, 2–4 points ($n = 476$)	27 (NS)
Help from social network[2]	None ($n = 786$)	20
	Help for one activity ($n = 293$)	30
	Help for 2+ activities ($n = 168$)	45 ($p<0.0001$)

[1] One point is given for three or more monthly contacts with (a) children, (b) siblings, (c) other kin, and (d) friends.
[2] One point is given for each of the following activities provided by children, kin, or friends: cleaning, cooking, washing, shopping, personal care, and minor repairs/maintenance.
NS, not significant.

Table 12. Characteristics of high versus low users of services and respondents in need of services

Variable	Characteristics of high users compared to low users	Characteristics of respondents with unmet needs compared to no unmet needs
Geographical area	NS	NS
Household composition	Single[3]	Single[2]
Social class	NS	NS
Household income	Low[1]	Low[1]
Social network contacts	NS	NS
Help from spouse	NS	NS
Help from social network	High[1]	NS
Satisfaction with social relations	Dissatisfied[3]	Dissatisfied[3]
Self-assessed health	Poor[3]	Poor[3]
Chronic ailments	>2[3]	>2[3]
Hearing ability	Impaired[2]	Impaired[1]
Physical symptoms	>2[3]	>2[3]
Psychological symptoms	>2[3]	>2[3]
ADL	Low functional ability[3]	Low functional ability[3]
Daily activities performed	Low[3]	Low[1]

[1] $p = 0.05$; [2] $p = 0.01$; [3] $p = 0.001$; NS = Not significant.

Appendix 3: The pathways study—population and method (Denmark)

First, we interviewed key decision makers: directors of social services departments, managers and supervisors of domiciliary care, general practitioners, hospital staff involved in the discharge of elderly patients, and those who make decisions about residences for the elderly. They were interviewed twice, with a year's interval between, about general policy principles and about options and barriers in their systems. Twenty-four respondents were involved in this study. The data collection took the form of open-ended interviews guided by a list of issues. The interviews were conducted by two of us (P.D. and B.E.H).

Second, we identified four key points ('junctions') at which important decisions about the care of elderly are made and in which several professional groups or service agencies are involved:

- decisions about domiciliary care (only new and major cases, i.e., at least 4 hours of home help and/or combination of home nurse and home help);
- discharge from long-term stay in hospital;
- decisions about change of residence (nursing home, service flat);
- cases in which the general practitioner plays an important role in mediating between services or between the elderly and the service system.

At each of these junctions, we identified consecutive patients/clients, 70 years old or more, who on the basis of informed consent agreed to participate. In these cases we made three-party interviews including (a) the elderly client/patient, (b) if relevant, the primary care-giver, and (c) one or more key professional care-givers or decision makers. The interviews were generally speaking made two to four weeks after the relevant discharge/decision. If the situation was not settled by the time of interviewing we carried out a follow-up interview with the clients a few weeks later.

The study population

The study involved 111 cases described by 211 interviews, but 36 cases were never completed because of death, hospitalization, or practical obstacles. The material thus includes 75 cases described by 172 interviews

(73 interviews with elderly clients/patients, 93 with professional care-givers or decision makers, and 9 with primary care-givers).

The cases included were meant to be consecutive, but this criterion did not always work. We are aware of a few cases which should have been included but were not. We selected only cases that were admitted, i.e., successfully referred. We are not aware of any cases referred to domiciliary care but not admitted, and we believe there are either no or insignificant numbers of such cases. Entry into domiciliary care in Denmark is unrestricted, but elderly people who enter the system without a need will be discharged quickly.

The interviews

The data were collected by personal interviews guided by a schedule with a mix of standardized and open-ended questions and with the opportunity of elaborating the interview when important issues were brought up. All these interviews are made by one of us (P.D).

The interviews included data on basic demographic factors, social network and social support, psychological resources, functional ability, utilization of health and social services, the event which initiated the decision process, the process itself as described above, its outcome, and the respondents' evaluation of solutions and unsolved problems.

Data analysis

We have organized the data by the grounded theory method. Moreover, we identified ideal types of case trajectories (ideal types of decision processes), and made qualitative evaluations and descriptions of the outcome of the cases and of factors promoting and hindering a successful outcome. The final, qualitative analysis of the material has not yet been carried out.

This section includes only cases in which home-help provision was an important issue (53 cases described by 122 interviews). The presentation is a summary of the completed, preliminary analysis.

Appendix 4: Home-help referrals—typical trajectories (Denmark)

'Ideal-type analysis' serves as descriptive illustration of what happens in cases that we regard as typical. We describe three kinds of ideal types, one which we regard as a normal, one which we regard as a poor and one a successful trajectory. Moreover, these cases illustrate the way in which various parties engage in the decision.

Example of 'normal' trajectory in a home-help case

Reason for application for home help: Fall resulting in fractured ankle; hospitalized for 4 weeks, discharged without rehabilitation. Never had help before.

Decision: Gets 7 hours home help per week plus equipment.

Functional ability: Unable to move outdoors and to undertake domestic tasks. Poor hearing.

Household and social network: Living alone. Frequent contacts with family who are unable to help with daily activities.

Psychological resources: Feeling old now, otherwise no problems.

Health problems: None except the actual problem caused by the broken ankle.

Knowledge of service provision options: None

Alternative solutions considered: None except home help and equipment.

Who was involved in the decision: Hospital staff and home-help manager.

The *client's evaluation* of the decision/solution: Could not be better.

Unsolved problems: None, but lack of help immediately after discharge.

Interviewer assessment of this category of case: Usually discongruencies in the clients' and the professionals' description of functional ability, psychological resources and unsolved problems (indicating insufficient communication). Often unsolved problems.

Example of 'poor' trajectory in a home-help case

Reason for application for home help: Stroke, 4 weeks in hospital, discharge after insufficient rehabilitation.

Decision: Gets 10 hours home help per week plus weekend help plus equipment.

Functional ability: Able to carry out some personal hygiene, unable to do everything else.

Household and social network: Living alone; contact with children who are unable to provide daily help.

Psychological resources: Poor.

Health problems: Chronic asthma; cataract; wheelchair-bound.

Knowledge of service provision options: None.

Alternative solutions considered: Has considered service flat him/herself; has not discussed it with anybody.

Who was involved in the decision: Hospital staff plus home-help manager.

The client's evaluation of the decision/solution: Unhappy about changing home helpers. Lacks help for gardening.

Unsolved problems: Getting out of doors now and then. Changing home helpers. Gardening.

Interviewer assessment of the category of cases: Complicated cases. Poor communication. Clients with poor psychological resources. Unfinished solutions.

Example of 'successful' trajectory in a home-help case

Reason for application for home help: Fall resulting in hip fracture. Unable to put weight on the legs after the hospitalization. No help prior to this.

Decision: Gets 3 hours home help per day plus meals-on-wheels plus equipment, and gardening assistance.

Functional ability: Unable to do anything. Poor vision and poor hearing.

Household and social network: Living alone. Close and frequent contact with one relative and one friend.

Psychological resources: Strong.

Health problems: Arthritis; almost blind, impaired.

Knowledge of service provision options: Knows of services available.

Alternative solutions considered: Nursing home, which he/she does not want.

Who was involved in the decision process: Hospital staff, close relative, home-help manager.

The client's evaluation of the decision/solution: Very happy.

Unsolved problems: None.

Interviewer assessment of this category of cases: Good communication between the professionals and between the professionals and the client; the client him/herself plays the central role in the decision.

Appendix 5: Background data from the UK

Table 1. Types and sources of domiciliary care for elderly people (see also Table 4.1)

Activities	Who delivers	Who provides
Personal care: feeding, dressing, mobility, bathing	Auxiliary nurses	NHS, a few private schemes
	Community-care assistants	Social services (enhanced home helps)
	Occupational therapy	Both NHS and Social Services, depending on area
Chiropodists	NHS, private provision	
Home-making: cleaning, laundry, cooking, shopping, etc.	Home helps	Social services, a few private schemes
	Domestic helper	Private (not common for elderly)
	Meals-on-wheels	Social services and voluntary organizations
	Volunteers	Voluntary organizations, usually for specific tasks like gardening
Nursing: injection, bandaging, medication	Community nurses	NHS, a few private schemes
Surveillance:		
Case management	Health visitors	NHS (health needs only)
	Social workers	Social services)
Routine	Night-sitting service	Social services, voluntary organization (respite); NHS (terminal)
	Street warden schemes	Mostly voluntary organizations
	Alarm systems	Social services, some private schemes
	Sheltered housing	Local authorities, voluntary organizations, and private schemes
Socialization	Volunteers	Voluntary organizations
	Day centres	Social services[1] and voluntary organizations

[1] Services such as home helps can be provided to help relieve isolation, though this is not a primary function

Table 2. Extent of provision of relevant services (1985)[1]

	London	Metropolitan counties	Shire counties	Wales	England and Wales
Home helps[2] (staff)	8.7	9.9	5.9	8.0	7.3
Meals service[3] (meals per week)	214	122	108	112	126
Day centres[4] (places)	10.6	7.0	3.6	9.5	5.6
District nurses[5] (staff)	2.1	2.1	2.1	2.1	2.1
Auxiliaries (staff)	0.5	0.5	0.5	0.5	0.5
Other community nurses (staff)	3.3	3.3	3.3	3.3	3.3
Population 65+	1 031 500	1 650 000	4 525 900	448 900	7 656 000
Per 1000 population aged 75+					
Home helps[2] (staff)	20.0	24.2	13.7	19.3	17.1
Meals service[2] (meals per week)	493	296	254	272	296
Day centres[4] (places)	24.4	17.1	8.4	25.5	13.3
District nurses[5] (staff)	4.9	4.90	4.9	5.0	4.9
Auxiliaries (staff)	1.3	1.3	1.3	1.3	1.3
Other community nurses (staff)	7.9	7.9	7.9	8.0	7.9
Population 75+	446 900	677 700	1 935 000	185 500	3 245 100

[1] Figures in this table are based on the total provision of each service, regardless of the age group to which it is provided.

[2] Home helps: England from DHSS *Local authority social services statistics: staff of local authority social services departments at 30 September 1985, England*; Wales from Welsh Office/Y Swyddfa Gynreig *Health and personal social services statistics for Wales/Ystadegau lechyd a gwansanaethau cymdeithasol personol: Cymru*, No. 13 1986, Table 3.24.

[3] Number of meals supplied (including luncheon clubs) from CIPFA *Personal social services statistics 1985–86 actuals*, column 196 (scaled up to take account of missing data).

[4] Places at day centres in England, by region, from DHSS Personal Social Services Local Authority statistics *Adult training centres for the mentally handicapped and day centres for the mentally ill, elderly and the younger physically handicapped, at 31 March 1985*, England CA/F85/8, Table B, combining places at day centres for elderly and places at mixed centres. Places at day centres in Wales from Welsh Office/Y Swyddfa Gymreig *Activities of social services departments: year England 31.3.85/ Gweithgareddau adrannau gwasanaethau cymdeithasol: blwyddyn yn diweddu 31.3.85*, Table 3.2, places at day centres for elderly persons and places at mixed centres.

[5] Total number of nurses working in the community in England from DHSS *Health and personal social services statistics for England 1987*, Nursing and Midwifery staff: analysis of work and grade, Table 3.16. Wales from Welsh Office/Y Swyddfa Gymreig *Health and personal social services statistics for Wales/Ystadegau lechyd a gwasanaethau cymdeithasol personol: Cymru*, No. 13, 1986, Table 3.10, Nursing and midwifery staff, by DHA. These totals have been divided between different grades according to the proportions of nurses working in the community in England and Wales who are (i) district nurses, (ii) auxiliaries, and (iii) all other categories (from Dunnell and Dobs [1980]. *Nurses working in the community*, OPCS Social Survey Division, Table 11.2).

Table 3. Beneficiaries—how are the services distributed?

Percentage of people aged 65+ currently receiving services, by region

	London	Metropolitan counties	Shire counties	Wales	England and Wales
Home helps	10.7	10.7	8.6	9.1	9.3
Meals service	6.7	6.2	5.9	5.1	6.0
Elderly day centre	6.4	5.9	5.1	2.5	5.3
District nurse or auxiliary	3.8	3.7	5.6	6.1	5.0
Health visitor	1.2	0.5	1.7	1.5	1.4
n =	420	730	2038	198	3386

Percentage in each age group currently receiving domiciliary services

	Age groups (years)					
	65–69	70–74	75–79	80–84	85+	All 65+
Home help	1.5	5.7	10.7	22.4	34.2	9.3
Meal service	2.8	4.0	6.2	11.8	18.6	6.0
Elderly centre	3.6	5.2	5.8	8.2	6.5	5.3
District nurse or auxiliary	2.4	2.1	5.7	10.0	18.2	5.0
Health visitor	0.4	0.7	2.2	2.4	4.3	1.4
n =	(1028)	(987)	(760)	(380)	(231)	(3386)

Number of home-help hours received per week, by age group

	Aged 65+ (%)	Aged 75+ (%)
2 or less	56	55
3–6	38	38
More than 6	5	6
n =	285	220

Frequency (per cent) of use of the various services by clients aged 65+

	Home helps	Provided meals	Day centre	District nurse or auxiliary
Nearly every day	9	36	3	11
2–3 times a week	35	59	29	16
Once a week	50	3	54	29
Less often	7	1	14	44
n =	309	91	174	168

Table 3. (*cont.*)

	Home helps	Provided meals	Day centre	District nurse or auxiliary
Frequency (per cent) of use of the various services by clients aged 75+				
Nearly every day	10	34	2	11
2–3 times a week	37	62	34	15
Once a week	46	4	51	28
Less often	6	–	12	46
n =	239	79	90	123

Overlap of services—percentage who receive home-help services and home-nursing services

	Age 65+	Age 75+
Neither	87	76
Home help only	7	13
Home nursing only	3	6
Both	3	5
n =	3386	1371

Figures throughout Table 3 are from a special analysis of the 1985 General Household Survey. Sample sizes are indicated. For further information, see OPCS (1989) *General Household Survey 1986*, Chapter 12.

Table 4. Expenditure on health and personal social services—England and Wales

Gross expenditure on people aged 65+

	1965/6		1975/6		1985/6	
	absolute £m	as % of GNP	absolute £m	as % of GNP	absolute £m	as % of GNP
Community care						
Home help[1]	12.4	0.04	87.7	0.09	299.2	0.10
Day centres[1]	–	–	12.7	0.01	103.4	0.03
Meals[1]	–	–	16.0	0.02	57.0	0.02
Home nursing[1]	5.7	0.01	–	–	60.6	0.02
Family practitioner services[3]	13.0	0.04	132.0	0.14	911.0	0.30
Institutional care						
Residential homes:						
Local authority[1]	49.3	0.15	249.0	0.26	644.9	0.22
Private and voluntary[4]	–	–	66.3	0.07	588.5	0.19

Table 4. (*cont.*)

	1965/6		1975/6		1985/6	
	absolute £m	as % of GNP	absolute £m	as % of GNP	absolute £m	as % of GNP
Hospitals:						
Mental health/ psychogeriatric[5]	29.7	0.09	170.8	0.18	582.6	0.19
Geriatric[5] } Acute, etc.[5] }	201.9	0.63	84.0	0.09	287.4	0.09
			993.1	1.03	3949.8	1.29
Private nursing[4]	–	–	–	–	333.0	0.12
Total gross public expenditure on health and personal social services for the elderly[6]	–	–	–	–	7225.1	2.35
GNP	31 930		96 690		306 160	

Dashes signify unavailable data.

Total gross public expenditure (£m) on health and personal social services (all age-groups)[7]

	1965/66	1975/76	1985/86
Health services	–	3570	14 942
Personal social services	–	649	3 005
TOTAL	1188	4219	17 947

[1] From DHSS and Welsh Office *Health and personal social service statistics* for relevant year. Home help, day centres, and residential home expenditure adjusted to allow for proportion of places used by elderly, based on CIPFA *Local health and welfare statistics* and *Personal social services statistics—actuals* for the relevant year. These services are mostly paid for by the state but a small proportion is recovered through charges to clients (usually means tested).

[2] 1965/66 figures for Great Britain from *Ministry of Health report 1965*, Tables 44 and 57. Total expenditure multiplied by proportion of patients who are aged 65+ and scaled down proportionally to England and Wales population. 1985/86 figures from *Health and personal social services statistics for England 1987*: unit expenditure on nurses and midwives (Table 2.10) × total number of district nurses (Table 6.7), multiplied again by proportion of patients who are aged 65+, and scaled up to England and Wales population. This is a free service.

[3] Includes general practitioner, dentistry, ophthalmic, and pharmaceutical services. Costs are estimated for the elderly on the basis of usage of general practitioner services as follows. 1965/66 expenditure from HMSO *The National Plan—1965*, Table 20.2, multiplied by the proportion of all general practitioner consultations for patients aged 65+ from OPCS *Morbidity statistics from general practice 1970/71*, Table 5. 1975/76 expenditure from HMSO *Public expenditure to 1979/80*, Table 2.11, multiplied by proportion of all general practitioner consultations for patients aged 65+ from OPCS *1981–1982 morbidity statistics from general practice: third national study*, Table 16(1). 1985/6 from HMSO *The Government's expenditure plans 1989–90 to 1991–92*, Chapter 14: *Department of Health*, CM614, Tables 14.19 and

Table 4. (*cont.*)

14.20. Figures scaled to England and Wales population where necessary. Family practitioner committee services are usually free to the elderly.

[4] Estimated from average charge per resident, given by PSSRU Discussion Paper 563 (1989) *PSSRU/CHE survey of residential and nursing home: costs and charges*. Number of residents of residential homes (1975 and 1985) from DHSS Personal Social Services Local Authority statistics RA/85/2 *Residential accommodation for elderly and younger physically handicapped people: all residents in local authority, voluntary and private homes*, year ending 31 March 1985, England, tables C, E, and 1.01. Number of residents of nursing homes (1985 only) from PSSRU DP 564. Although these services are charged directly to the client, in practice about one half of these costs are met by the state through social security arrangements.

[5] Revenue expenditure for 1965 from DHSS *Health and personal social services statistics for England 1974*, Tables 2.7 and 2.8 (figures for mental health scaled to allow for medical salaries), multiplied by the proportion of beds used daily by persons aged 65+ from Ministry of Health and General Register Office *Report as hospital in-patients enquiry for the year 1966*, Part 1, Table 12. Revenue expenditure for 1975 from DHSS *Health and personal social services statistics for England: 1987*, Table 2.6, and from Welsh Office *Health and personal social services statistics for Wales 1978*, Table 2.03, multiplied by the proportion of beds used daily by those aged 65+ from DHSS, OPCS and Welsh Office *1975 Hospital in-patients enquiry: main tables* (acute, etc.), and DHSS *In-patients statistics from the mental health enquiry for England 1975*, Table B22.1 (Mental Health). Revenue expenditure 1985 from same sources as for 1975 (Wales: 1987 edition), multiplied by the proportion of beds used daily by patients aged 65+ from DHSS, OPCS *1985 hospital in-patient enquiry: main tables*, Table 1 (acute, etc.), and DHSS statistical bulletins 2/2/88 and 2/3/88 *Results of the mental health enquiry 1986* (Mental Health). The services are free to patients.

[6] From HMSO *The Government's expenditure plans 1989–90 to 1991–92*, Chapter 14, *Department of Health*, Chart 14.4 (average unit costs), for 1986/7, multiplied by appropriate populations, and deflated to 1985/6 prices. This figure slightly exceeds the total of other services listed partly due to the different basis of calculation and partly due to the omission of minor services from the main table.

[7] 1965/66 from *The National Plan—1965* CMND 2764, Table 20.2. 1975/76 from *Public expenditure to 1979–80*, Table 2.11. 1985/86 from *The Government's expenditure plans 1989–90 to 1991–92*, Chapter 14, *Department of Health*, Table 14.1, and Chapter 17, *Wales*, Table 17.5. 1965/66 and 1975/76 are based on GB totals scaled down according to population of England and Wales.

Appendix 6: Background data from France

Table 1. The development in the number of elderly people aged 60 or over in institutions (from INSEE data)

	1962		1975		1982	
	N[1]	(%)	N[1]	(%)	N[1]	(%)
Social institution	201	(2.8)	320	(3.9)	302	(4.0)
Psychiatric hospital[2]	34		39		34	
General hospital[2]	–		25[3]		60[3]	

[1] Number in thousands.
[2] For more than 6 months.
[3] Usually in a long-stay hospital ward.
[4] Plus 88 000 in sheltered housing.

Table 2. The main services for elderly people that come to the home

Activities	Services
Domestic tasks	Home-help services[1]; ± repair services[4]; ± social worker[2]
Personal care	Home-nursing services (SSIAD)[1]; Meals-on-wheels[3]; ± 'Life Auxiliary'[2]; ± independent nursing[2]
Technical care	Independent nursing[2], physiotherapy, chiropody, etc.[2]
Surveillance	Home warden[4]; + tele-alarm[3]
Socialization	Voluntary visitor[4]
Improvement of housing	Association for improving housing[2]

[1] Specific statutory service.
[2] Non-specific statutory service. 'Life auxiliaries' is a special service for disabled people, sometimes used by elderly people.
[3] Local, regulated service.
[4] Local, non-regulated service.

Table 3. Home helps in 1986 according to the beneficiaries, the number of hours and the expenditure of the various funders. (Source: Ministry of Solidarity, Health and Social Protection 1988.)

Funder	Number of beneficiaries (thousands)	Number of hours (millions)	Expenses (FF) (billions)
Social welfare	127[1]	25.3	1.75
General old-age insurance scheme[2]	272	28.6	1.3
Other insurance schemes[3]	105	8.9	0.7
TOTAL	504	62.8	3.7

[1] Of whom 4000 beneficiaries receive cash benefit instead of service in kind.
[2] This is the largest insurance scheme and includes salaried workers in trade and industry. It covers about two-thirds of pensioners.
[3] For example, for civil servants, miners, each of which have their own insurance scheme.

Table 4. Regional variations in the percentage of beneficiaries of home helps financed by the general old-age insurance schemes. (Source: National Office for Old Age Insurance for Salaried Workers 1978, 1988.)

Regions	1977	1987
Bordeaux	2.9	5.6
Clermont-Ferrand	2.1	3.9
Dijon	2.4	4.6
Lille	3.6	5.1
Limoges	3.2	4.3
Lyon	3.7	4.8
Marseilles	2.3	3.5
Montpellier	3.3	5.0
Nancy	2.3	4.5
Nantes	3.2	5.4
Orléans	2.9	4.6
Paris	2.0	3.3
Rennes	2.5	3.2
Rouen	2.2	4.0
Strasbourg	2.0	4.9
Toulouse	3.5	5.5
TOTAL	2.7	4.4
Number of beneficiaries	131 000	270 000

Table 5. Development in the number of hours received by beneficiaries of home help financed by the general old-age insurance scheme in 1977 and 1987. (Source: National Office for Old Age Insurance for Salaried Workers 1977, 1988.)

Number of hours per month	1977	1987
	% beneficiaries	% beneficiaries
<16 hours	42.0	58.0
16–30 hours	53.5	39.0
>30 hours	4.5	3.0
TOTAL	100	100

Table 6. Beneficiaries of home-help and home-nursing services by age (total number, from all funding sources). (Source: Ministry of Solidarity, Health and Social Protection 1988; National Office for OAISW 1988.)

Age groups (years)	Home helps	Home nursing
60–64	0.4	0.05
65–69	2.7	0.1
70–74	4.1	0.2
75–79	8.1	0.5
80–84	11.7	1.1
85+	14.3	2.2
TOTAL 65+	6.9	0.6
75+	10.4	1.0

Table 7. Percentage of people aged 65 years or over, living at home and confined to bed or armchair, according to the help received. (Source: Gauthier and Colvez 1989.)

Source of help	Hte. Normandie[1] (1978–1979) (n = 30)	Ile de France (1982) (n = 22)	Rhône-Alpes (1986) (n = 60)
Professional or volunteer	3.6	26.3	45.0
Member of the family	82.1	94.7	85.5
Neighbourhood/friend	14.3	5.3	8.3

[1] Elderly people reported only the most frequent source of daily help.

Table 8. Percentage of elderly people of 65 years or over having one (or several) disability/ies without being confined to bed, according to the help received. (Source: Gauthier and Colvez 1989.)

Source of help	Whole population		Population living alone	
	Ile de France (n = 534)	Rhône-Alpes (n = 1121)	Ile de France (n = 241)	Rhône-Alpes (n = 511)
Professional or volunteer	27.7	34.5	40.3	50.1
Member of the family:				
of the same age	31.1	21.8	2.1	2.9
younger	39.7	52.9	46.5	49.5
Neighbourhood/friend	22.8	17.5	39.0	26.2

Appendix 7: Background data to the Berlin study

Each questions starts: 'Are you able . . .'

ADLE—elementary activities

—to move outdoors?
—to walk between rooms?
—to use stairs?
—to walk at least 400 m?
—to carry a heavy load, e.g., a shopping bag with 6 full bottles for 100 m?
—to use the lavatory?
—to wash and bathe yourself?
—to dress and undress?
—to get in and out of bed?
—to do your own cooking?
—to feed yourself?
—to cut your toe-nails?
—to do light housework (wash dishes)?
—to do heavy housework (clean windows, general house cleaning)?

ADLI—instrumental activities

—to make phone calls (including to find out the number in a directory and to dial)?
—to shop for groceries and clothes?
—to get to distant public offices and facilities?
—to use public transport (to go by bus, underground, train, and taxi)?
—to take prescribed medicine?
—to handle money?
—to complete forms and applications (at post office, bank, etc.)?
—to walk or go by public transport to a medical doctor (without any help)?

The answer categories are:
—without difficulty
—with difficulty but without help
—not unaided
—not possible

Fig. 1. Activity of daily living (ADL): selected items.

Table 1. Need for support in selected activities of daily living among elderly men and women in various age groups

Level of support needed	% of each age (years) group			
	70–74	75–79	80–84	85–89
Men				
None	75	48	39	22
Low	20	48	44	40
High	5	4	17	38
TOTAL (= 100%)	44	46	46	55
Women				
None	50	47	25	7
Low	44	41	46	62
High	6	12	29	31
TOTAL (= 100%)	54	51	59	70

Table 2. Need for external support among elderly men and women of different ages

Level of external support needed	% of each age (years) group			
	70–74	75–79	80–84	85–89
Men				
None	98	87	83	69
Low	2	13	17	20
High	0	0	0	11
TOTAL (= 100%)	44	46	46	55
Women				
None	66	55	50	27
Low	28	35	36	47
High	6	10	14	26
TOTAL (= 100%)	54	51	59	70

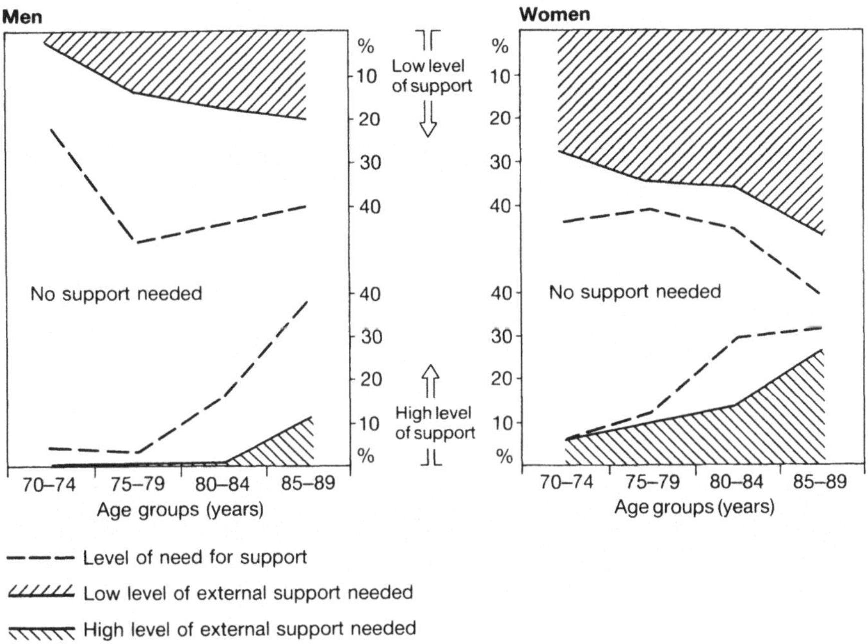

Fig. 2. The extent of need for support in relation to age and household structure.

Table 3. Use of community-based nursing care[1] in the course of one year (follow-up survey) by elderly men and women of different ages

	Age range (years)							
	71–75		76–80		81–85		86–90	
Use	*n*	%	*n*	%	*n*	%	*n*	%
Men[2]								
Yes	1	2.6	3	7.9	3	8.1	3	7.3
No	37	97.4	35	92.1	34	91.9	38	92.7
TOTAL	38	100	38	100	37	100	41	100
Women[3]								
Yes	2	3.9	4	8.3	9	18.4	18	32.1
No	49	96.1	44	91.7	40	81.6	38	67.9
TOTAL	51	100	48	100	49	100	56	100

Weighted data: average utilization within the general population = 10 per cent.
[1] Including home nursing, home care, home help.
[2] Non-significant differences according to age.
[3] Highly significant differences according to age.

Appendix 8: Background data from Israel

Table 1. Developments in the composition of the elderly population of Israel, 1970–1999. (Source: Statistical Abstract of Israel Central Bureau of Statistics (1971–1988).)

	Population (in thousands)							Percentage of growth		
	1970	1980	1988	1989	1990	1995	1999	1970–1979	1980–1989	1990–1999
TOTAL	202.7	338.2	395.0	402.4	409.7	434.4	462.3	67	21	13
Age group (years)										
65–74	144.7	229.7	234.9	237.5	240.0	260.9	264.3	59	4	10
65–69	83.2	126.7	129.4	134.7	140.0	137.7	141.3	52	10	1
70–74	61.5	103.0	105.5	102.8	100.0	123.2	123.0	67	−3	23
75+	58.2	108.5	160.1	164.9	169.7	173.5	198.0	87	56	17
Sex										
Men	100.1	159.3	179.9	182.2	184.4	192.0	204.4	59	16	11
Women	102.6	178.9	215.1	220.1	225.1	242.2	257.8	74	25	15
Ethnic origin										
Asia-Africa	53.2	75.5	102.4	106.3	110.2	131.8	159.5	42	46	45
Europe-America	132.3	242.5	267.5	270.4	273.2	270.6	263.6	83	13	−4
Non-Jews	17.2	20.2	25.1	25.7	26.2	31.8	39.2	17	30	50

Table 2. Estimates of disability among the elderly population of Israel, 1980–2000

	Population (in thousands)						Percentage of growth	
	1980	1988	1989	1990	1995	2000	1988–2000	1988–1995
Number of disabled in ADL[1]								
TOTAL	31.5	42.4	43.6	44.8	49.3	55.9	32	16
In the community[2]	25.6	33.6	34.5	35.4	39.1	44.6	33	16
In long-term care institutions[3]	5.9	8.8	9.1	9.3	10.2	11.3	28	16
Number of persons requiring help with home-making (in the community)[4]	122.7	150.8	153.9	157.0	169.7	184.7	22	13
% disabled in ADL[5]	9.3	10.7	10.8	10.9	11.3	12.1		
In the community[6]	7.8	8.8	8.9	9.0	9.4	10.1		
In long-term care institutions[5]	1.7	2.2	2.3	2.3	2.3	2.4		
% disabled in home-making[6]	37.5	39.7	39.8	39.9	40.7	41.7		

[1] Including persons requiring assistance with at least one of the following basic ADL functions: bathing, eating, dressing, continence control.
[2] Based on constant disability rate by age, sex and ethnic origin.
[3] Distribution between institutions and community based on the assumption that current institutionalization rates by age, sex, and ethnic origin are constant.
[4] Including persons requiring at least one hour per week of assistance in basic household tasks *and* there is no other person in the household able to perform these tasks.
[5] Percentage of disabled out of total number of elderly people in community and institutions.
[6] Percentage of disabled in the community out of total number of elderly people in the community.

Table 3. Extent of personal-care services in Israel by source of financing, 1981–1989

			1988–89	
	1981	1984	First implementation stage	Full implementation stage
Number of recipients[1]				
TOTAL	3 043	4 874	7 444	16 246
National Insurance Institute			–	13 734[3]
Ministry of Labor and Social Affairs	645	1 399	1 754	1 782
Ministry of Health	520	945	–	–
General Sick Fund	1 878	2 530	5 690	1 730
Percentage of recipients of total population aged 65+ in the community	0.9	1.4	2.0	4.2
Average weekly hours per recipient				
TOTAL	4.2	5.6	8.8	9.3
National Insurance Institute	–	–	–	10.3
Ministry of Labor and Social Affairs	5.5	3.8	2.8	2.9
Ministry of Health	5.9	6.6	–	–
General Sick Fund	2.6	6.2	10.7	6.2

[1] Total number of recipients does not include self-referral elderly to Matav Association (see Table 5) and other private agencies.
[2] Those who receive both personal-care and home-making services are listed here as personal-care recipients.
[3] In addition, approximately 150 are receiving cash benefits; a further 650 persons received care in day centres for the elderly, some of whom also received some personal care at home.

Table 4. Extent of home-making and prepared meals services, Israel, 1981–1989

	1981	1984	1988–89: First implementation stage	1988–89: Full implementation stage
Home-making				
Total number of recipients	8 002	10 138	10 304	7 418[1]
Ministry of Labor and Social Affairs	8 002	10 138	10 304	7 418
Percentage of recipients of total population aged 65+ in the community	2.5	2.9	2.7	1.9
Average weekly hours per recipient		1.0	2.5	2.8
Prepared meals				
Number of recipients	3 155	3 500	3 500	3 500
Percentage of recipients	1.0	1.0	0.9	0.9

[1] This figure is biased downward because home-making services are provided to recipients of personal care under CLTCI who are not reported as a separate service by the National Insurance Institute and therefore could not be included in this table.

Table 5. Extent of personal-care services by source of financing since the full implementation of the CLTCI law, 1989

	Recipients: Absolute numbers	Recipients: %	Hours of care/month: Absolute numbers	Hours of care/month: %	Monthly cost: $[3]	Monthly cost: %	Weekly hours per recipient
TOTAL[1]	17 074	100	714 040	100	3 968	100	9.4
Ministry of Labour and Social Affairs	1 782	10	23 156	3	114	3	2.9
General Sick Fund	730	4	20 012	3	90	2	6.2
National Insurance Institute	13 734[2]	80	629 529	88	3 524	89	10.3
Self-referral to Matav Association	828	5	41 343	6	240	6	11.3

[1] The total number of recipients does not include the personal care provided to self-referrals by private providers (not Matav).
[2] See footnote 1 in Table 3.
[3] In thousand US$.

Table 6. Extent of personal care provided by the Matav Association by source of financing, 1989

	Recipients		Hours of care/month		Monthly cost		Weekly hours per recipient
	Absolute numbers	%	Absolute numbers	%	$[1]	%	
TOTAL[1]	7 020	100	283 712	100	1 771	100	9.1
Ministry of Labor and Social Affairs	1 223	17	14 672	5	79	4	2.7
General Sick Fund	448	6	11 497	4	62	4	5.8
National Insurance Institute	4 521	64	216 200	76	1 390	78	10.8
Self-referral to Matav Association	828	12	41 343	15	240	14	11.3

[1] In thousands $.

Table 7. Recipients of CLTCI law by age. (Source: Morgenstin *et al.* 1989.)

Age (years)	%
60–64	4
65–69	11
70–74	16
75–79	25
80–84	22
85+	22

Table 8. Home-making services financed by the Ministry of Labor and Social Affairs, March 1989

District	Number of recipients	Recipients as % of elderly in the community	Number of hours	Number of weekly hours per recipient	Monthly cost ($)
TOTAL	7 418[1]	1.9	90 657	2.8	377 025
Jerusalem	679	1.9	8 639	2.9	36 516
North	1 078	2.7	12 684	2.7	53 101
Haifa	1 064	1.6	11 894	2.5	49 626
Central	1 631	2.2	21 613	3.0	88 314
Tel Aviv	1 665	1.2	21 638	2.9	90 233
South	1 301	4.1	14 189	2.5	59 235

[1] These elderly people live in 6005 households.

Table 9. Professional home-nursing visits provided by the General Sick Fund (1988)

District	Number of elderly recipients	Elderly recipients as % of the elderly in the community	Number of home visits	Number of home visits per elderly recipient
TOTAL	10 739	2.8	43 051	4.0
Jerusalem	638	1.8	2 469	3.9
North	1 339	3.4	4 724	3.5
Haifa	1 998	3.1	8 120	4.1
Central	2 675	3.7	11 244	4.2
Tel Aviv	2 736	2.0	11 287	4.1
South	1 353	4.4	5 207	3.8

Table 10. The development of the professional home nursing by the General Sick Fund, 1981–88

Year	1981*	1985	1988	Growth between 1981–88 (%)
Number of elderly recipients	7424	9961	10 739	45
Elderly recipients as percentage of the elderly in the community	2.3	2.7	2.8	22
Number of home visits	38 943	42 431	43 051	11
Number of monthly home visits per elderly recipient	5.2	4.3	4.0	−23

* Based on estimates.

Table 11. Comparison between needs and existing personal-care services for 1980–1988, prior to the implementation of CLTCI law

	1980		1983		1988[5]	
	Thousands	%[1]	Thousands	%[1]	Thousands	%[1]
Total disabled in ADL in the community[2]	25.6	7.8	28.4	8.1	33.6	8.8
Disabled in the community: require formal services[3]	10.8	3.3	11.9	3.4	14.4	3.8
Recipients of formal services[4]	3.3	1.0	5.1	1.5	9.1	2.4
Percentage coverage of unmet needs for formal services		31		43		63
Percentage of recipients out of total disabled population		13		18		27

[1] Percentages of those aged 65+ in the community.
[2] Including persons requiring assistance with at least one of the following basic ADL functions: bathing, eating, dressing, continence control.
[3] Including persons requiring at least one hour per week of assistance in basic household tasks, with no other person in the household able to perform these tasks.
[4] Recipients of formal services include elderly referred by public agencies and self-referrals to Matav Association.
[5] For two years before the complete implementation of CLTCI, funds were transferred under CLTCI to the Ministry of Health and Social Affairs and to the General Sick Fund in order to expand the network of services until final implementation of personal benefits in April 1988. Thus comparison of coverage before and after CLTCI should be made with 1983.

Table 12. Comparison between needs and existing personal-care services after the full implementation of the CLTCI law 1989

	Thousands	Percentage[1]
Total disabled in ADL in the community	34.5	8.9
Total recipients:	17.1	4.4
Financed by the National Insurance Institute	13.7	3.5
Financed by others	3.4	0.9
Percentage of recipients among the total disabled population		50

[1] Out of those aged 65+ in the community.

Table 13. Public expenditure in Israel on institutional care and home care, 1988. (Source: Beer and Factor 1989.)

	Monthly public expenditure[1]	%
Total expenditure	13 186	100
Institutional care	8 743	66
Home care	4 443[2]	34

[1] In thousand US$.
[2] Includes only the expenditure on the two main services provided: personal care and home-making.

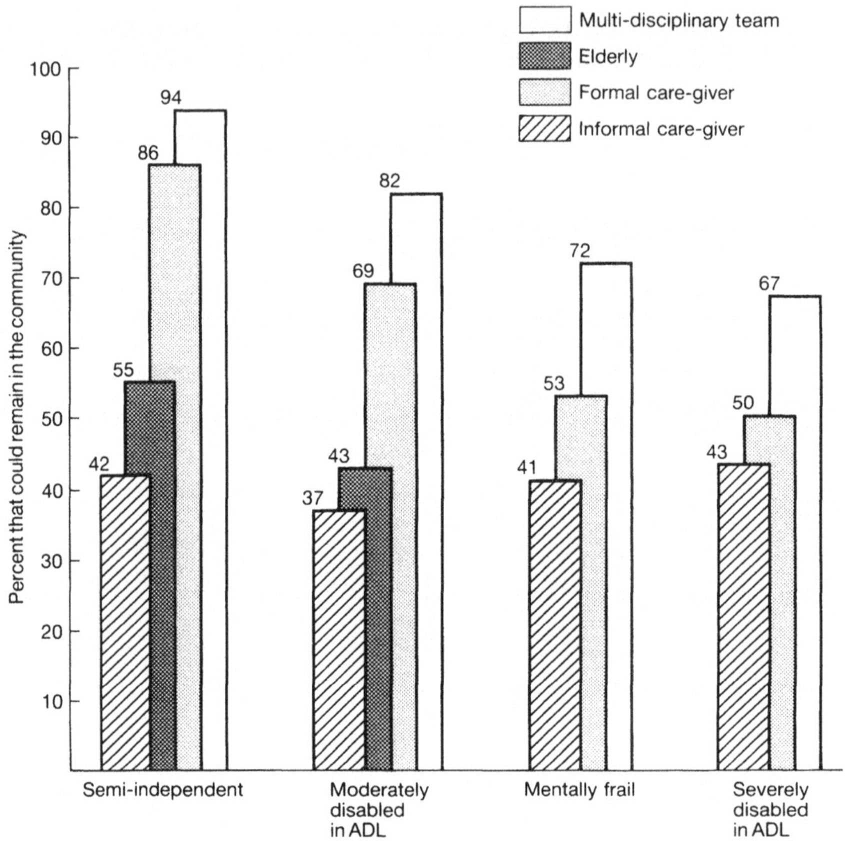

Fig. 1. Elderly people on approved waiting-lists for institutionalization who could remain in the community, by type of informant; in the two right-hand columns the opinions of the elderly people are not presented because functional or mental incapacity prevented many from being interviewed (after Habib and Naon 1987, see Chapter 7 references, p. 187).

Appendix 9: Examination of the need for help from others in care of the elderly (Questionnaire)[1] (Israel)

Please indicate only *one* option for each function. The nurse will note the functional level in the appropriate box. Points will be coded and scored up by the claims official. Please describe who provides assistance in each function.

a. Mobility in the home: **Points**

- ☐ Bedbound; unable to get out of bed on his own or to take a few steps — 1
- ☐ Uses wheelchair and needs help in transferring to and from wheelchair or in manipulating chair — 1
- ☐ Uses wheelchair but transfers and manipulates chair independently — 0.5
- ☐ Mobile with or without mechanical aid, but needs help of another person in walking or in getting up — 0.5
- ☐ Independent with mechanical aid (walker, cane) — 0
- ☐ Walks freely — 0

Description of functional ability and help needed: (indicate who helps and if no help is available)

____

____

b. Dressing: **Points**

- ☐ Needs full or extensive help in dressing — 1
- ☐ Needs some help (shoes, socks, buttoning, lacing, attaching orthopaedic appliances) ____________ — 0.5
- ☐ Dresses without help ____________ — 0

Description of functional ability and help needed (indicate who helps and if no help is available)

____

____

____

c. Washing: **Points**

- ☐ Needs full assistance in washing, in bed, bath, or shower ____________ — 1.5
- ☐ Needs active help in some washing activities ____________ — 1
- ☐ Needs help in shaving/ washing hair — 0.5
- ☐ Needs encouragement/ presence in bathroom, but not active assistance ____________ — 0.5
- ☐ Washes without help — 0

Description of functional ability and help needed (indicate who helps and if no help is available)

____

____

____

d. Feeding and drinking: **Points**

- ☐ Needs full feeding (including liquids and feeding-tube) — 1.5
- ☐ Needs partial help in eating or drinking — 1

- ☐ Needs help in eating, cannot even help himself to bread, hot or cold drink, cannot warm up his own food, forgets to eat if he isn't reminded 0.5
- ☐ Complete blindness (if not included in any of the above items) 0.5
- ☐ Eats and drinks without help 0

Description of functional ability and help needed (indicate who helps and if no help is available)

____

____

____

e. Continence: **Points**

- ☐ Incontinence both in fecal and urinary functions, does not care for himself, is totally dependent on others ____________ 3
- ☐ Incontinent in either the fecal or urinary functions during day and night hours, does not care for himself, is totally dependent on others ____________ 2
- ☐ Uses bathroom but needs extensive help (in mobility, dressing, personal hygiene after use) ____________ 1.5
- ☐ Uses bathroom or pot/bottle, but needs help ____________ 1
- ☐ Uses bathroom or pot/bottle but needs some assistance 0.5
- ☐ Is partially incontinent and does not care for himself ____________ 0.5
- ☐ Continent, or independent in using bathroom or aids (changes his own bag, etc.) 0

Description of functional level and help needed (indicate who helps and if no help is available)

____

____

____

f. The need for supervision at home:

1. Assessment of an orientation of the elderly: nurse is requested to indirectly determine during interview whether person knows where he lives, birthdate, father's name, doctor's name, etc. In addition, nurse is asked to ascertain during the interview whether the person understands basic ADL activities and find his way around the house (bathroom, kitchen, etc.).

____

____

____

2. Description of behaviour during visit (co-operative, passive, quiet, aggressive, etc.)

____

____

____

3. Reported incidents or accidents during past three months (kind and frequency of incident, and source of information)

____

____

____

4. Actual provision of supervision (reported on basis of description of daily routine or other sources)

____

____

____

g. Nurse's decision on supervision: **Points**

- ☐ Person endangers himself or his environment when left alone. Constant supervision of another person at home is required. 6.5
- ☐ Requires supervision in performing ADL activities (scored only if the person received at least 2.5 points in above ADL examination).[2] 0
- ☐ Does not endanger himself or others when left alone. 0

Notes

[1] Procedures for use of assessment tool are described in detail in a manual for the nurse.
[2] i.e., person was already determined eligible on the basis of the need for supervision in ADL activities and therefore does not receive additional points for supervision.

Appendix 10: Background data from Italy

Table 1. Number of clients by classification in the Italian regions.

Regions	Classification of clients														
	Nuclear families	% of total helped	Handicapped	% of total helped	Disabled	% of total helped	Elderly	% of total helped	Receiving psychiatric services	% of total helped	Citizens in need	% of total helped	Classification unspecified	% of total helped	Total helped
North															
Liguria	103	7.44	45	3.25	58	4.19	1156	83.5	21	1.51	–	–	–	–	1 383
Valle d'Aasta	5	4.31	–	–	1	0.86	107	92.2	3	2.58	–	–	–	–	116
Lombardia	62	0.36	6	0.03	49	0.28	489	2.8	23	0.13	3	0.01	16 360	96.2	16 992
Trentino-Alto-Adige	842	29.3	1	0.03	75	2.61	498	17.3	18	0.62	15	0.52	1 422	49.5	2 871
Friuli-Venezia Giulia	5	0.19	–	–	102	4.07	450	17.9	20	0.79	133	5.31	1 794	71.6	2 504
TOTAL North	1017	0.04	52	0.21	285	1.19	2700	11.3	85	0.35	151	0.63	19 576	82.0	23 866
Centre															
Umbria[1]	–	–	–	–	–	–	–	–	–	–	–	–	–	–	–
Marche	9	2.32	3	0.77	7	1.80	320	82.6	–	–	3	0.77	45	11.6	387
Lazio	–	–	–	–	7	6.93	94	93.0	–	–	–	–	–	–	101
TOTAL Centre	9	1.84	3	0.61	14	2.86	414	84.8	–	–	3	0.61	45	9.22	488
South and islands															
Abruzzo	10	2.32	2	0.46	1	0.23	105	24.4	2	0.46	–	–	310	72.00	430
Campania	200	18.70	10	0.93	4	0.37	387	36.3	9	0.84	–	–	456	42.70	1 066
Puglia	365	6.96	50	0.95	98	1.87	3921	74.8	47	0.89	406	7.75	350	6.68	5 237
Sicilia	–	–	–	–	–	–	9	100	–	–	–	–	–	–	9
Sardegna	55	18.40	–	–	1	0.33	199	66.7	–	–	–	–	43	14.4	298
TOTAL South and islands	630	8.94	62	0.88	104	1.47	4621	65.6	58	0.82	406	5.76	1 159	16.40	7 040
Overall total	1656	5.27	117	0.37	403	1.28	7735	24.6	143	0.45	560	1.78	20 780	66.1	31 394

[1] The Authority for the region of Umbria, which participated in the research, did not give information on classifications and on numbers of clients.

Table 2. Types of services and number of authorities offering them

Geographical areas	No. of authorities replying	Home-making	Personal care	Laundry	Food provision	Meals-on-wheels	Linen & clothing	Heating	Furnishing & bedding	Water, heating, lighting	Sanitary facilities	Rebuilding work	Redecorating	Rent contribution	Administrative work	Escorted visits	Telephone installation	Providing literature	Radio, TV, etc.	Organizing recreation	Facilitating recreation	Education	Nursing help	Home medical tests	Rehabilitation	Night cover	Administration of health care	Delivering medicine	General medical help	Monthly financial help
North																														
Liguria	8	8	6	8	6	3	4	4	2	3	2	3	3	5	7	6	4	1	1	2	–	2	3	4	3	1	5	4	4	1
Valle d'Aasta	2	2	2	2	1	1	1	1	1	1	1	–	1	–	2	2	–	–	–	2	–	1	2	1	1	–	2	2	–	–
Lombardia	7	7	7	7	3	5	4	3	3	4	2	1	4	5	7	5	4	3	1	4	3	3	7	6	5	3	7	6	2	1
Trentino-Alto-Adige	10	10	10	9	4	6	2	1	1	1	1	–	1	1	10	8	2	–	2	4	1	3	6	6	3	–	7	8	4	–
Friuli-Venezia Giula	5	5	5	5	2	5	2	2	3	–	–	–	2	1	5	4	1	–	–	4	1	–	4	4	–	1	5	5	–	1
TOTAL North	32	32	30	31	16	20	13	11	10	9	6	4	11	12	31	25	11	4	4	16	5	9	22	21	12	5	26	25	10	3
Centre																														
Umbria[1]	1	1	1	1	–	1	–	–	–	–	–	–	–	1	1	1	–	–	–	1	–	–	1	1	–	–	1	1	1	–
Marche	5	5	5	2	3	2	3	4	3	4	–	1	3	5	5	5	3	–	–	4	2	2	3	3	2	1	4	3	2	–
Lazio	3	2	2	1	–	1	–	–	–	–	–	–	–	2	2	2	–	1	–	1	–	–	1	1	–	–	1	2	1	–
TOTAL Centre	9	8	8	4	3	4	3	4	3	4	–	1	3	8	8	8	3	1	–	6	2	2	5	5	2	1	6	6	4	–
South and islands																														
Abruzzo	7	6	6	4	2	3	2	5	1	2	1	–	1	3	5	6	3	1	–	4	–	2	4	2	3	2	5	4	1	1
Campania	6	4	4	3	2	3	2	–	2	3	1	1	1	2	6	5	2	–	–	4	2	2	2	2	1	–	4	2	1	–
Puglia	27	25	23	18	10	15	8	4	7	5	2	5	12	13	27	23	4	3	2	15	6	6	21	10	8	–	23	25	7	–
Sicilia	1	–	–	1	–	1	–	–	–	–	–	–	–	–	1	1	–	–	–	–	–	1	1	–	–	–	1	–	–	–
Sardegna	6	6	5	4	–	4	1	3	1	2	2	2	4	–	4	4	–	2	1	3	1	1	4	1	1	–	4	4	2	–
TOTAL South and islands	47	41	38	30	14	26	13	12	11	12	6	8	18	18	43	39	9	6	3	26	9	12	32	15	13	2	37	35	11	1
Overall total	88	81	76	65	33	50	29	27	24	25	12	13	32	38	82	72	23	11	7	48	16	23	59	41	27	8	69	66	25	4

Appendix 11: A translation of an LIER assessment form (the Netherlands)

Indication form II / Punch draft LIER system / Tasks home-help service

(National intake and documentary system)

Name of client ________________	Name of institution:
Residence: ________________	________________
Address: ________________	________________
Ref. no. ________________	Telephone: __________

Card sort / Institution number / Family no. / Date / Code hh / District

I EXECUTIVE WORKER

1. Household help
   a. organization household activities
   b. meals
      — breakfast/lunch
      — preparing dinner
      — cooking
      — laying the table
      — doing the dishes
   c. clothing/linen
      — washing
      — ironing
      — clothing
      — mending
   d. maintenance house/household effects
      — light chores
      — heavy chores
   e. shopping
      — daily
      — periodically
   f. plants/pets

2. Care as regards:
   a. children (babies, tiny tots, toddlers)
      — bathing, changing, dressing, helping with feeding
   b. adults
      — body care (washing, hair)
      — helping to dress/undress and get in/out of bed
      — helping with eating
      — help with physical exercise in and about the house
      — supervision of carrying out medical instructions and use of medicines
      — nursing/rehabilitation at home

3. Supervising/social
   a. run household
      financial/administrative affairs
   b. keep children busy
      guiding children
      raising
   c. atmosphere-creating tasks/replacing hostess
   d. working visit to externally nursed person
   e. observation
      listening
      mental support
   f. helping to change
      — household tasks
      — care/caring tasks
      — supervising/social tasks

II HOME-HELP ORGANIZER

Supervising care
Instruction
Make a person wake up to his/her problems
Helping to change
Supporting/coping with problems
Relegating
Co-operation

Advice as regards frequency working contact with:

— client system	1 × per __ weeks
— executive worker	1 × per __ weeks

III ALLOCATION EXECUTIVE WORKER/HOURS

Indicated help
  1 = specialized home carer
  2 = home carer
  3 = home carer for the aged
  4 = home help
  5 = home help for the aged
  6 = alpha
  7 = ____

Help allocated (see above)

Motivation at deviation
  1 = indicated quality not available
  2 = personal qualities prevail
  3 = organizational limitation
  4 = ____

Indicated number of hours:
  number of times of help per week (frequency)
  from: __h to __h
  from: __h to __h

Number of hours allocated:
  number of times of help per week (frequency)
  from: __h to __h
  from: __h to __h

Motivation at deviation:
  1 = due to factors inside institution
  2 = due to factors in client system
  3 = __

Expected duration of care:
  __ weeks (X) = up to 1 month
  __ months (Y) = from 1–6 months
  __ months (Z) = more than 6 months

1* = taking over
2* = helping

Index

abilities, *see* disabled; functional ability
access, *see* entry
ACRE, *see* Age Care Research Europe
activities
  of daily living, functional status and the cross-national perspectives 248, 256
    in Germany 133–4, 325, 326
    in Israel 159, 166, 248, 329
    in the Netherlands 225–6, 227–8, 229
    see also functional ability
  of helpers/carers/services, *see* tasks
administration/management
  in Belgium, of health/social services 17–18
  cross-national perspectives 277, 278, 279
  in Italy 207–8
  see also organization
age
  data relating to
    in Belgium 300
    cross-national perspectives 254–6
    in Denmark 255, 304
    in England and Wales 255, 317
    in Germany 326, 327
    in Israel 327, 332
    in the Netherlands 216–17, 255
  of persons receiving home help 254–6
Age Care Research Europe (ACRE) study 3–6, 261, 262, 292
  Denmark and the 46–9
  in practice 4–6
  rationale 3–4
aged, the, *see* older people
alarm systems in France 110–11
allocation of home care 261–72
  in Belgium 28–36, 267–8, 269
  criteria for 263–6; *see also* assessment
  cross-national perspectives 261–72
  in Denmark 60, 268, 269, 271
  factors affecting 266–70
  in the Netherlands 344
alone, living, *see* living alone
alpha care/help in the Netherlands 218–19, 253
amount, *see* quantity
application (for home help)
  in Denmark 49, 59
  in Italy 197
  successful, *see* clients
assessment
  of home-care measures, cross-national perspectives 273–6
  for home help/support
    cross-national perspectives 263–7, 281
    in Denmark 84
    in England and Wales 84–5, 87
    in Germany 133, 135
    in Israel 172, 181–2, 337–9
    in the Netherlands 219–20, 224, 281
    service co-ordination and 87
  for nursing home 52
  of unmet needs, in Israel 171–2
  see also reassessment
assistance, *see* help; payments
assistants, family-help/home-help/domestic
  categorization by respondents, in Germany 154
  qualifications and training
    in Belgium 22
    in Italy 196
Association for Planning and Development of Services for the Aged in Israel (ESHEL) 162
attitudes/viewpoints/opinions
  of professionals 143–50, 263, 268–70
  of users/clients 150–2, 274
Audit Commission for England and Wales 66–7, 81, 89
authorities, local/regional, *see* local authorities
AWBZ (Exceptional Medical Expenses Scheme, Netherlands) 213, 217, 220, 224, 233, 282

Baden-Württemberg 131
bathing, capacity for, in Denmark 306
Belgium 11, 15–37, 242–92 *passim*, 299–301
beneficiaries, *see* clients
benefits in Israel 166–7, 180–1
  in-kind 181–1
  level 182–3
  see also claims; payments

Berlin (West) 122, 131–43, 257, 266, 276, 325–7
Britain, Great (UK) 12, 63–98, 242–92 *passim*, 315–20
budget 266–7
  cross-national perspectives 266–7
  entitlement vs. 266–7
  in Israel 177–9
  see also costs; expenditure; funding
bureaucracy in care allocation in Germany 145–6, 266

capacities, functional, *see* functional ability
Care Benefits Act (Germany) 138–9, 153
Care of the elderly—needs and barriers (Freie Universität of Berlin) 152
carers
  as clients 262
  informal, *see* informal care
  professional
    attitudes of 268–70
    in Belgium 33–4
    in France 111
    preferences for care and actual care obtained by 33–4
case finding, service co-ordination and 87
case management 76, 87–8, 90, 92–3, 95
cash, payments/assistance in
  in France 100, 112
  in Israel 166–7, 180–1
Catholic Pensioners Union (Belgium) 27, 29
Catholic Sickness insurance (Belgium) 27
centralization of service provision
  in Israel 183–5
  in Italy 194
centres
  community care, in Germany 140–3, 143, 148, 151
  day and social
    in Denmark 42
    in Italy 202, 206
  home-care service
    in Belgium 26
    in Italy 197, 198, 199, 206
charging and paying for home help
  in Denmark 48–9
  in England and Wales 71
  in the Netherlands 215, 216, 232–3
chronically ill/frail persons, care of
  in Denmark 52
  in Germany 124, 126, 143, 150, 153
  in Israel 160, 170
  in the Netherlands 216, 219
churches
  in Belgium 27
  in Germany 122, 127, 129
claims in Germany
  entitlement 136–40
  mechanisms 143–52
  see also benefits; cash; payments
cleaning help 24, 27–36
  allocation 23–4, 28–9
  in Belgium 24, 27–36
  cross-national perspectives 253
  decisions/decision-making on 31–6
  in Denmark 306
cleaning services 24
  in Belgium 24, 28–9
  home help and, relation between 24
clients/beneficiaries/recipients/target populations/users
  attitudes/viewpoints of 150–2, 274
  carers as 262
  for cleaning services, in Belgium 24
  for home help/care
    in Belgium 21
    cross-national perspectives 246–8, 254–9
    in Denmark 45–9, 304, 305–9
    in England and Wales 72, 78–81, 83–4, 90, 94, 317–18
    in France 105, 106–8, 109–10, 322–4
    in Germany 141, 150–2
    in Israel 165–6, 168, 169
    in Italy 198, 199, 340
    in the Netherlands 220, 225–6, 232–3
  policies relating to 246–8
CNAVTS (National Office for Old Age Insurance for Salaried Workers, France) 106, 107, 322, 323
collaboration/co-operation/co-ordination/integration (concerning services)
    cross-national perspectives 252, 285–6
  in Denmark 60, 252, 286
  in England and Wales 77–8, 86–9, 91, 92, 94–5, 286
  in France 113–14
  in Germany 144–5
  in Israel 170–1
  in Italy 202–3, 208
  in the Netherlands 221, 232
  see also fragmentation
collaborative research 4–5
Commission for the Study of the Problems of Old Age (France) 100, 101
communal housing in Italy 204
communes in Denmark 41–2
Communist Party, Italian 191, 211
community care (and community services)
  in Denmark 302
  in England and Wales 67, 76–7, 77, 86, 318

in Germany 140–3, 148–9, 327
centres for 140–3, 143, 148, 151
home care vs. 6–8
in Israel 164, 174–5
in Italy 204
local authorities and 67
in the Netherlands 221–4
Community care: an agenda for action 67
Community Care Bill (1990, UK) 282
Community Long-Term Care Insurance (CLTCI) and the CLTCI law 160, 162–4, 165–85 *passim*, 248, 291, 331, 332, 334
community nurses/nursing services
co-ordination with other services 77
in England and Wales 76–7, 77
in Germany 119, 128
Community Services and the Social Production of Welfare 96
competitive tendering in England and Wales 95–6
complementarity of care in the Netherlands 226–8
Conservative (Tory) government (UK) 67, 268, 283, 284, 288, 291
conservative welfare states 287, 290
contacts with other services, *see* collaboration
continence, assessment in Israel 338
contributions by client, *see* charging
conversation 260–1
co-operation, *see* collaboration
co-ordination, *see* collaboration
corporatist (conservative) welfare states 287, 290
costs
cross-national perspectives 289–90
in England and Wales 94
in Germany 138–9
in Israel 178
in the Netherlands 222, 233
see also charging; expenditure; funding; payments
coverage, extent of, as function of need for services 171–4
cross-national analysis of services 9, 10, 237–95
cross-national research 4, 5

day centres, *see* centres
decentralization of service provision
in Israel 183–5
in Italy 194
decisions/decision-making (on services) 6, 262–6
cleaning help, in Belgium 31–6
cross-national perspectives 262–7, 293
on home help 262–6
in Belgium 31–6, 265
in Denmark 49–59, 59–60, 60, 264–5
in Italy 202, 209, 210, 266
problems and, *see* problems
deinstitutionalization 274–5
delivery, *see* provision and delivery
demand/request for services/help 257–8
in Belgium 33–4
cross-national perspectives 257–8
in Israel 176–7, 258
in Italy 196–9
see also application
dementia, senile, in Italy 201, 210
demographic aspects
in Belgium 299
in Denmark 306
in Israel 157–9
Denmark 11, 38–62, 242–92 *passim*, 303–14
départements (in France) 100, 105, 109, 110–11, 112, 114
destinational outcomes for recipients of community social services in England and Wales 85
development of home-care/home-help services, historical, *see* historical development
disabled/handicapped people (and disability)
in England and Wales 71, 79, 82
in France 106–7
in Israel 159, 166, 172, 173, 182–3, 329
in Italy 192, 205
long-term care, *see* long-term care
in the Netherlands 225–6, 226–8
see also functional ability
discharge from hospital 52
discontinuity in care provision in Germany 139, 151
disruptions in care provision in Germany 151–2
distribution of services, cross-national perspectives 273–4
District Health Authorities in England and Wales 76, 77–8
district nurses/nursing
in England and Wales 76–7
in the Netherlands 221, 232
Division of Aging of the Ministry of Labor and Social Affairs (Israel) 161–2
doctors, *see* general practitioners; physicians
domestic assistance allowance in England and Wales 71
domestic assistants, *see* assistants

domestic difficulties, targeting related to, in England and Wales 82
domestic tasks in France 111, 321
Domiciliary Care Project (UK) 96
dressing capacity, assessment in Israel 337
drinking capability, assessment in Israel 337–8
duties, *see* tasks
dying, care of the 52

earnings, *see* income
East Anglia, home-help staffing in 74
East Midlands, home-help staffing in 74
eating capability, assessment in Israel 337–8
economic collaboration between agencies 60
  in Belgium 299–301
economic factors
  in home-care policies 289–90
  in Israel 157–9
  see also charging; costs; expenditure; funding; payments
elderly people, *see* older people
elementary activities of daily living, in Germany 325
eligibility
  assessment, in Israel 181–2
  criteria
    in Israel 165–6, 168, 169
    in Italy 188–9
  see also entitlement
England (as part of UK) 12, 63–98, 242–70, 315–20
entitlement to services/benefits 266–7
  budget vs. 266–7
  cross-national perspectives 266–7
  in Israel 163, 176–80
  see also eligibility
entry/access to home-help services
  in Denmark 51–3
  in England and Wales 76
  in Israel 177–9
environmental issues 294
equipment in Denmark 42
ESHEL (Association for Planning and Development of Services for the Aged in Israel) 162
estimation, *see* assessment
examination, *see* assessment
Exceptional Medical Expenses Scheme (AWBZ, Netherlands) 213, 217, 220, 224, 233, 282
exit from home-help services 51–3
expenditure
  in Belgium 301
  cross-national perspectives 289–90
  in Denmark 302
  in England and Wales 73, 318–20
  in France 105, 107–8, 322
  in Israel 335
  in the Netherlands 215, 216, 222–3
  see also budget; costs; funding

families/relatives
  cross-national perspectives 241, 258, 283–4
  financial incentives for, in England and Wales 112
  policies and their impact on 241, 283–4
  role
    in Germany 126–7, 129
    in Israel 159, 160–1
  services for 241, 242, 258–9
    in the Netherlands 216, 219
  see also informal care
Family Allowance Office (France) 112
family-help assistants, qualifications/training 22
Federal Social Assistance Act (Germany) 138
feeding capability, assessment in Israel 337–8
finances, *see* costs; expenditure; funding
Flanders 15–37, 269, 272–3
Flemish region 17–26
flexibility of home help
  in Denmark 51, 60
  in England and Wales 90
fragmentation (separation) of services 251, 281–2, 285–6
frail persons, *see* chronically ill; long-term care
France 11, 99–117, 321–4
frequency of home help
  in Belgium 21–2
  in England and Wales 317–18
functional ability/disability/capacity 247–8, 254–6
  cross-national perspectives 247–8, 254–6
  in Denmark 3–6, 47, 306, 307
  in Germany 132–6, 247–8
  in Israel 159, 166, 181–2, 248
  in the Netherlands 220, 225–6
  policies relating to 247–8
  see also activities; disabled
funding/financing
  cross-national perspectives 267–8, 277, 278, 279
  home care
    in Belgium 22–3, 267–8
    in England and Wales 70–1, 78

in France 100, 101, 102, 108–9, 112
in Germany 136–40
in Israel 165–6, 168, 169, 179–80, 330, 331
joint 78
in the Netherlands 215, 217–18
provision and, separation of 267–8
research 5
see also expenditure; investment
future prospects for home care 292–5

gap filling 93
'gate-keepers' 139–40, 149
gender-related data
in Belgium 300
in Denmark 304
in Germany 326
in Israel 327
General Household Survey (UK, 1985) 78, 79, 257
General Inspectorate of Social Affairs (France) 106
general practitioners
cross-national perspectives 262–3, 269–70
decisions (referral, etc.) by 147, 147–8, 262–3, 269–70
in Germany 145, 147, 147–8
General Sick Fund (Israel) 160, 162, 166, 167, 172, 183, 333
Genoa 190–209, 247, 250, 257, 266, 292
Germany 11, 118–56, 242–92 *passim*, 325–7
Government and government agencies
in Belgium 301
in England and Wales 65–6, 67, 71, 72, 268, 283, 284, 288, 291
in Israel 159–86 *passim*
local, *see* local government
in the Netherlands 214, 215, 224, 233, 291
see also specific agencies/political parties and political factors
grants in France 101
Great Britain (UK) 12, 63–98, 242–92 *passim*, 315–20
Griffiths report 67, 79, 88, 89, 95, 96, 282, 291
Groot-Antwerpen area 27–9
Growing Old in the Future 101–2
growth
policies without (in 1980s) 278–9
without policies (in 1960s and 1970s) 278–85

handicap, *see* disabled; functional ability
health (well-being)
criteria of, cross-national perspectives 247–8
home help and its effects on 85
health insurance, *see* insurance
health-related care, other forms of care and, relevance of distinction between 256–7
health services
administration 17–18
in Belgium 17–18, 301
co-ordination with home-help services 86–8
cross-national perspectives 243–5, 285, 294
in Denmark 302
in England and Wales 65, 86–8, 95–6, 318–20
in Germany 124
home care as an alternative to 243–5
in Israel 171
in Italy 203
social and, separation 285
see also National Health Service
health visitors, in England and Wales 76–7
help/support
cleaning, *see* cleaning help
disabled people lacking, targeting related to, in England and Wales 82
external, in Germany 134–6, 138, 326
home, *see* home help
informal, see informal care
kind received, cross-national perspectives 259–61
need for, *see* need
requests for 33–4
see also tasks
helpers, home, *see* home helpers
hierarchies of services and service systems in Germany 119, 125–7
historical development of home-care/home-help services
in Denmark 38–40
in England and Wales 64–8
in France 99–103
in Germany 119–22
in Israel 161–2
in Italy 190–2, 193–4, 207, 209
in the Netherlands 214–17
Holland 12, 213–35, 242–92 *passim*, 342–4
home(s), *see* housing *and specific types of homes (e.g. nursing homes)*
home care, definition/concept of 8–9, 284–5
home help (major and specific references)
allocation 28–36, 60, 84–5

home help (*continued*)
amount/frequency of 21–2
application for, *see* application
assessment for, *see* assessment
assistants, *see* assistants
in Belgium 16–23, 27–36
charging for, *see* charging
cleaning services and, relation between 24
co-operation/collaboration with other services, *see* collaboration
cross-national perspectives 254–63
decisions on, *see* decisions
definition 9, 16–23
in Denmark 38–62, 305–9
in England and Wales 69–91
flexibility, *see* flexibility
in France 104–8, 322–4
funding, *see* funding
historical development of services, *see* historical development
in Israel 161–9
kinds of 8–9
need for, *see* need
organizers
in England and Wales 70, 76, 89
in the Netherlands 213–34, 343
pathways into/through/out of services for, *see* entry; exit; pathways
provision, *see* provision
strengths and weaknesses of services 50–1
home helpers
categorization by respondents, in Germany 154
cross-national perspectives 249
part-time, in the Netherlands 219
tasks
in Belgium 20
in Denmark 44–5, 303
in England and Wales 80–1, 315
in France 106, 321
in the Netherlands 218, 228
home-making 8, 9
cross-national perspectives 253
in Denmark 44
in England and Wales 69, 315
in Germany 123, 125, 126, 126–7, 127, 130–1
in Israel 167–81, 175–6, 331, 332, 333, 334
in the Netherlands 227, 228, 230
hospital(s)
admissions to 276
prevention/reduction 137, 147–8, 244, 275
in Germany 137, 147–8, 244, 276
cross-national perspectives 240–1, 244, 275, 276
decisions (referral, etc.) by 148–50, 263
discharge from
in Denmark 52
in Germany 146–7
in Israel 175
in Italy 203
in the Netherlands 231–2
doctors in, *see* physicians
expenditure on, in England and Wales 319
policies and their impact on 240–1, 244, 275, 276
social service departments in, in Germany 149–50, 154
hours of service, *see* time
household
income, in Denmark 306
structure/composition
in Denmark 306
in England and Wales 80
in Germany 134, 137–8
support from, in Germany 131
housewife, home help as a stand-in for, in the Netherlands 218
housework
cross-national perspectives 260
in Germany 131
in the Netherlands 342
housing/homes
in Denmark 39–40
in France 111–12
in Italy, communal 204
in the Netherlands 221–2, 231
see also specific types of homes (e.g. nursing homes) and institutions
Humberside, home-help staffing in 74

illness, chronic, *see* chronically ill; long-term care
income
criteria, cross-national perspectives 246–7
household, in Denmark 306
service use and, in the Netherlands 226
testing, *see* means testing
incontinence, assessment in Israel 338
informal care/support 245–6
in Belgium 33–4
cross-national perspectives 241, 245–6, 258–9, 262, 283–4
decisions by persons giving 262
in England and Wales 79, 91, 92, 94
in France 112–13
in Germany 129, 131, 132–6, 137–8

in Israel 160–1, 245–6
in the Netherlands 226–30, 231
policies and their impact on 241, 245–6, 283–4
preferences for care of and actual care obtained by persons giving 33–4
see also families/relatives
information
agencies' need/requirement for
in Israel 170
in the Netherlands 232
decisions based on, in Italy 202
on law, in Israel 177
INSERM 107
institutionalization 274–6
cross-national perspectives 244–5, 274–6
in England and Wales 85, 86
in Israel 336
prevention of 85, 86, 244–5, 274–6
institutional services/care (residential/nursing homes, etc.)
cross-national perspectives 241, 243–5, 274–6
in Denmark 41, 274–6 *passim*, 302
in England and Wales 318–19
in France 321
home/community services vs. 7–8, 164, 174–5, 204, 221–4, 243–5, 274–6
in Israel 164, 174–5, 336
in Italy 193, 195, 203, 203–4, 209, 210, 211
in the Netherlands 221–4, 225, 232, 274–6 *passim*
policies and their impact on 241, 243–5, 274–6
see also hospitals; nursing homes; residential care
instrumental activities of daily living
in Germany 325
in the Netherlands 225–6, 227–8, 229
insurance (health/sickness/old age/social)
in Belgium 25, 27, 29
cross-national perspectives 280
in France 101, 108, 322, 323
in Germany 119, 122–3, 125, 127, 138, 139, 150, 257, 267, 280
in Israel 159–60, 163, 177, 183, 280; *see also* Community Long-Term Care Insurance; National Insurance Institute
in the Netherlands 213
integration, see collaboration/co-operation/co-ordination
interviews in the Danish pathways study 311
investment, direct provision and, ratio 93–4
Israel 12, 157–87, 242–92 *passim*, 327–36
Italy 11–12, 188–211, 242–92 *passim*, 340–1

job definition, restricting 145
joint services, *see* collaboration
junctions (key points) in service system 6, 311

key points in service system 6, 311

labour, division of, disruption resulting from 151
Landelik Indicatie en Registratiessysteem (LIER, National Intake and Documentary System) 220, 224, 342–4
Laroque report 100, 101
law, *see* legislation
legislation and the law
in Denmark 40–1
in England and Wales 64, 70, 282
in Germany 123–4, 125, 138, 138–9
in Israel, *see* Community Long-Term Care Insurance law
in Italy 193, 208
Liberal sickness insurance organization (Belgium) 27, 29
liberal welfare states 287, 288, 290
LIER (Landelik Indicatie en Registratiessysteem) 220, 224, 342–4
life, quality of, home help in relation to, in Denmark 48, 308
linkages, *see* collaboration/co-operation/co-ordination
living alone
in Denmark 305, 306
in England and Wales 79
in the Netherlands 227
Local Government Training Board (UK, 1988) 91
local/regional authorities
in Denmark (= communes) 41–2
in England and Wales 67, 71, 73–6, 79, 81, 83–4
in Italy 193, 195, 340–1
local/regional government/municipalities
in England and Wales 65–6
in France 105
see also départements
London, inner and outer, services and staffing in 75, 316, 317

long-term care of chronically ill/disabled/ frail persons 275
cross-national perspectives 275
in Germany 143, 150
in Israel 160

Maintien à domicile 99–117
Making a reality of community care 66–7
Malben 161
management
case 76, 87–8, 90, 92–3, 95
of services, *see* administration
managers, service, in Belgium 20, 21
Managing services for the elderly more effectively 66
Managing Tomorrow 91
marital status
in Belgium 300
in Germany 134
see also spouses
market mechanisms, privatization and increased reliance on 283
Matav Association (Israel) 167, 332
Maternity and Child Welfare Act (UK, 1918) 64
meals, home-delivered, in Israel 168–9, 331
means/income testing
in Germany 124
in Israel 166
men, *see* gender-related data
mental health service in Italy 203
Midlands, home-help staffing in 74
Ministry of Health (Israel) 159, 160, 166, 183
Ministry of Health (UK) 64, 70
Ministry of Health, Welfare and Culture (Netherlands) 213, 217
Ministry of Labor and Social Affairs (Israel) 159, 160, 161–2, 165, 168, 170, 172, 332, 333, 335
Ministry of/for (National) Solidarity (France) 106, 108
Ministry of Social Affairs (Israel) 167
Ministry of Social Welfare (Israel) 181
Ministry of Solidarity, Health and Social Protection (France) 322, 324
mobility
assessment, in Israel 337
handicaps, in the Netherlands 225–6
monitoring (of needs/services), service co-ordination and 87–8
moral incentives, policy and 277, 278, 279
municipalities, *see* local government

National Conference on the Retired and the Elderly (France) 103
National Health Service
in England and Wales 65, 95–6, 291
in Italy 203
National Health Service Act (1946, UK) 64, 70
National Insurance Institute (Israel) 160, 166, 167, 172, 177, 184
National Intake and Documentary System (Landelik Indicatie en Registratiessysteem, LIER) 220, 224, 342–4
National Office for Old Age Insurance for Salaried Workers (CNAVTS, France) 106, 107, 322, 323
National Union of Associations for Care and Services in the Home (France) 103
need(s) (for assistance/help) 256–8
cross-national perspectives 256–8, 263–7
in Denmark 304, 305, 306–8, 309
in England and Wales 82, 83
in France 107
in Germany 132–6, 141, 150, 152–3, 326
in Israel 171–2, 182–3, 256, 333–5
in Italy 201–2, 257
resources and, matching of, *see* targeting
unmet 171–2, 201–2, 256–7, 306–8, 309
see also demand; help
Netherlands 12, 213–35, 242–92 *passim*, 242–4
north of England, home-help staffing in 74
Northrhine-Westphalia 128, 129
north-west of England, home-help staffing in 74
nurse (and nursing), professional
community, *see* community nurses
district, *see* district nurses
home 8, 9, 25
in Belgium 25
cross-national perspectives 249, 252, 274
in Denmark 41–2
in England and Wales 69, 76–7
in France 108
in Germany 119, 120, 121, 125, 126, 127, 128–9, 139, 274, 327
in Israel 169, 181, 183, 333
in Italy 195, 203
in the Netherlands 220–1
interfaces/co-operation with other services 77, 86–7, 203, 221, 232, 252
specialized, in Germany 119
nursing activities/care, home-help/care and
in Denmark 44
overcoming barriers between 251–2

nursing homes
  cross-national perspectives 241, 243
  in Denmark 41, 52
    assessment for 52
    temporary admission to 42
  in the Netherlands 221–2, 223–4
    temporary admission to 221
  policies and their impact on 241, 243
  see also institutional services/care

Old Age Insurance (France) 322, 323
  'general regime' of 106, 107–8
older people, policies for
  future prospects 294–5
  impact 241
  trends in 16–17
opinions, *see* attitudes
organization (of services) 251–4
  in Belgium 18, 253
  cross-national perspectives 251–4
  in England and Wales/UK 65–6, 254
  in France 104–5, 108–9
  in Germany 127–9, 140–3, 141–3, 151, 252
  in Israel 165, 167, 168, 169–71, 181, 183–5, 253
  in Italy 193–5, 206, 207, 251
  in the Netherlands 224, 253
  see also administration
organizers, home-help, *see* home help
outcomes of home help 85–6
overlap of services in England and Wales 317–18

packaging, service, service co-ordination and 87
part-time helpers in the Netherlands 219
pathways to home-help services
  in Denmark 49–50, 59, 310–11
  in England and Wales 76
paying, *see* charging
payments/assistance/reimbursements
  in France 100, 112
  in Germany 124, 137–8
  in Israel 166–7, 180–1
  see also benefits; claims
pensions
  in Denmark 302
  in Israel 158
perceptions, *see* attitudes
personal care 8, 9
  cross-national perspectives 253, 260, 261
  in Denmark 44
  in England and Wales 69, 72, 94, 260, 315
  in France 321
  in Israel 164–7, 170, 172, 175–6, 178, 330, 331, 332, 334
  in the Netherlands 227, 228, 230
Personal Social Services Research Unit Domiciliary Care Project (UK) 96
personnel, *see* staff
physicians, hospital
  decisions (referral, etc.) by, in Germany 148–9, 263
  viewpoints of, in Germany 148–9
pillarization, organizational principle of, in the Netherlands 224
planning of care/running of service
  in England and Wales 87
  in Israel 171
  in Italy 206, 207–8
  service co-ordination and the 87, 171
policies 240–95
  aims 240–8
  in Belgium 16–17, 18–19
  cross-national perspectives 240–95
  in Denmark 59–60
  in England and Wales 71–3, 89, 95–6
  factors affecting 285–92
  in France 100–3
  in Germany 119–31
  growth without (in 1960s and 1970s) 278–9
  without growth (in 1980s) 278–85
  impact of 240–1
  implementation, factors affecting 285–92
  in Italy 192–3, 208
  in the Netherlands 224–33, 233
  for older people, trends, *see* older people
  in practice 248–72
  services arriving before or after 242
  trends in 273–95
policy measures 277–8
political factors
  cross-national perspectives 286–9, 290–2
  in England and Wales 67, 71, 268, 288, 291
  in France 102
  in Italy 191, 292
  in the Netherlands 233–4, 291
  in welfare ideologies 286–9
  see also government
priorities, service, in Germany 125–7
private services 283
  in Belgium 18
  co-ordination with other services 78, 88
  cross-national perspectives 283
  in England and Wales 70, 78, 88, 95, 283
  in France 100, 105
  in Germany 138, 142, 144, 153, 283
  in Israel 167
  in Italy 195, 204, 208–9, 283

privatization, cross-national perspectives 283
problems
in the decision-making process
solution of 55, 56–7, 58
unsolved 57–9
in Denmark 47–9, 56–7, 58
in Israel 171–2
in Italy 200, 201–2
professional carers, *see* carers
professionalizing of home help 253–4
professional nurses, *see* nurses
providers
attitudes/viewpoints of 268–70
cross-national perspectives 268–70
in Germany 143–6
organization of, *see* organization
provision and delivery of help/care 240–61
aims 240–8
in Belgium 18–26, 267–8, 292–3
cross-national perspectives 240–61, 267–8, 273–4, 292
in Denmark 42–4, 57, 60, 268, 292
in England and Wales 69–78, 93–4, 315, 316
funding and, separation of 267–8
in Germany 129–31, 136–43, 293
investment in relation to 93–4
in Israel 164, 164–75, 183–5
in Italy 198, 199, 202
in the Netherlands 217–20
patterns of 248–61
policies on, *see* policies
quantity of 248–51
see also tasks
psychiatric nurses in England and Wales 76–7
psychogeriatric nursing homes
in Denmark, assessment for 52
in the Netherlands 223–4
Public Centre for Social Welfare (Belgium) 18, 27

qualification(s)
of family- and home-help assistants, in Belgium 22
for home care, *see* eligibility; entitlement
quality of life, home help in relation to, in Denmark 48, 308
quantity
of home help 21–2
of provision 248–51
questions/questionnaires (on need for help)
in Germany 325
in Israel 337–9

reassessment
lack of 259
service co-ordination and 87–8
recipients of home help, *see* clients
referral 146–50, 262–3, 269–70, 312–14
cross-national perspectives 262–3, 269–70
in Denmark, trajectories 312–14
in Germany, viewpoint of agencies responsible for 146–50
regional government, *see* local/regional authorities; local/regional government
rehabilitation 269
reimbursements, *see* payments
relatives, *see* families
replacement of one service by another (substitution) in the Netherlands 225, 226, 230–2
request for services/help, *see* application; claims; demand
research
collaborative 4–5
cross-national 4, 5
design 5
funding 5
strategies 4
see also Age Care Research Europe
residential care
cross-national perspectives 241, 243–5, 275–6
in Denmark 41
in Italy 193, 203, 204, 209
policies and their impact on 241, 243–5, 275–6
see also institutional services/care
resource(s)
in England and Wales, case management and 93
in Italy 205
needs and, matching of, *see* targeting
respite care in Denmark 42
respondents in case study in Denmark 53–4
RIZIV (State Institute for Sickness and Invalidity Insurance, Belgium) 25

Scotland 262–3, 264, 270–1, 271
Seebohm Report 65–6
selectivity in care provision in Germany 139
senile dementia in Italy 201, 210
separation (fragmentation) of services 251, 281–2, 285–6

service(s)
historical development, *see* historical development
needs and, matching of, *see* targeting
policies arriving before or after 242
types 9; *see also specific types and resources*
use of 248–61
service centres 26
service managers in Belgium 20, 21
sex, *see* gender
sharing of responsibilities, *see* collaboration
sheltered housing in the Netherlands 221, 222
shopping 260
sickness insurance, *see* insurance
single persons, *see* living alone
social assistance in Germany 138
social centres, *see* centres
socal-democratic welfare states 287, 288
social insurance in Israel 163, 177, 183
social isolation in England and Wales 79
Socialist Party, Italian 191
Socialist sickness insurance organization (Belgium) 27, 29
socialization
in Denmark 44
in England and Wales 69, 315
in France 111
in Italy 205, 206, 211
social network characteristics, home help in relation to, in Denmark 48, 307, 308
Social Security Act in Denmark (1973) 40
social security payments in England and Wales 71
Social Services Inspectorate (England and Wales) 72, 81, 89
social services and social welfare
in Belgium 17–18
co-ordination with other services 86, 252
cross-national perspectives 243–5, 252, 270, 280–1
in Denmark 302
doctors' interest in/knowledge of 263
in England and Wales 67, 74–5, 76, 86, 95
in Germany 119, 123–4, 149–50, 154, 280–1
health services and, separation 285
home care as an alternative to 243–5
in Israel 170, 171, 181
see also welfare
social support by home helpers 261
social workers
in Belgium 20
co-ordination with home-help services 86
in Israel 170, 181, 183
in Italy 196
socio-economic trends in Israel 157–9
south of England, home-help staffing in 74
south-west of England, home-help staffing in 75
soutien à domicile 102
spending, *see* expenditure
spouses, care by 259; *see also* marital status
staff (personnel) and staffing
in Belgium 22
in England and Wales 73, 74–5
in France 106, 108–9
in Germany 142, 143, 144, 151–2
in Israel 165, 167, 168, 169, 182
in Italy 195–6
in the Netherlands 217–19
training, *see* training
see also carers *and specific types of staff*
State Institute for Sickness and Invalidity Insurance (Belgium) 25
strengths of home-help services 50
structure of home-help services
in Denmark 50–1, 60
in England and Wales 70
strengths and weaknesses in 50–1
subsidiarity, principle of, in Germany 126, 127
substitution by home-help service in the Netherlands 225, 226, 230–2
supervision
in France 110–11
in Israel 338
in the Netherlands 227, 228, 230, 343
support, *see* help
surveillance in England and Wales 69, 315
system(s), service
hierarchies of, in Germany 119
policies and 285–6, 291, 293

tailor-made care in the Netherlands 218
talking (conversation) 260–1
target clientele/population, *see* clients
targeting (= matching of needs to resources) 281–2
cross-national perspectives 281–2
in England and Wales 72, 81–4, 90, 91–2, 254, 282
in France 197
tasks/duties/activities
cross-national perspectives 259, 259–61
of the elderly, in the Netherlands 218, 228
of home helpers, *see* home helpers
of home-help services/organizations
in England and Wales 64, 315
in France 321
in the Netherlands 218, 259
of informal carers 259
in the Netherlands 218, 228

technical care in France 111, 321
telephone alarm systems in France 110–11
tendering, competitive, in England and Wales 95–6
Thames region, home-help staffing in 74
Thanet Community Care Project 93, 94
time allowances/limitations/considerations
  cross-national perspectives 250, 260, 261
  in Denmark 303
  in England and Wales 81, 84, 317
  in France 105, 107–8
  in Germany 145
  in the Netherlands 216, 219, 344
  for personal care 260
trade and industry policies in England and Wales 95–6
training
  in Belgium 22
  in England and Wales 73
  in Germany 146
  in Italy 195, 196, 207
twenty-four hour home care in Denmark 41, 42

United Kingdom 12, 63–98, 242–92 *passim*, 315–20
use (of services] 248–61
  cross-national perspectives 248–61
  in Denmark 304
users, of services, *see* clients

Vieillir Demain 101–2
views/viewpoints, *see* attitudes
visitors, health, in England and Wales 76–7
volunteers/voluntary services 242
  co-ordination with other services 78, 88–9
  in England and Wales 70, 78, 88–9
  in Israel 161
  in Italy 194–5, 211

Wales (as part of UK) 12, 63–98, 242–92 *passim*, 315–20 *passim*
  home-help staffing in 75
washing capabilities
  in Denmark 306
  in Israel 337
weaknesses of home-help services 50–1
welfare 286–9
  social, *see* social services and social welfare
  traditions/ideologies, cross-national perspectives 286–9, 290
well-being, home help and its effects on 85
Westphalia 128, 129
West Midlands, home-help staffing in 74
women (in the family), role of 259
  in Israel 159
  see also gender
Women's Royal Voluntary Service 89

Yorkshire, home-help staffing in 74

The manufacturer's authorised representative in the EU for product
safety is Oxford University Press España S.A. of El Parque Empresarial
San Fernando de Henares, Avenida de Castilla, 2 - 28830 Madrid
(www.oup.es/en or product.safety@oup.com). OUP España S.A. also acts
as importer into Spain of products made by the manufacturer.
Printed and bound by CPI Group (UK) Ltd, Croydon, CR0 4YY
14/09/2026
02216286-0005